Cultures of Wellbeing

Cultures of Wellbeing
Method, Place, Policy

Edited by

Sarah C. White
*Professor of International Development and Wellbeing,
University of Bath, UK*

With

Chloe Blackmore
Researcher, University of Bath, UK

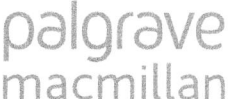

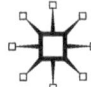

Selection and editorial matter © Sarah C. White and Chloe Blackmore 2016
Individual chapters © Respective authors 2016

All rights reserved. No reproduction, copy or transmission of this publication may be made without written permission.

No portion of this publication may be reproduced, copied or transmitted save with written permission or in accordance with the provisions of the Copyright, Designs and Patents Act 1988, or under the terms of any licence permitting limited copying issued by the Copyright Licensing Agency, Saffron House, 6–10 Kirby Street, London EC1N 8TS.

Any person who does any unauthorized act in relation to this publication may be liable to criminal prosecution and civil claims for damages.

The authors have asserted their rights to be identified as the authors of this work in accordance with the Copyright, Designs and Patents Act 1988.

First published 2016 by
PALGRAVE MACMILLAN

Palgrave Macmillan in the UK is an imprint of Macmillan Publishers Limited, registered in England, company number 785998, of Houndmills, Basingstoke, Hampshire RG21 6XS.

Palgrave Macmillan in the US is a division of St Martin's Press LLC, 175 Fifth Avenue, New York, NY 10010.

Palgrave Macmillan is the global academic imprint of the above companies and has companies and representatives throughout the world.

Palgrave® and Macmillan® are registered trademarks in the United States, the United Kingdom, Europe and other countries.

ISBN 978–1–137–53644–0

This book is printed on paper suitable for recycling and made from fully managed and sustained forest sources. Logging, pulping and manufacturing processes are expected to conform to the environmental regulations of the country of origin.

A catalogue record for this book is available from the British Library.

Library of Congress Cataloging-in-Publication Data
Cultures of wellbeing : method, place, policy / edited by Sarah White, Senior Lecturer, University of Bath, UK, Chloe Blackmore, Researcher, University of Bath, UK.
   pages cm
   ISBN 978–1–137–53644–0 (hardback)
 1. Interpersonal relations.   2. Well-being.   I. White, Sarah, 1963– editor.   II. Blackmore, Chloe, 1985– editor.
HM1106.C85 2015
158—dc23   2015027912

To my family of origin:
'Yes to life' Margaret
'Glass three quarters full' Kathryn
and Barrie, who even in late dementia can still sometimes
engage himself and us with a conspiratorial wink

Sarah, Bath 2015

Contents

List of Illustrations ix

Preface xi

Notes on Contributors xv

1 Introduction: The Many Faces of Wellbeing 1
 Sarah C. White

Part I Mixed Methods

2 Enquiries into Wellbeing: How Could Qualitative Data Be Used to Improve the Reliability of Survey Data? 47
 Laura Camfield

3 Measuring National Wellbeing: What Matters to You? What Matters to Whom? 66
 Susan Oman

4 Staying Well in a South African Township: Stories from Public Health and Sociology 95
 Emer Brangan

5 Economics and Subjectivities of Wellbeing in Rural Zambia 118
 Sarah C. White and Viviana Ramirez

6 'The Weight Falls on My Shoulders': Close Relationships and Women's Wellbeing in India 144
 Shreya Jha and Sarah C. White

Part II Qualitative Research

7 The Dynamics of Relational Wellbeing in the Context of Mobility in Peru 175
 Rebecca Huovinen and Chloe Blackmore

8 Tensions in Conceptualising Psychosocial Wellbeing in Angola: The Marginalisation of Religion and Spirituality 198
 Carola Eyber

9 Picture This: Visual Explorations of Wellbeing in a
   Landmine-Contaminated Landscape in Cambodia   219
   Gabrielle Davies

10 Authorised Voices in the Construction of Wellbeing
   Discourses: A Reflective Ethnographic Experience in
   Northern Mexico   240
   Juan Loera-González

11 Historical Reconstruction and Cultural Identity Building
   as a Local Pathway to 'Living Well' amongst the Pemon of
   Venezuela   260
   Iokiñe Rodríguez

Index   281

Illustrations

Figures

1.1	The construction of wellbeing knowledge	3
1.2	Plot of wellbeing approaches in public policy	7
5.1	Inner wellbeing	122
6.1	Gulabi's domain scores, pivot graph, 2011 and 2013	159
9.1	The home of one of the villagers	221
9.2	Cambodian noodles	230
9.3	Tin of money	231
9.4	Rice fields	232
9.5	Going to the fields	232
9.6	The road through the village	234
9.7	Cattle	235
11.1	Location of Canaima National Park	262

Tables

2.1	Focus-group data to inform taxonomy and selection of indicators	59
3.1	Question 1: What things in life matter to you? From Questionnaire 1	69
3.2	A summary of question 1: What things in life matter most to you? From Questionnaire 2	70
3.3	A summary of Questionnaire 1 from the ONS MNW debate consultation: Tick-box responses compared to 'Other' free-text field responses	71
3.4	A summary of Questionnaire 2 from the ONS MNW debate consultation: Tick-box responses compared to 'Other' free-text field responses	72
3.5	A summary of categories from secondary thematic analysis of free-text field usage	84
3.6	A summary of themes coded from secondary thematic analysis of free-text field usage from question 1, Questionnaire 2	86
5.1	Items from factor analysis that measured six domains of inner wellbeing	128

5.2 Descriptive statistics: Happiness and inner wellbeing 129
5.3 Pearson's correlation: Inner wellbeing and happiness 130
5.4 Linear regression analysis of happiness over inner wellbeing 130
5.5 Correlation of economic status indicators and IWB domains 131
5.6 Regressions of IWB domains over economic status and control variables 132
6.1 Close relationship items in round one fieldwork (2011) 151
6.2 Close relationship items in round two fieldwork (2013) 152
6.3 Gulabi's domain scores, 2011 and 2013 159

Boxes

11.1 The ideal vision of the future for the Pemon from Kumarakapay 268
11.2 The type of society that the Pemon of Kumarakapay want to have 270

Preface

At a conference recently, I was explaining to an eminent economist the approach to wellbeing set out in this book. He listened courteously and then asked, 'Does this have any empirical application?' 'That depends,' I responded, 'on what you mean by "empirical".' 'Well,' he waved his hand expansively, 'measurement'.

The identification of the empirical (which the dictionary defines as 'based on, concerned with, or verifiable by observation or experience') with measurement dominates much of the recent writing on wellbeing, especially in psychology and economics. Sample sizes may be large but the data are thin, comprising numerical scores by which people rate their emotional experience or satisfaction with their lives. This casts a huge shadow over the very different ways that people may identify what is important for them to live well and the work they put into bringing this about. The aim of this book is to investigate that shadow.

The title, *Cultures of Wellbeing*, is thus intended to celebrate the diversity of, and to call for greater intercultural dialogue about, what matters for people to live well together. At a time of unprecedented movements of refugees into and across Europe, what wellbeing means, whose wellbeing counts and how wellbeing may be promoted more inclusively and effectively are issues of pressing importance to policy. This volume presents evidence and thinking to inform these debates. It draws on primary research in marginalised communities in different places: Africa (Angola, Zambia, Ethiopia and South Africa); South and South-East Asia (Central India and Cambodia); Latin America (Venezuela, Peru and Mexico); and on a national survey in the UK. It also reflects on different aspects of life: health and physical activity; religion; migration; child poverty; entrepreneurship and economic life; marriage and family relationships; landmine impact; and the politics of community and identity.

But *Cultures of Wellbeing* doesn't only refer to the different understandings and experience of wellbeing across the world. It also relates to the first word in our sub-title: *Method*. We argue that research methods have their own 'cultures' in terms of taken-for-granted assumptions about the way the world is, key terms and reference points, criteria for truth, and core routines, rituals and practices – the 'rules of the game'. Different methodologies do not simply highlight different aspects of wellbeing; they play an active role in generating different kinds of data and analysis, and so ultimately in constituting quite distinct accounts. Part I of the book investigates this directly, as its mixed method studies explore how qualitative (narrative-based) and quantitative (numerical) data may support, complement, contrast or conflict with each other. Part II focuses on qualitative studies, but similarly considers how the data were constituted differently according to how researchers entered 'the field', who they were (and were perceived to be), how research relationships developed over time and how different methods – such as asking people to take photos and describe what they showed – enabled different kinds of understanding to emerge. The book closes by describing how an outsider-conceived study was transformed to become a means for community self-reflection and mobilisation, so blurring the distinction between researcher and researched.

Across the differences of place and method, the chapters in this book share a common orientation towards the exploration of meaning and social practice. As such, we follow others in identifying an overall approach of 'relational wellbeing' to complement and challenge the dominant constructions of psychological or subjective wellbeing. We hope that this volume will contribute to the advancement of relational wellbeing into a more robust and widely used approach. The evidence presented here questions taken-for-granted oppositions between subjective and objective, science and politics, mind and body, love and money, people and environment. Perhaps most critical is the argument that the 'home' context of wellbeing is not the individual, but the collective or relational. At its simplest, this means that 'my wellbeing' includes – at least – the wellbeing of those who are close to me. More ambitiously, it suggests that wellbeing does not 'belong' to individuals at all, but is produced through interaction with others and the context in which wellbeing is experienced.

Putting relationality at the centre makes wellbeing political with both a small and a large 'p'. At the regional, national (or supra-national) level, the politics of relational wellbeing become not the marshalling of 'happiness' indicators, but the debate about which types of policy – and what values underlying these – best enable a society and polity to flourish. Politics with a small 'p' means recognising that ideologies of 'good lives' can exclude and discipline; they cannot simply be taken at face value. The task of wellbeing research is not to parrot the normative statements of relatively empowered actors. Rather, it is to investigate the complex terms that must be negotiated and forms of practice undertaken as men and women, young people and adults, those in mid-life and those who are older, wealthier and poorer, people from majority and minority ethnic groups, people of different nationalities and people with differing kinds of abilities engage with each other in the work of producing wellbeing.

The immediate roots of this book lie in two workshops, held in Bath in October 2013 and in Oxford in January 2014, as part of the Wellbeing and Poverty Pathways research project, funded by the Economic and Social Research Council (ESRC) and the Department for International Development (DfID) under the Joint Scheme for Research on International Development (Poverty Alleviation) grant number RES-167-25-0507 ES/H033769/1. First drafts of most of the chapters were presented at these events and the Oxford conference was enlivened by a stimulating keynote speech by David Hulme of Manchester University.

More broadly, the book represents well over a decade's work on wellbeing at the University of Bath and from the wider community we have gathered on the way. This began in 2002 with the Wellbeing in Developing Countries (WeD) ESRC research group, which spanned five years and involved country teams in four countries (Bangladesh, Ethiopia, Peru and Thailand). Work on wellbeing at Bath continued through research on religion in India and Bangladesh under the DfID-funded Religions and Development (RaD) programme based at the University of Birmingham (2005–2010); collaborations in action research projects with NGO partners; extensive engagement with the capability approach; the first MSc in Wellbeing in International Development and Public Policy; and a host of PhD projects on wellbeing, several of which are represented in this volume.

My thanks for contributing to the thinking that has made this volume possible thus go first to my colleagues at Bath who participated in the WeD programme and have continued as vital wellbeing conversationalists since: James Copestake, Séverine Deneulin, Joe Devine and Susan Johnson. Thanks also to former colleagues, Pip Bevan, Laura Camfield, Mark Ellison, Ian Gough and particularly – of course – Geof Wood. Special thanks go to Allister McGregor, Director of WeD, who has played a pivotal role in shaping the trajectory of research on wellbeing and international development.

Second, I am grateful to my colleagues in Wellbeing and Poverty Pathways who have extended and expanded my understanding of wellbeing in so many ways: Stanley O. Gaines Jr. of Brunel University for leading quantitative data analysis and his endless patience in explaining statistics to me; further quantitative support from Andrea Baertl-Helguero,

Antonia Fernandez and Viviana Ramirez; Nina Marshall as communications and administrative officer, with Xaroula Kerasidou, Fiona Remnant and Lizzie Spencer providing backup. Thanks also to Jane Millar for her help in shaping up the research proposal and to our remarkably understanding case officer, Lyndy Griffin of the ESRC. My thanks also to our excellent country-based teams. In Zambia, Joseph Kajiwa was the lead researcher and our general guide. He was supported by Stephen Kalio, Kelvin Matesamwa, Jonnathan Mtonga and Goodson Phiri. In India, special thanks are due to Sulakshana Nandi, Chaupal and Gangaram Paikra for supporting the research and to our local team of peer researchers: Pritam Das, Usha Kujur, Kanti Minjh and Dinesh Tirkey. Lastly, and most profoundly, my thanks to Shreya Jha, who has proved an extraordinary research colleague and inestimable friend.

Ideas presented here have gestated through panels on wellbeing at Development Studies Association conferences since 2003, and I am grateful to presenters and attendees for their input, especially my co-convenor for many years, Neil Thin of Edinburgh University. Students on the MSc in Wellbeing have provided vital stimulation to develop our ideas, as have the PhD students who provide the intellectual lifeblood at Bath, as elsewhere. In particular, I have been privileged to work with Asha Abeyasekera, Emer Brangan, Gabrielle Davies, Oscar Garza, Elizabeth Graveling, Tigist Grieve, Mikaela Luttrell-Rowland, Sorcha Mahony and Viviana Ramirez.

For guidance regarding economic aspects of wellbeing, and for her friendship, I am grateful to Uma Kambhampati of the University of Reading. For insightful discussions of development, and her unfailing concern for my personal wellbeing, heartfelt thanks to Eleanor O'Gorman.

As I close, I want to thank all the contributors who have made this volume such a rich and stimulating collection of studies, and for being so timely and good-natured in preparing and revising their chapters. Finally, this book would not have been possible without the unstinting hard work, attention to detail and good humour of Chloe Blackmore, who organised the Bath workshop and supported me throughout the editing process. Any errors, needless to say, are all my own.

Sarah C. White
Bath, September 2015

Contributors

Chloe Blackmore holds a master's degree in wellbeing and human development from the University of Bath. She is interested in notions of responsible and sustainable wellbeing, which she has most recently pursued through a PhD thesis on global citizenship education using qualitative methods. She is currently researching and evaluating educational initiatives in this field.

Emer Brangan started her working life as a clinical scientist in the NHS, but in 2002 moved into the social sciences by way of a master's degree in international development. Thereafter she spent two years project managing medical humanitarian intervention in DR Congo and Ethiopia. Since 2011, she has been based at the University of Bristol, working in health research and teaching. Her research interests include inequality and inequity, social determinants of health, ontology and epistemology in public health, and concepts of wellbeing.

Laura Camfield trained as an anthropologist, but now works collaboratively using qualitative and quantitative methods and training others in their use. Her current focus is on enhancing the quality of cross-national methodologies used to collect qualitative and quantitative data on poverty and vulnerability (funded by an Economic and Social Research Council (ESRC) comparative cross-national research grant). She has published widely on methodology, specifically in relation to mixing methods to improve the quality of surveys and measures.

Gabrielle Davies has lived and worked in various countries around the world and has an esoteric employment history that ranges from international development to international business. Currently residing in academia, her research interests include wellbeing, particularly in post-conflict society, socio-ecological relations and the dynamic relationship between people and planet and participatory and visual research methods. Her doctoral research explores how the presence of landmines affects the wellbeing of local people in Cambodia.

Carola Eyber works as a senior lecturer at the Institute for International Health and Development, Queen Margaret University. She has over 15 years' experience of research, policy and development practice with displaced populations in various settings predominantly in sub-Saharan Africa. Her main research interests are psychosocial wellbeing in conflict and poverty settings, child protection and local approaches to promoting resilience, healing and coping with adversity.

Rebecca Huovinen has recently completed her doctorate ('Mobile Lives in Peru: The Dynamics of Relational Anchoring') in the Department of Social and Policy Sciences, University of Bath. She was previously a research administrator for the Wellbeing in Developing Countries ESRC Research Group and completed a one-year placement with the WeD-Peru team.

Shreya Jha is a research officer at the University of Bath. Based in Delhi, her current work concerns wellbeing and poverty in Zambia and India. She is a qualitative researcher and has a particular interest in how operational models of wellbeing can be integrated into development practice.

Juan Loera-González is an anthropologist with a PhD in development studies from the Institute of Development Studies (IDS), University of Sussex, a master's degree in social anthropology and an MA in poverty and development. His academic interests are local understandings of wellbeing, poverty dynamics, persistent ethnic inequality and mechanisms of resistance in Mexico, Chile and other Latin American countries. He is currently a postdoctoral researcher at the Interdisciplinary Center for Intercultural and Indigenous Studies in Chile.

Susan Oman is a doctoral researcher at the ESRC Centre for Research on Socio-Cultural Change (CRESC), University of Manchester. Her Arts and Humanities Research Council (AHRC)-funded inter-disciplinary research interrogates the cultural politics of wellbeing, on which she has delivered a number of papers at international conferences. She teaches cultural policy and politics and currently leads a unit called 'Performing Research' at the Royal Central School of Speech and Drama.

Viviana Ramirez is a doctoral candidate in the Department of Social and Policy Sciences, University of Bath. She holds an MSc in wellbeing and human development from the same institution and a bachelor's degree in economics from the Universidad de las Americas Puebla, Mexico. Wellbeing is her main field of expertise, focusing on its theoretical and methodological foundations, the role of relationships and relationality and the use of mixed methods research. Other research interests include happiness, the capabilities approach, social policy and development. She has participated in blog publications including the United Nations Research Institute for Social Development's (UNRISD) Think Piece Series and Wikiprogress America Latina, and recently contributed to a book published jointly by the Universitat de Barcelona and the Educo Foundation.

Iokiñe Rodríguez holds a research post in the Anthropology Centre at the Venezuela Institute for Scientific Research (IVIC) working on the articulation of knowledge systems for sustainable development and environmental conflict transformation. She has worked extensively in Canaima National Park, Venezuela, as part of inter-disciplinary and multi-institutional research teams studying environmental conflicts and helping to strengthen the capacity of the Pemon indigenous people to enter into dialogue about environmental change and sustainable development with other park actors.

Sarah C. White is Professor of International Development and Wellbeing at the University of Bath. Her research explores the tensions between local experience and global policy narratives, with a particular emphasis on culture and social identities. Since 2002, the main focus of her research has been wellbeing in developing countries, most recently through an ESRC/DFID (Department for International Development) grant in India and Zambia, *Wellbeing and Poverty Pathways*, 2010–14. Her edited book *A Practical Guide to Wellbeing Assessment* was published in 2014.

1
Introduction: The Many Faces of Wellbeing[1]

Sarah C. White

Introduction

In her novel *Regeneration* (1998), Pat Barker presents the following reflection of the neurologist and anthropologist W. H. R. Rivers (1864–1922) on his fieldwork in the Solomon Islands:

> I thought I'd go through my usual routine, so I started asking questions. The first question was, what would you do with it if you earned or found a guinea? Would you share it, and if so who would you share it *with*? It gets their attention ... and you can uncover all kinds of things about kinship structure and economic arrangements, and so on. Anyway, at the end of this ... they decided they'd turn the tables on me, and ask me the same questions. Starting with: What would *I* do with a guinea? Who would I share it with? I explained I was unmarried and that I wouldn't necessarily feel obliged to share it with anybody. They were *incredulous*. How could anybody live *like that*? And so it went on, question after question.... They were rolling round the deck by the time I'd finished. And suddenly I realized that *anything* I told them would have got the same response ... it would all have been *too bizarre*. And I suddenly saw that their reactions to my society were neither more nor less valid than mine to theirs. And do you know that was a moment of the most *amazing* freedom. I lay back and I closed my eyes and I felt as if a ton weight had been lifted.... It was the *Great White God* de-throned, I suppose. Because we did, we quite unselfconsciously assumed we were the measure of all things. That was how we approached them. And suddenly I saw not only that we weren't the measure of all things, but that *there was no measure*.
>
> (Barker 1998: 212, excerpted)

2 Many Faces of Wellbeing

As at once a neurologist and anthropologist, W. H. R. Rivers seems ideally suited as a guide into qualitative, mixed method, intercultural research into wellbeing. This passage is redolent of the experience of wellbeing as something that 'happens' – first interactively, in the stimulation of intercultural exchange, shared conversation, laughter and insight, and second internally, in the release of being de-centred, letting go of the need to judge and assess. At the heart of the episode is Rivers' recognition of the many ways of being, with his own society no more providing a universal standard than does any other. Striking also is his sense of liberation at escaping the need to 'measure'. Finally, the sense of dislocation he describes – and embraces – may echo a common experience amongst those who research wellbeing, given the multiplicity of influences on it and the extensive range of its possible interpretations.

This book provides a distinctive collection of empirical studies of wellbeing in diverse contexts, predominantly in the Global South. 'Cultures of wellbeing' refers first to diversities in social and cultural constructions of wellbeing, and the need for analysis of and dialogue between them. It further suggests that wellbeing is produced through social and cultural (including political, economic and environmental) practice. In addition, it draws attention to the distinct cultures in different traditions of research, materialised in their routinised practices, techniques and technologies, norms and assumptions, structures and social organisation, and what they hold sacred. This connects to the second major theme, that of method. The concern here is first to challenge the dominance of quantitative methods and illustrate the contribution of qualitative and mixed methods approaches to the study of wellbeing. Second, we emphasise the significance of methodology in shaping *all* accounts of wellbeing. Both culture and methods relate in turn to the third theme of place. This points to the situated nature of both 'lay' and 'expert' understandings of wellbeing, and suggests that space and place constitute critical dimensions of wellbeing that deserve much greater attention. Finally, the underlying context of the contributions in this volume is concern for the ways that wellbeing has been, and may be, adopted as a focus in policy and practice.

As described below, there are multiple accounts of wellbeing in policy and multiple ways in which the concepts which underlie these are construed. Atkinson (2013: 138) notes that a common response to this diversity is to argue for standardisation, an agreed set of indicators or tools which can be used for constructing authoritative accounts. Our interest in this book is rather different. While different contributors adopt different outlooks and lines of argument, as a collective,

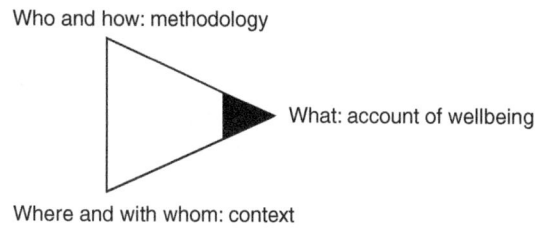

Figure 1.1 The construction of wellbeing knowledge

the volume proposes a shift of focus away from *what wellbeing is*, to exploring *how accounts of wellbeing are produced*. We thus explore the relationships between three key elements of wellbeing research: *what* is claimed (accounts of wellbeing); *how* research is undertaken and by whom (researcher identity, cultural and disciplinary assumptions and methods of enquiry producing data and their analysis); and *where and with whom* the research takes place (place and cultural and socio-economic context) (see Figure 1.1). Practical challenges in generating robust data come together with differences in researchers' underlying philosophical assumptions regarding epistemology (what can be known and how can it be known, including what it means to do cross-cultural research) and ontology (what actually *is*, including conceptions of personhood and wellbeing or happiness).

Each of the chapters thus considers the ways that discipline, method, and/or local culture, socio-economic structure and place shape constructions of wellbeing. Across the volume as a whole, the reification of wellbeing as a 'real thing' that people may 'have' is resisted. Instead, the argument is advanced that constructions of wellbeing are intrinsically connected to the places in which they are generated and the research methods by which they are produced.

The framework of the book is deliberately comparative. Geographically, the chapters span communities across Africa (Angola, Zambia, Ethiopia and South Africa), South and South-East Asia (Central India and Cambodia), Latin America (Venezuela, Peru and Mexico) and the UK. They draw on different disciplines, including international development, public health, anthropology, sociology and psychology. They focus on different aspects of life: health and physical activity; religion; migration; economic life; family relationships; landmine impact; and the politics of community and identity. Finally, they present and reflect on different methodological approaches, including a national survey, mixed methods, ethnography and a variety of visual and participatory methods. The case studies are organised into two sections. The first five reflect on mixed methods approaches, the second five on qualitative methods. Together, they highlight the complementarities and tensions between quantitative and qualitative methods, issues of reliability in self-reported data, the importance of grounding questions with locally relevant examples, and the scope for person-centred approaches which allow people to talk about what is important for their own wellbeing in their own words.

The purpose of this introductory chapter is threefold. First, it aims to locate this volume in relation to the wider field of wellbeing in policy contexts and the key concepts and methods which this involves. Second, it reflects on the key methodological terms and issues which structure these debates. Third, it introduces the case-study chapters, and describes how they relate to the broader field and how they advance the argument of the volume as a whole.

The field of wellbeing

The ubiquity of references to wellbeing and the diffusion of meanings they bear means any attempt to summarise the field must inspire some trepidation. What perhaps unites contemporary work on wellbeing is the conviction, expressed in many ways, that it is possible to bring wellbeing about intentionally, through a combination of will and technique. Most immediately this is seen in the multitude of publications of the 'manage yourself, manage your life' variety promoting self-help psychology, health, spirituality, exercise, diet and lifestyle as a means to self-advancement. But it is also evident in public policy, as voluntary organisations, local councils, national governments and multi-lateral organisations increasingly identify the advancement of wellbeing as their stated objective and statisticians promise new measures which can quantify 'how people think about and experience their lives' (Organisation for Economic Co-operation and Development [OECD] 2013: 3).

The diversity, volume and velocity of increase in references to wellbeing suggest a cultural tide that sweeps together a range of different interests and agendas. Its association with health and harmony holds the promise of a release from the tensions of modern life, a hope of re-balancing and revival. Its appeal to 'science' – predominantly statistics but more recently neuroscience – reflects the longing for authority and robust foundations for action. Politically, wellbeing gives voice to desires for an alternative, a new moral economy, a counterweight to the excesses of capitalism in a world where the promise of socialism no longer seems credible. Its claim to put people's own perspectives at the heart of policy-making promises more democratic processes, or even empowerment. Its positive charge offers a corrective to tired old problem-focused policy-making, encouraging people to express their aspirations rather than rehearse their deprivations. Paradoxically perhaps, the stress on personal experience also fits well with the individualist ideologies of late capitalism and their faith in the pursuit of happiness through choice in consumption.

As the paragraph above suggests, much of the energy driving the wellbeing agenda derives from the Global North and those already in a position of relative material advantage. Is it simply a problem of late modernity searching for its soul, a moral reflux in societies which have gorged on excess and sought salvation through consumption? What is the value of this agenda in the Global South, where people surely have more immediate, material concerns to contend with?

This is a serious question. There is without doubt a danger that countries and communities in the Global South have foisted on them an inappropriate agenda derived from elsewhere; the history of international development is full of such examples (e.g. Cooper and Packard 1997, Crush 1995). The chapters in this volume identify several ways in which the dominant approaches to wellbeing need to be challenged or discarded in order to understand lived experience in Asia, Africa and Latin America. There is also a danger that the South – or the East – is invoked in a nostalgic projection of 'the good life'. Romance with 'the world we have lost' is as central to the self-identification of modernity and development as is the disparagement of 'traditional societies' (Grossberg 1996). It is precisely because of our sensitivity to such patterns of discursive dominance that we argue the need for more in-depth, qualitative studies which express what wellbeing does – and does not – mean for particular people in particular places, as a way to open up a fuller and more balanced dialogue.

The next section introduces four 'faces' of wellbeing in public policy. Before discussing these, however, it is necessary to consider how happiness fits in. There is no clear answer to this. Some writers talk exclusively of wellbeing, some only of happiness and others mix and match between the two. Across the literature as a whole, happiness generally appears as a narrower concept, a component of wellbeing, sometimes identified with 'subjective wellbeing' (SWB) (though this fit is far from perfect or consistent, as discussed below). Happiness tends to be identified more with emotion or feelings, and with the individual, while wellbeing may include 'objective' elements – such as standard of living, access to health care or education – in addition to 'subjective' elements –

such as satisfaction with life. Wellbeing has a more established trajectory as a shared objective for community or polity (e.g. Collard 2006). However, happiness is also applied to collectivities, as in the archetypal 'happy family', and initiatives like 'Happy City' show that happiness is not limited to applications at the individual level (http://www.happycity.org.uk/). In general, happiness is viewed as the more controversial concept, more ideological for its critics, more challenging of prevailing orthodoxies for its advocates. Although our primary orientation is towards wellbeing, we acknowledge that wellbeing and happiness form part of the same cultural complex. Our approach is therefore to explore the ways that different authors use the terms, rather than seeking to draw a definitive line between the two.

Accounts of wellbeing in public policy

This section identifies four 'faces' of wellbeing and happiness in public policy. The first takes a macro approach, using wellbeing to broaden the scope of issues for government attention and specifically to move beyond a sole or primary emphasis on economic growth as the marker of progress. The second focuses on personal wellbeing, aiming to get individuals to take action to promote their own health and happiness. The third concerns the economic concept of utility and involves using subjective measures of happiness or satisfaction to evaluate policy and programme effectiveness. The fourth poses fundamental questions of the current political, economic and social settlements.

The boundaries between these are porous and sometimes fuzzy. The intention is not to draw hard and fast lines between them, but to offer a grid which can be used to map out some key areas of difference in this rather fluid field. The grid focuses particularly on two dimensions. First, does the approach involve subjective or objective dimensions of wellbeing? Second, does it concern the substantive content of wellbeing, or does it primarily involve using measures of wellbeing as a means to evaluate something else? Before proceeding, it is worth taking a little time to explain how I am using these terms.

The division between 'objective' and 'subjective' dimensions of wellbeing is contested, as discussed below. For the moment, though, we adopt a simple definition. Objective dimensions of wellbeing are those that in principle can be verified by an external observer. Quality of housing, level of education or income would be examples. Subjective dimensions of wellbeing are those that are interior to the person him or herself – thoughts and feelings – where in principle the individual is the ultimate authority (see Gasper 2010, for a more extended discussion). In practice, in social science research, both kinds of data are generally gathered through self-report, either verbally or through a written or online survey. Both kinds of data are thus open to dissimulation, as people say they have one house when in fact they have two, or say they are happy when in fact they are sad. As discussed below and in Camfield (this volume), self-reported data are also very sensitive to the instruments that are used to collect them. This is one of the ways that the simple distinction between objective and subjective begins to unravel.

In public policy, the current interest in wellbeing takes two forms. For some, wellbeing is a substantive concern. This prompts questions like, what does wellbeing mean to different kinds of people and what promotes or inhibits wellbeing? For others, wellbeing, and specifically SWB, is primarily of interest as a means to evaluate something else. In this approach, how happy or satisfied people say they are provides an indicator of the success of a policy or style of government. While some approaches are at one extreme and some at the other, overall this difference is more a matter of emphasis than a complete contrast. A substantive concern with wellbeing may also be the basis of evaluation.

Figure 1.2 maps the four faces of wellbeing in public policy and the key concepts that underlie them on this grid of subjective–objective,

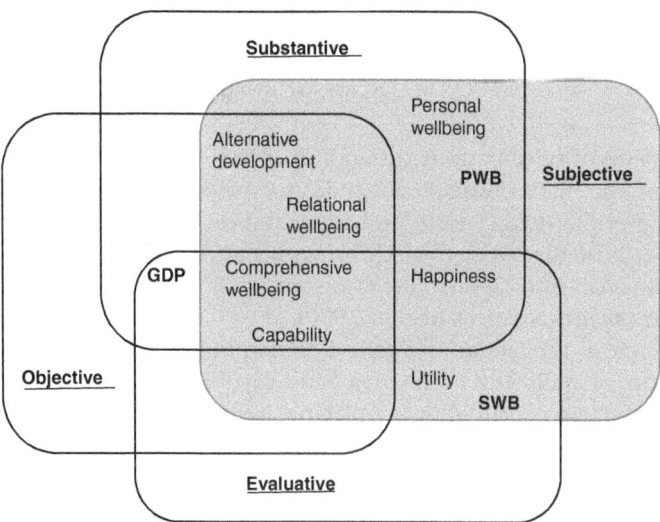

Figure 1.2 Plot of wellbeing approaches in public policy

substantive–evaluative axes. The darker rectangle identifies the approaches that include a subjective dimension, which are the main focus of this volume. The diagram is explained further in relation to the specific concepts and approaches in the discussion below.

Comprehensive wellbeing

Comprehensive wellbeing is the most established approach to wellbeing in public policy. It is commonly referred to in shorthand as 'beyond GDP' (Gross Domestic Product). It comes at the centre of our grid of wellbeing approaches (Figure 1.2), involving both objective and subjective indicators and being used in both evaluative and substantive ways.

Comprehensive wellbeing typically comprises three key elements. The first is breadth, the promotion of a broad range of indicators 'not just economic growth' to measure societal progress. The second is relevance, the claim that statistics should reflect 'what really matters to people' (see Oman, this volume). The third is the increasing inclusion of subjective alongside objective elements. The Report of the Commission on the Measurement of Economic Performance and Social Progress, better known as the Stiglitz Report, which was presented to President Sarkozy of France in 2009, is an influential example. As the following quotation makes clear, the issue of measurement is key to this agenda:

> Another key message, and unifying theme of the report, is that the time is ripe for our measurement system to *shift emphasis from measuring economic production to measuring people's well-being*.
> (Stiglitz *et al.* 2009: 12, original emphasis)

The claims of novelty notwithstanding, in fact the limitations of using GDP as the main development indicator have long been recognised. Quality of life (QoL) health and social indicators have been gathered since at least the 1960s (Noll 2011) with national surveys such as the Scandinavian and German welfare surveys, British Social Trends and French *Données Sociales* since the 1970s.

The most influential theoretical underpinning of comprehensive accounts of wellbeing is Amartya Sen's capability approach. This has made a major contribution to placing wellbeing on the global economics and international development agenda. It has also been widely adopted in other disciplines, such as education. The concept of capability developed as a critique of measuring standards of living either by what people have (commodities) or by the pleasure or happiness they derive from these (utility) (Sen 1983). Instead, capability focuses in a more active way on the person, in terms of 'the ability to do various things by using that good or those characteristics' (Sen 1983: 160). Capabilities then occupy an intermediate space between an overly material focus on goods, income and commodities and an overly subjective focus on happiness or satisfaction, potentially comprehending and going beyond both. Capabilities constitute 'the alternative combinations of things a person is able to be or do' (Sen 1993: 30). These 'valued functionings' – to use Sen's term – range from the basic needs for human life, such as being adequately nourished, to more psychological and relational factors, such as 'achieving self-respect or being socially integrated' (Sen 1993: 31). Although the approach was developed in part as a reaction against the emphasis on happiness/utility in economics, Sen counts the ability to be happy amongst 'important functionings', but without pre-eminence (Sen 1993: 37). He also emphasises agency and freedom as both prerequisites for and constituents of wellbeing. These may also be in tension: Sen (2009: 290) gives the example of Gandhi's hunger strike during the struggle for Indian independence to illustrate how people may have reason to pursue goals that undermine their individual wellbeing.

While its newness may be over-stated, the inclusion of subjective indicators of life satisfaction within broader measures of comprehensive wellbeing has experienced a major upsurge. The OECD reported in 2013 that the UK, France, Italy, the United States, the Netherlands, Japan and South Korea are following established examples like Canada, Australia and New Zealand in either measuring or planning to measure SWB at a national level. The democratic aspiration is evident in the style, such as the informal labels on the categories of the UK Office for National Statistics' (ONS) 'Wheel of Wellbeing', which include 'Our relationships', 'What we do' and 'Where we live' (ONS 2014).

Along with the heightened profile of national wellbeing statistics, there has been an increase in global indices that mix objective and subjective measures in ranking countries according to different criteria of 'progress'. The World Values Survey led the way in 1981. Intended more directly to challenge the dominance of GDP in public policy, the United Nations Development Programme (UNDP) launched in 1990 the Human Development Index (HDI), succeeded by the Multi-dimensional Poverty Index (MPI) in 2010 (Alkire and Foster 2011). Both the HDI and MPI are calculated on the basis of objective assets or achievements.

Other indices that mix objective and subjective measures of wellbeing include the New Economic Foundation (NEF)'s 'Happy Planet Index' (2006 onwards), the OECD's Better Life Index (2011 onwards), the

Legatum Institute's 'Prosperity Index' (2010 onwards), HelpAge International's Global AgeWatch Index and the Social Progress Imperative's Social Progress Index (both launched in 2013).[2] Although these indices appear similar to one another and draw largely on the same sources of data, they differ in the particular indicators chosen and the ways these are combined to form the domains which are used to tell the main story. Each index therefore represents a series of political choices, from the choice of issues on which to generate data, to the selection of what will be the key indicators amongst these, to the ways these indicators are combined and labelled.

Personal wellbeing

Personal wellbeing stresses behaviour change. Policies aim directly to promote individual wellbeing, assuming the individual is responsible for him or herself. The archetype here is health policy, where the public are encouraged to eat more healthily, exercise more, drink and smoke less (see Brangan, this volume).

A well-known example is NEF's widely cited *Five Ways to Wellbeing* (Thompson et al. 2008). Developed with UK government funding, the brief was 'to devise a set of actions that enhance an individual's personal well-being' explicitly ruling out 'actions oriented at the societal or governmental level' (Thompson et al. 2008: 3–4). The recommendations (Connect, Be Active, Take Notice, Keep Learning and Give) thus all target individual behaviour. On our grid, personal wellbeing appears to the upper right, in the overlap of subjective and substantive approaches (see Figure 1.2).

Happiness is central to the understanding of personal wellbeing. The measurement of happiness and its promotion as a policy target are at the core of positive psychology, launched in the USA in 1998, with the aim of focusing on good mental health and personal strengths against the tendency to emphasise mental illness and dysfunction. In the UK, Layard (2006) has used happiness scholarship to advocate increased government spending on counselling and mental health. Over time, however, a primary focus on happiness tends to shift to a broader wellbeing agenda. Thus in 2011, Seligman published a new book, *Flourish*, which advocated a broader 'wellbeing theory' which added relationships and achievement to the elements of 'authentic happiness' he identified earlier (positive emotion, engagement and meaning). The difference, Seligman (2011: 25) claims, is that wellbeing 'cannot exist just in your own head' but brings in objective as well as subjective dimensions: 'a combination of feeling good and having meaning, good relationships, and accomplishment'. Interestingly, for both Layard and the later Seligman, the promotion of personal wellbeing is cast as a social, not simply individual, project (see also Biswas-Diener 2011). However, the strong undertow of individualism in their core disciplines of psychology and economics means that the social is conceived primarily as contributing to individual wellbeing or (also) as the sum of individual wellbeings. The individual remains the unit of analysis.

The link between personal happiness and public policy is also being made at the international level. As the global standard-bearer for the promotion of Gross National Happiness (GNH), it is the government of Bhutan that has taken the concept the furthest.[3] GNH has its basis in an apparently throwaway comment by the king of Bhutan in 1972, which was taken up by two Canadians and worked into a questionnaire. Both the idea and the measures of GNH have been re-worked many times since, making it a truly 'glocal' project, which seeks to meld ecological awareness and Bhutanese 'wisdom' together with standard development and Western 'science of happiness' scholarship. 'Happiness: Towards a New Development Paradigm', produced by 'an international expert working group' for the government of Bhutan in December 2013, exemplifies this mix (NDP 2013). It includes standard development concerns with living standards, health and education, alongside environmental sustainability and the values of service, interconnectedness and co-operation. Creating the right living conditions will not in itself secure wellbeing, it claims. Instead, 'the inner transformation of our own mind-sets and behaviours is as important for happiness as the transformation of these outer conditions of wellbeing' (NDP 2013: 34). It therefore includes 'happiness skills ... drawn creatively from human historical experience, wisdom traditions, and modern science' (NDP 2013: 20) as a vital complement in 'transforming those conditions towards higher human potential' (NDP 2013: 36).

The history of GNH is in many ways indicative of the trajectory of happiness in public policy: it tends to transform into the broader 'comprehensive' face of wellbeing. This is evident in the United Nations (UN) (2011) 'happiness resolution'. Having declared itself *'Conscious* that the pursuit of happiness is a fundamental human goal' (UN 2011, emphasis in the original), the UN goes on to locate happiness and wellbeing in the context of 'sustainable development' and 'the need for a more inclusive, equitable and balanced approach to economic growth'.

Utility

A central aspect of the excitement around measures of SWB in policy circles is the promise that they offer a direct indicator of utility, which can be used as a measure of policy or programme effectiveness. In Figure 1.2 it thus appears to the lower right, in the overlap between subjective and evaluative approaches. The OECD Statistics Office provides a strong example, though it is careful to stress that subjective indicators should not replace, but can 'complement other measures' (OECD 2013: 36). The OECD (2013: 36) explains:

> being grounded in peoples' [sic] experiences and judgements on multiple aspects of their life [sic], measures of subjective well-being are uniquely placed to provide information on the net impact of changes in social and economic conditions on the perceived well-being of respondents.

There are two aspects to this claim. The first is that SWB can provide a direct link to the real effect of a policy on people's experience, so one can evaluate not just whether a policy has achieved its aims, but what this has meant for people's happiness or QoL. The second is that SWB can provide a single, composite impact measure by which policy makers can compare the relative effect of different kinds of intervention such as health versus housing, or inflation versus unemployment. According to the OECD (2013: 37–43), SWB can aid policy evaluation, helping for example in cost–benefit analyses to assign a value to life events such as marriage, divorce, or unemployment and can be used to predict behaviour, such as the Arab Spring[4] or employees' likelihood of seeking alternative employment. In addition, they claim, it can help guide individual decision-making, giving people better information on what will actually make them happier, as against what they perhaps erroneously believe will do so.

The argument of this volume raises considerable doubt as to whether such claims are credible. At this point, however, what is important to recognise is the frame that enables them to appear so. This derives from the totemic place that the notion of 'utility' occupies in economics. The pre-eminence of utility, or the happiness or satisfaction that people derive from their needs or desires being met, dates back at least as far as Bentham's classic utilitarian formula that pronounced the good to be 'the greatest happiness of the greatest number'. The difficulty was that no direct measure of utility was available and philosophical objections were raised to the notion of comparing levels of utility between different people (Collard 2006). As a result, in their search for robust, 'objective' measures of utility, economists have widely adopted proxies such as 'revealed preferences', which focus on the choices people actually make (Samuelson 1938). At their simplest, such proxies assume that utility can be measured in terms of what people are willing to pay for particular goods or services. Crudely speaking, the higher the prices paid, the greater the utility that is revealed. Since wealthier people can satisfy a greater range of higher value preferences, this means logically that the utility (or satisfaction, or happiness) that they can derive should be greater than that of poorer people. Wealthier countries (i.e. those with higher GDP[5]) should similarly be able to satisfy more needs and desires and so provide a higher level of utility to their citizens.

Graduated response scales as direct subjective measures of happiness and satisfaction seem first to have been used in a study of women's sex lives in 1920 (Angner 2011: 6). Happiness and satisfaction questions have appeared since 1930 in educational psychology and in 1960 in studies of mental health (Angner 2011). By the 1960s, some data were available that showed life satisfaction on a national basis. The assumption that rises in GDP would lead to increased happiness could thus be tested. The results both confirmed and confounded previous expectations (Easterlin 1974). As predicted, within a given country, wealthier people tended to report themselves happier than did those who were poorer. But across countries, differences in average levels of wealth were much smaller than those by economic status within countries, and there was not the same clear association between happiness and wealth overall (Easterlin 1974: 106, 108). In addition, within a country – the United States – increased GDP per capita over time did not correspond with rising levels of happiness. Rather, Easterlin (1974: 121) argued, 'the growth process itself engenders ever-growing wants' which in turn become drivers of further growth into the future.

The 'Easterlin paradox' sparked a major debate that evolved into a new sub-discipline, 'the economics of happiness'. While the form of the debate is technical, involving the statistical manipulation of national datasets, its core is moral and political, with SWB standing for utility as a definition of the good. Some contributors use Easterlin's findings to argue that life is more than money, to advocate happiness as a policy target and urge going 'beyond GDP', as described above. Other scholars dispute Easterlin's findings and/or extend the focus to consider how happiness is affected by other issues such as 'freedom', provision of state welfare, human rights or levels of inequality (e.g. Alesinaa et al. 2004, Rothstein 2010, Veenhoven 2000). There remains considerable controversy about the results. Carol Graham (2011: 16–21) suggests that this derives substantially from differences in the methods employed: the sources of data, the questions used, the countries surveyed and the measure of income used, as well as 'real' differences such as rates of economic change and changing aspirations. There are also more fundamental conceptual and methodological questions about the mapping of SWB at a national scale. These include whether it makes sense to map 'real' GDP figures against constructs of (fixed end) happiness scales, which by definition cannot continue to rise. Methodological issues are discussed further in the section on SWB below.

Development alternative

The fourth face of happiness and wellbeing in public policy poses an alternative set of values. At a minimum, this questions what is 'good growth', suggesting the economy should be developed only in ways that serve human fulfilment and are environmentally sustainable. Stronger versions argue that what matters is not economic growth but economic sufficiency. More political versions emphasise social justice and may sponsor some form of solidarity economy, involving smaller, self-managed units of production with egalitarian forms of management and an orientation towards fair trade and environmental sustainability. More personal versions emphasise quality of life in the home and community and may counsel disengagement and self-reliance. There are many forms of each and many initiatives which combine both aspects. Religious motivation is quite common. In Figure 1.2 this approach appears at the upper centre. It considers wellbeing in substantive terms and tends to dissolve the distinction between subjective and objective.

Worldviews of indigenous (or 'Fourth World') peoples have been very important in inspiring visions of an alternative to 'business as usual' capitalist development. While these are diverse and polyvocal (Fabricant 2013), they tend to have various underlying orientations in common. These include an emphasis on oneness, with humanity as part of nature and social relations intertwined with the natural environment. For some in Peru, Ecuador and Bolivia, this goes as far as rejecting the nature/culture divide and seeking to include 'earth-beings', such as mountains, as persons with rights to political inclusion (De La Cadena 2010). The orientations also tend to be systemic, cyclical or reciprocal rather than linear, and they typically emphasise place and particularity rather than aspiring for 'global' universality (see Davies, this volume). This can lead to some very radical and challenging assertions about the locatedness of knowledge. Rasmussen and Akulukjuk (2009), for example, contrast the way that Inuit learn environmental knowledge experientially with English-language patterns of learning which detach students from their environment, and ask:

> Shouldn't environmental studies at universities be teaching the languages and epistemologies of the people Indigenous to the particular biocultural region under study?
>
> (Rasmussen and Akulukjuk 2009: 286)

It is in Latin America that indigenous views of wellbeing have achieved the greatest political influence. Most widely known as *buen vivir*, which is translated as 'living well together',[6] representations of indigenous cosmologies have given form to rights-based struggles against the dominance of traditional political elites, the United States and neo-liberal capitalism. In Ecuador and Bolivia, they have been officially recognised and incorporated in new national constitutions (see Rodríguez, this volume). In theory at least, this means new attention is paid to the claims of the natural world and environmental sustainability, there is political acceptance of the need for greater redistribution and state welfare programmes, and recognition is given to the collective rights of marginalised peoples to inclusion within a pluri-cultural and plurinational state (Radcliffe 2011). The translation into practice is complex. The economies of both Ecuador and Bolivia remain heavily dependent on mining, oil or gas extraction, with high environmental costs. There are also different views of what it means to 'live well together' between and within indigenous groups (Artaraz and Calestani 2014, Loera-González, and Rodríguez, this volume). There are serious conflicts of interest between people by geographical location and occupation, and between policies in prioritising protecting the environment or financing social welfare or providing water and sanitation to the urban poor (Fabricant 2013). And for any country it is not clear how far a radically different economic model can be implemented, given high levels of need in the population, daily political challenges in reforming state structures and the power of global economic structures and relationships (Radcliffe 2011).

Summing up

This section has presented four different 'faces' of happiness and wellbeing in public policy. In practice, as noted above, the distinctions between these approaches are not clear-cut. Encouragement towards greater personal wellbeing frequently appeals to the same visions of wholeness and harmony that animate alternative development approaches. Measures of national progress that go 'beyond GDP' increasingly include SWB alongside indicators of health and education. Strong advocacy of happiness tends to morph over time into a broader concern with personal or comprehensive wellbeing. This fluidity and porosity between different understandings of happiness and wellbeing can be seen as both a strength – linking back to a common core motivation – and a weakness – the terms lack clarity and definition. Part of the explanation for this permeability is that the different faces of wellbeing draw on a common fund of concepts. The next section discusses the most prominent of these.

Key concepts: Psychological and subjective wellbeing, and happiness

This section introduces the two concepts that underlie much of the promotion of happiness and subjective dimensions of wellbeing in public policy: SWB and psychological wellbeing (PWB). The lack of fixity within the field means that there is not a perfect match between concept and application, but there is nonetheless a predominant association that can be discerned between SWB and utility, and personal and psychological wellbeing. The section closes with a critical reflection on happiness as a project of the self.

Subjective wellbeing

SWB is the predominant approach to measuring happiness and wellbeing in contemporary public policy. While it may be incorporated within accounts of personal and of comprehensive wellbeing, its core orientation is towards utility. The great attraction is its slimness, or parsimony, as it assesses the level of pleasure, happiness or satisfaction rather than its substantive content. SWB thus asks simply 'how happy' people are; it does not concern itself with how that happiness is defined or what its basis might be.

SWB is not only conceptually light, it is the most methodologically straightforward approach to apply. At its simplest, it may be measured through a single question asking people how happy they are with their lives as a whole. While the term 'happy' may be used, such questions more precisely concern life satisfaction. For greater reliability, a number of items may be combined. Examples include Diener *et al.*'s (1985) five-item Satisfaction with Life Scale (SWLS)[7] and the Personal Wellbeing Index (PWI) of satisfaction across eight life domains (International Wellbeing Group 2006).[8] The Gallup World Poll (launched in 2005) provides the most influential source of data on SWB in public policy at present. This asks people to locate their lives now and where they expect to be in five years' time on a ladder on which rung number ten is the 'best possible life for you' and zero is 'the worst possible life for you' (Gallup n.d.).[9]

Although these are all measures of life satisfaction, they are not all the same. Attention in the SWLS is on the self and individual aspirations. The PWI includes subjective assessments of 'objective' factors – standard of living, health, personal relationships, safety, etc. There is also a substantive difference between the interior-oriented exercise of reflecting on one's own happiness and the exterior-oriented exercise of ranking one's life against other possible lives. While these differences may seem matters of detail, they can significantly affect results. Gallup's approach is the one that correlates most closely with income, both across individuals and across countries. This leads Kahneman and Deaton (2010: 16492) to suggest it is the 'purest' measure. I would argue, instead, that the 'ladder of life' encourages people to think of their lives in economic terms.[10] The heat generated by the Easterlin paradox indicates the political sensitivity of questioning the association between economic growth and human happiness. It is thus a matter of concern that the favoured measure of life satisfaction is the one that has the strongest in-built bias towards an economic frame.

Amongst psychologists, SWB is often construed as a composite of (cognitive) life satisfaction and (affective) 'affect balance', or the extent to which people experience positive versus negative emotions (e.g. Diener 2000). Emotion-based assessments of happiness correlate much less closely with economic status than does life satisfaction (e.g. Diener et al. 2010, Graham 2011). Means of assessing emotions span the methodological spectrum, from asking people to describe the emotional content of various episodes in their lives; through counting the frequency of emotions classified as 'positive' and 'negative' over a given period (e.g. Watson et al. 1988); to 'experience sampling' which seeks to capture immediate ratings of emotions as they are experienced (e.g. Larson and Csikszentmihalyi 1983); to observation of frequency of smiling (Nettle 2005); to brain imaging (e.g. Berridge and Kringelbach 2011). Stiglitz et al. (2009: 147) identify experience sampling as the 'gold standard' in measuring hedonic experience.[11] This is based on the logic that 'true' accounts of emotions are given at the time of the experience, recall and reflection distorts. This may be disputed, of course, as it assumes feelings are simple and transparent to the self and discounts the human activity of 'needing to make sense of' emotions. Such attempts to control for 'subject effects', leading ultimately to faith in external observation of facial or brain activity, reflect, I believe, an existential anxiety generated for quantitative researchers working with a positivist epistemology on subjective data – they need to try to make it objective. I discuss this point further in the section on 'Constructing wellbeing knowledge' below.

Cross-cultural analysis of SWB also reveals some cultural differences in how people assign scores. Diener *et al.* (2000), for example, find that (white) Americans tend to give higher average scores than do East Asians, particularly when it comes to 'global' life satisfaction, as opposed to domain-specific measures. The authors relate this to a 'positivity disposition' which varies between cultures. Others might attribute it instead to differences in the strength of the ideology of happiness and positivity on the one hand, and norms of modesty or self-deprecation on the other (see e.g. Ahmed 2010, Held 2002). Whatever the diagnosis, it clearly shows that SWB scoring is not culture-neutral, but influenced by social norms and values.

While SWB's focus purely on self-assessment may bring an attractive simplicity, it is also subject to significant conceptual critique. The first is that what gives you pleasure may not be good for you, so the notion of wellbeing should include not just what feels good (at the time) but what *is* good in some intrinsic way. This rehearses debates that go back to the ancient Greeks about hedonic (pleasure-oriented) versus 'eudaemonic' (virtue or fulfilment) views of the good life. In my view, this critique is misdirected. We simply do not know the basis on which people rate their 'happiness' in life, except when the measures are quite narrowly focused on emotion or affect. For 'global happiness' or life-satisfaction questions, it is at least as likely that people are basing their ratings on eudaemonic as hedonic criteria. Somewhat ironically for the measure which has put happiness on the global policy agenda, the 'happiness' of SWB has no substantive content: it functions simply as a marker of subjective success in life.

The second critique concerns the use of SWB in policy. This is the 'happy peasant' issue – that people may state that they are happy even in very grim circumstances, making happiness a very equivocal indicator. Sen (1983: 160) suggests one aspect of this, as he states that poor people's expressions of happiness may simply reflect 'a cheerful disposition'. Also, as Ehrenreich (2009: 170) amongst many others points out, in contexts of inequality, emphasising satisfaction carries an inherently conservative weighting. High satisfaction may signify the low aspiration of internalised oppression, rather than the experience of positive fulfilment many people identify with happiness. This issue of adaptation also throws into question the practical use of SWB measures in project or policy evaluation. Adaptation concerns the way frames of reference shift with altered circumstances, meaning that objectively higher standards of living will not necessarily be reflected in increased levels of satisfaction, or vice versa (see Clark ed. 2012).

A third critique questions the robustness of data on SWB. This suggests that apparently global 'satisfaction with life' responses may be heavily influenced by contextual factors, such as the happenchance of mood, the weather or an immediate 'feel-good' trigger like finding a coin on the photocopier just before being asked about life satisfaction (Schwarz and Clore 1983). The common response to such objections is that with a large enough sample such effects will be evened out. But what if the 'framing' effect is provided by the questionnaire itself? In a paper suggestively subtitled, 'How the Questions Shape the Answers', Schwarz (1999) suggests that there is an intrinsic relationship between the instruments used to gather self-reported data and the information they produce (see also Camfield, this volume). Drawing on a wide range of research in psychology, Schwarz (1999: 93) argues:

> Unfortunately, self-reports are a fallible source of data, and minor changes in question wording, question format, or question context can result in major changes in the obtained results.

For satisfaction measures, people need to bring to mind not just the object itself – such as one's marriage, in the case of marital satisfaction – but also a standard against which to evaluate this (Schwarz 1999: 100). Deaton's (2012) study of levels of SWB in the United States during the economic crisis of 2008 to 2010 provides evidence of this. He found that the effect of the economic crisis on SWB, even at its worst, was 'dwarfed' by the effect of changes in the order in which questions were asked (in particular, shifting questions about politics to just before questions on life evaluation) (Deaton 2012: 23). While this issue is typically discussed in terms of technique and reliability, it has a more interesting conceptual dimension, as it points to the essentially relational and situated character of subjective data.

There is also the danger of manipulation of SWB measures if they come to be seen as politically significant. Frey and Gallus (2013: 207) thus caution against the political pitfalls of adopting a happiness index as a key measure of government success, warning:

> the Index will be systematically distorted due to the incentive for citizens to answer strategically and the incentive for government to manipulate the Index in its favour.

This again raises epistemological issues. In drawing attention to the fact that these data are produced by knowing subjects who might have an interest in a particular kind of result, it calls into question claims of 'happiness science' that invoke a natural science paradigm where data are simply available to direct observation and not affected by the fact of being observed. These issues concerning the underlying philosophical assumptions of this research are discussed further below.

The final point concerns what kind of subject is being construed in SWB. There seems an underlying – probably unconscious – motif of the market as the model of society. This is perhaps why SWB surveys look so similar to market research: they can be seen to position people as consumers rating their satisfaction, with their lives as the item to be consumed. Ironically, despite SWB's stress on the individual, the person as the subject who judges or feels is ultimately dissolved. The data are the 'choices', feelings or perceptions registered as scores, detachable and detached. This objectification of subjective data through breaking their relationship to the perceiving subject is a necessary preliminary before quantitative analysis. The chapters that follow show some of the interesting results that emerge when qualitative research enables that relationship to be restored (e.g. Camfield, Brangan, White and Jha, this volume). Here, the main point to note is that SWB may not be as light or culture-free as it appears: it comes with its own underlying set of values and view of the person and how it should be construed.

Psychological wellbeing

PWB links most closely with the personal face of wellbeing in policy contexts. Its underlying model of wellbeing is organic, evoking notions of health, in either literal or metaphorical terms. The close connections between health and wellbeing are strikingly evident in the World Health Organization's (1946) definition:

> Health is a state of complete physical, mental and social well-being and not merely the absence of disease or infirmity.[12]

Scholars of PWB are committed to a eudaemonic approach which sees wellbeing in terms of functioning and fulfilment and a life well lived. Ryff (1989: 1070) thus draws attention to 'the important distinction between the gratification of right desires and wrong desires'. Her six domains of PWB[13] aim to bring a longer history of humanistic psychology to bear on empirical investigation and clinical application

(Ryff 1989, Ryff and Keyes 1995).[14] Ryan and Deci (2001) consider that PWB results from the achievement of three basic psychological needs: autonomy, competence and relatedness. They thus recognise SWB as one possible indicator of positive psychological health, but only one. More importantly, 'assessments of self-actualization, vitality, and mental health...assess well-being conceived of as healthy, congruent and vital functioning' (Ryan and Deci 2001: 147).

There is no single authorised scale for self-determination theory (SDT), but a range of questionnaires developed for different purposes. Ryff's full questionnaire has 84 items (14 per domain) but this can also be reduced to nine items per domain.[15] By contrast, the Warwick–Edinburgh Mental Wellbeing Scale (WEMWBS) (Secker and Stewart-Brown 2007) comprises just 14 questions (or seven in the short version) about mood, energy and cognitive functioning. As a framework, this does not reflect the same ambitions to theorise wellbeing but instead comes closer to a conventional, diagnostic understanding of mental health, with a more positive spin. This perhaps reflects its origins in a partnership with the Scottish National Health Service (Tennant *et al*. 2007).

The main critiques of PWB approaches concern their claims to universality. Ryff is highly vulnerable here, as both her characterisation of the domains and the items to test them are steeped in the values of North American culture. They thus reward strong statements of individualism – 'I judge myself by what I think is important, not by the values of what others think is important'; control – 'In general, I feel I am in charge of the situation in which I live'; continuous personal growth – 'I think it is important to have new experiences that challenge how you think about yourself and the world'; openness in relationships – 'I find it difficult to really open up when I talk with others'[16]; actively pursuing one's own sense of purpose in life – 'I am an active person in carrying out the plans I set for myself'; and positive self-assessment – 'I like most aspects of my personality.'

While Ryan and Deci have worked hard to maintain that their three psychological needs are indeed universal, SDT similarly rests on a strong, liberal humanist, universalist model of the human being:

> people's happiness and well-being are inseparable from their experience of personal and motivational autonomy in pursuing freely chosen life-goals, actions, and behaviors. We consider this axiom to be universal and applicable to people from all cultural communities.... The feeling of autonomy and self-determination is what

makes us most fully human and thus most able to lead deeply satisfying lives – lives that are meaningful and constructive – perhaps the only lives that are worth living.

(Chirkov *et al.* 2011: 1)

The SDT argument for cross-cultural applicability rests on its definition of autonomy, which is argued to be quite distinct from independence and so not tied to more individualist cultural settings. The opposite of autonomy, SDT theorists argue, is heteronomy, or being denied choice by another. If one personally identifies with the values of one's group and therefore chooses to follow them, this constitutes the exercise of autonomy. Miller *et al.* (2011) have tested this with matching sets of North Americans and Hindus in India and confirm both that choice or autonomy is important for satisfaction and that people can experience a sense of choice in contexts where they also feel a sense of duty – doing their duty can be felt to be a positive experience. Reflecting the importance of close attention to routinised practices, however, Miller *et al.* (2011: 58) point to problematic coding in widely used SDT questionnaires. These interpret references to duty as indicating an absence of choice or autonomy, and so implicitly identify autonomy with individualism, against the stated views of SDT theorists.

PWB also faces an important political critique. Ahmed (2010: 12) sounds a caution about the notions of 'higher' and 'lower' forms of wellbeing which are characteristic of eudaemonic approaches. These are highly vulnerable to class, ethnicity and gender bias, such that 'hierarchies of happiness may correspond to social hierarchies'.

Questioning happiness

As noted above, Sen has presented a consistent and trenchant critique of promoting happiness as the goal of development policy (e.g. Sen 1983, 1993, 2009) and others have recently reinforced this (Nussbaum 2012, Stewart 2014). As described already, in practice, this does not seem as serious a concern as it might appear – even approaches that begin with happiness have a strong tendency to shift into a broader concern with wellbeing. In this section, therefore, I take a different tack, and consider criticisms of the promotion of happiness as an ideology of the self.

As already remarked, it has long been recognised that statements of happiness cannot stand in any simple way as evidence of having a good life. Some people are by nature happier and/or more content than others. Some religious and cultural scripts countenance acceptance of one's lot in life, while others value struggle and striving. Some cultures reward modesty and temperance in expressions of self, others positivity and self-affirmation. People adjust expectations upwards and downwards according to what they experience. This may have quite contradictory consequences. On the one hand, it may result in the 'hedonic treadmill' (Brickman and Campbell 1971) where nothing is ever enough. On the other, it may lead to acceptance of inequality or oppression as natural or inescapable, or more positively, to an ability to make the best of very difficult circumstances.

The prevalence of these options is not simply random or a matter of idiosyncratic choice, but is rooted in – and contributes to – culture and political economy. The generation of inexhaustible desire is one of the engines driving the global capitalism of late modernity. This is expressed not only in the 'need' for ever expanded material consumption, but also in the way that the self comes to be viewed as itself a project to be worked on and re-worked over time, with an underlying promise of perfectibility (Craib 1994). Craib links this to the dominance of the market as a metaphor that governs how we think about social life (see also Sahlins 1976[17]). I note above that an implicit idiom of the market seems to underlie the concept and practice of SWB. Working in a market, Craib (1994: 30) points out, requires a certain kind of personal 'front', one that 'does not acknowledge what might be thought of as "defects" in the product'. This has implications for the representation of self through SWB indicators, discussed in the next section.

Ehrenreich (2009) presents an example of how happiness narratives can be used to discipline individuals' expression of self in her polemic against the dominance of positive thinking in the United States. In a particularly powerful chapter, she reflects on her own diagnosis of breast cancer, the way it provided a new merchandising opportunity with a plethora of teddy bears and pink bows, and the policing of her emotional response to it. Her expression of anger on a website brought rebuke from other women living with breast cancer. The 'healthy' response to cancer, and the only acceptable response, was to look for the positives, 'for her own sake', and with the (sometimes explicit) implication that negative thinking could inhibit a cure, or even be responsible for the cancer having developed in the first place. This emphasis on personal responsibility for (in this case physical) wellbeing is a very strong theme within 'personal wellbeing', as described above. Ehrenreich sees her experience as an encounter with 'an ideological force in American culture... that encourages us to deny reality, submit cheerfully to misfortune, and blame only ourselves for our fate' (Ehrenreich 2009: 44).

Sointu (2005) emphasises the public policy effect: that the increasing stress on personal responsibility for 'one's own wellbeing' may be linked to the retrenchment of the state and the removal of statutory welfare provision.

Ahmed (2010) contrasts the repeated emphasis on happiness as the object of desire with its ineffability, suggesting that happiness may simply stand as a marker for desire itself:

> If happiness is what we wish for, it does not mean we know what we wish for in wishing for happiness. Happiness might even conjure its own wish. Or happiness might keep its place as a wish by its failure to be given.
>
> (Ahmed 2010: 1)

If, as she goes on to remark a few pages later, 'Where we find happiness teaches us what we value' (Ahmed 2010: 13), the variability in views of happiness and wellbeing described in this volume should not surprise us: it directly reflects the different values and orientations of the commentators. Accordingly, Ahmed lays a powerful emphasis on the ideological character of happiness and the way it can serve to re-inscribe mainstream values and identities. Referring to bodies of feminist and anti-racist scholarship that have de-constructed notions of 'the happy housewife' and 'the happy slave', she points to the 'unhappy aspects of happiness'. These are the ways it can legitimise dominant social institutions and the forms of subordination they embody, as 'happiness is used to redescribe social norms as social goods' (Ahmed 2010: 2).

Craib's analysis speaks strongly to the promotion of happiness and SWB, despite not addressing it directly. In Craib's view, the self of late modernity is a false self, its alienation obscured by the stress on individual autonomy:

> My argument is that late modernity produces a fragmented and isolated self and a fragmentation of our experience of ourselves; this is masked with a vision of the omnipotent self-constructing self which maintains many of the phantasies of infancy into adult life.
>
> (Craib 1994: 166)

Drawing on his work as both social theorist and psychotherapist, Craib (1994) suggests that a major aspect of the human condition is the encounter with limits and the inevitability of disappointment.

Reflecting on the optimism and future orientation of both psychology and sociology, Craib (1994: viii) suggests:

> The first duty of the human sciences is perhaps to hold on to both sides of the equation: that life can be good and made better, and that life ends in the ultimate disappointment of death.

Craib's emphasis on the importance of adjusting to the limitations of life is strongly echoed in many cultural scripts across place and time. Jackson (2011: 61–62) provides one example, in his description of what wellbeing means amongst the Kuranko people of Sierra Leone:

> For Kuranko, it is how one bears the burden of life that matters, how one endures the situation in which one finds oneself thrown. Well-being is therefore less a reflection on whether or not one has realized one's hopes than a matter of learning how to live within limits. Singing, like Sira, on an empty belly.

Constructing wellbeing knowledge

Underlying the various accounts of wellbeing are significant differences in views of the research process, and indeed the world that it represents. Considered more closely, the straightforward contrasts between objective and subjective, qualitative and quantitative, paradoxically appear both much less clear-cut and more heavily loaded with differing sets of philosophical baggage. One of the strengths of mixed methods' enquiries is that they force (sometimes painful) reflection on personal investments in what counts as data and as theory, how analysis is done, how goals are defined, what techniques are employed, how the relationship between researcher and researched is understood and what is held as sacred and beyond question. This section maps out some of this terrain. This leads into an outline of relational wellbeing, the approach taken by most of the contributions to this volume, and an introduction to the empirical chapters that follow.

At the simplest level, quantitative methods involve the generation of numbers and their statistical analysis, while qualitative ones typically involve words and their interpretation. Similarly, in everyday speech, 'objective' means unbiased, or even true, while 'subjective' suggests biased, or even untrue. Conventional thinking tends to see a natural fit between the quantitative and objective ('facts'), and the qualitative and subjective ('feelings' or 'meanings'). In practice, things are not so straightforward. As seen above, quantitative methods predominate in wellbeing research even when the subject matter is subjective. Interview data can be analysed quantitatively, with key pieces of text or references or types of occurrence codified for comparison across cases to build a causal story. Numerical data may be analysed qualitatively, to explore what they reveal of a particular respondent or set of people (see also Camfield, Oman, Brangan, and Jha and White, this volume).

More significant than types of data and techniques of analysis are underlying differences in philosophies of research. Quantitative research tends to assume a positivist, empiricist or realist epistemology. Its paradigm of research is the natural sciences and the independent observation of objective data. Research design involves testing a hypothesis and is thus relatively fixed from the outset. It aims to simplify and standardise, especially through the use of numbers and measurement, reducing complex reality into a more manageable number of concepts or factors. It seeks commonality and comparability, favouring standard tools with a minimum of adaptation to context. It tends to test for linear, external relationships between variables and ideally demonstrates causality. It aspires to science, universality, generalisation and simplicity, and puts its faith in large numbers to overcome idiosyncratic differences and reveal hidden truths.

Qualitative research, by contrast, tends to assume a constructivist, interpretivist epistemology that emphasises the social construction of meaning and the value of seeking to understand the way research subjects see their world. Research design may be exploratory and inductive, allowing considerable flexibility to respond to new discoveries as the research develops. It emphasises particularity, variability and the complex inter-relations of various factors. Its orientation is towards quality rather than quantity, description rather than measurement. It emphasises power and process and researcher reflexivity. It aspires to depict accurately the particularities of the research context, putting its faith in rich description and in-depth analysis of specific cases.

A first step in becoming more self-conscious about the implication of methods in constructing accounts of wellbeing is to separate out the different elements involved. To explore this further, we return to W. H. R. Rivers in the Solomon Islands.

From Rivers' account it can be seen that the experience of wellbeing is essentially subjective, but it can be registered by quantitative and qualitative instruments. For Rivers, it began as cognitive insight: 'I suddenly saw that their reactions to my society were neither more nor less valid than mine to theirs.' This was accompanied by physiological sensation, 'I lay back and I closed my eyes and I felt as if a ton weight had been lifted.' If the instruments had been to hand, this would no doubt have registered measurably in levels of serotonin and images of brain activity. What is important to note is that *any* representation of this experience is just that, a representation. Neither medical instruments nor verbal descriptions can convey precisely the quality of the experience in itself. Words come closest, because they come most 'naturally' – it is through words that we try to make sense of what we are feeling to ourselves. Also, words engage the imagination and it is through imagination that we can begin to enter into the experience of others. Had an SWB researcher been present, he or she could perhaps have got Rivers to rate his feelings on a Likert scale (though I suspect Rivers would have resisted!). In this way, the experience could be *translated* into quantitative terms, but it is easy to see that it is not its home language: the 'translation' would have made it into something quite unlike itself, because its texture as an *experience* would have been removed.

Undertaking such close analysis makes evident the distinctions between what happens (the experience), the instruments that record it, the data they produce and the techniques of analysis that are applied. To preserve this recognition, it is helpful to talk about data being generated or constructed, rather than gathered. Data are not just lying about waiting to be picked up by a passing researcher, they are produced through the labour of research. Even something as tangible as housing, for example, has to be codified before it becomes data. What will be recorded? Quality of roof, of floor, material of construction, number of rooms, presence of outdoor space, tenure status...? There are always decisions about what variables matter, always marginal empirical examples which are difficult to classify.

The larger point this reveals is that research is a social process. Two aspects of this are noted above: Schwarz's (1999) work on the way questionnaires shape responses and Frey and Gallus' (2013) concern about the political manipulation of happiness scores if they are seen as significant markers of government success. A further dimension is the self-consciousness of respondents. This is recognised in psychology as 'social desirability bias', that people tend to give the responses that they think will make them look good. As Ahmed (2010: 5) points out, if happiness is what everyone wants, then to be asked how happy you are is a very loaded question. How you answer can affect not only how others see you, but also how you see yourself, and perhaps even how you feel. Each year I get my students to take one of the many SWB tests available online. Invariably the de-briefing involves several people saying how they wanted to go back and change their answers, 'because I am a very positive person and I didn't feel that the results I got reflected that'. These are online surveys where the results are visible only to the individual. The extent to which we nonetheless regulate our responses shows the weight that rating our happiness carries in our performance of self (Goffman 1959) – with ourselves in the front row, even if there is no one else in the audience.

While it is clearly mistaken simply to identify quantitative research with objective data and qualitative with subjective, there is nonetheless a discernible association that derives from their techniques and epistemologies. The stress on social construction in qualitative methods, the emphasis on the meanings carried even by the tangible and material, tends to give even the most concrete observation a certain subjective character. Many qualitative researchers, myself included, find it hard to refer to objective wellbeing without placing 'objective' in quotation marks. As Sahlins (1976: 168) puts it:

> No society can live on miracles.... None can fail to provide for the biological continuity of the population in determining it culturally.... Yet men do not merely 'survive'. They survive in a definite way.

Conversely, the logic of quantitative methodologies is to objectify their data, breaking the link to their subjects, discarding as unhelpful noise the specificities of cultural or personal meanings. The yen of quantitative researchers towards the objective, even though their material is subjective, shows in the search for external indicators of emotional states. This is what seems to underlie the OECD's (2013: 41) claim that measures of SWB can transcend the limits of people's own understanding, revealing the inner truth of how people are *really* doing, even beyond their 'conscious' thoughts and feelings.

> Most importantly, measures of subjective well-being provide information on the actual impact of an initiative on the respondent's subjective well-being, rather than the impact that the respondent consciously identifies.
>
> (OECD 2013: 41)

Perhaps most obviously, the longing for the objective amongst quantitative researchers of SWB is expressed in the repeated claims that there is now a 'science of happiness' (e.g. Diener 2000, Graham 2011, Layard 2006).

Towards a relational view of wellbeing

Relational wellbeing is an emergent concept that provides some major challenges to the dominant conceptions of wellbeing and the ways these have been mobilised in policy. It is the concept that underlies the positioning of wellbeing – or 'living well together' – as a political alternative to development. Rather than economics or psychology, relational wellbeing is framed by sociological, anthropological or geographical perspectives and is primarily qualitative in orientation. While it has yet to be categorised definitively, it can be discerned from the convergence of views of a number of scholars working quite independently. As such, there are many trends that are shared and some that have been developed by one specific scholar or group of scholars. This book is intended as a contribution to the advancement of relational wellbeing into a more robust and widely used concept.

The starting point of relational wellbeing is that notions of wellbeing are seen as socially and culturally constructed, rooted in a particular time and place (Atkinson et al. 2012). This makes it critical not to assume a 'universal' approach, but to investigate how wellbeing is understood by the people who are the subjects of research (see e.g. Atkinson et al. 2012, Calestani 2013, Fischer 2014, Jackson 2011, Jimenez ed. 2008, Mathews and Izquierdo 2008, Thin 2012). In the majority of cases, these 'local' concepts are relational in a second sense. Wellbeing is not seen as the property of individuals but as something that belongs to and emerges through relationships with others (Christopher 1999). This is particularly evident in studies outside the West, where people tend to lay greater emphasis on collective identities and relationships of (often unequal) reciprocity. Jackson (2011: 59), in his study of the Kuranko people in Sierra Leone, expresses this clearly in a passage commenting on Sen's capability approach:

> Because human existence is nothing if not *social and ethical*, fulfilment does not lie solely in our freedom 'to lead the kind of life [we have] reason to value'; it consists in our capacity to realize ourselves in relation to others.

While cultural forms clearly differ, it is worth noting that this sense of 'being-in-relationship' is also found in many of the everyday ways that ordinary people in the West talk about wellbeing, which are quite different to the abstracted and individualised approaches of much wellbeing scholarship.

In Figure 1.2, relational wellbeing appears in the upper centre area of the diagram, showing its interest in wellbeing is substantive, and it exists in the overlap between objective and subjective approaches. It is important to recognise how it differs from subjective and psychological wellbeing. Scholars of subjective and psychological wellbeing also recognise the importance of material sufficiency and security and good relationships for an individual's wellbeing, but they envisage this primarily in exterior terms, with wellbeing itself defined as intra-psychic. Thus economic or relational status might be calculated as an independent variable, having an *effect on* subjective or psychological wellbeing as the dependent variable (see also Ramirez forthcoming, White and Ramirez, Jha and White, this volume). In relational wellbeing, material, relational and subjective dimensions are seen as mutually imbricated and co-constituting (see Gough and McGregor 2007, White 2010). As White (2010) explains, the rice which is emblematic of Bangladeshi conceptions of wellbeing is thus not simply a source of calories, but is a condensed symbol of community – those you eat with and those you do not – love, identity, nourishment, entitlement and belonging. As in the quotation from Sahlins above, when seen like this, simple oppositions between 'objective' and 'subjective' wellbeing begin to dissolve.

A further aspect of relational wellbeing which distinguishes it from the other concepts is its stress on wellbeing as process. This perhaps remains to be fully explored and appears in a number of different forms. One is attention to life-course and the way that current understandings of wellbeing incorporate both reflections on the past and expectations of the future (Lloyd-Sherlock and Locke 2008, White 2002, Huovinen and Blackmore plus Rodríguez, this volume). Another is to frame wellbeing as something that *happens* rather than as a set state. An example would be the analysis of Rivers' experience in the Solomon Islands, which opens this chapter. A third approach is to emphasise the dynamic inter-relations between different components of wellbeing. McGregor (2007: 337) for example characterises wellbeing processes as 'involving the interplay over time of: goals formulated, resources deployed, goals and needs met, and the degree of satisfaction in their achievement'. Davies (this volume) stresses the iterative and systemic character of relations between people and the environment in her notion of 'wellbeing ecology'. Fourth, seeing wellbeing as process helps to recognise how (personal) wellbeing is increasingly invoked in self-management, or – as suggested above – implicated in the performance of self (Ahmed 2010,

Atkinson 2013: 140–141). Atkinson (2013) presents the most radical approach, in which wellbeing is detached from individualised subjects and inheres instead in assemblages of relationships amongst people and places and material objects and intangible aspects of places (such as atmosphere).[18] Wellbeing thus becomes profoundly situated and relational, located in 'the movement and clusterings of affect' that emerge at particular conjunctions of time and place (Atkinson 2013: 142).

Its awareness of complexity and emphasis on the social context may make relational wellbeing seem less 'policy-ready' than some other formulations. In fact, however, there are a number of ways in which relational wellbeing has clear practical implications.

Atkinson (2013: 139) suggests that the very fact that there is no precise or generally acceptable definition of wellbeing makes it valuable as a process tool. She describes how the process of discussing wellbeing, and the variability of concepts that this involved, was itself useful in formulating goals for local government action. This is one of the main ways that Wellbeing Wales used their 'sustainable wellbeing toolbox' (Thomas 2014). The reflections of other non-governmental organisations (NGOs) on their use of tools for wellbeing and QoL assessment similarly place a strong emphasis on the value of debate and discussion (White with Abeyasekera ed. 2014).

A relational wellbeing perspective also provides the grounds for policy critique. While there is much to be said for a wellbeing approach in policy, there is clearly the danger that it becomes simply the performance of a public relations exercise aimed at galvanising support through its 'people-friendly' form for established agendas and routines of policy practice. More concerningly, Ehrenreich's account of her experience of cancer shows that wellbeing narratives may be co-opted for very personal and invasive disciplining of the self. Addressing such issues is a political task and cannot be achieved through conceptual means alone. Nevertheless, the social and material grounding of relational wellbeing approaches provides them with better means to critique and resist. The primary technical and empiricist orientation of psychological and subjective wellbeing make them much more vulnerable to capture.

Brangan (this volume) states as follows the main policy message that arises from her research:

> Those interested in promoting health and preventing non-communicable diseases need to look upstream and beyond the sphere of health to consider how to create conditions conducive to the broader wellbeing within which health will more easily flourish.

While this reflects the immediate focus of her work in health, its general message of the need to look 'upstream' and beyond the specific policy focus summarises a theme that is common to many of the chapters presented in this book. This illustrates how the division drawn above between 'substantive' and 'evaluative' eventually breaks down: an evaluative tool that will result in improvements in policy and practice must ultimately be based in substantive understanding of the lives of the target population.

Atkinson (2013: 142) sums up as follows the ultimate implication for policy of relational wellbeing:

> A shift is demanded away from how to enhance the resources for wellbeing centred on individual acquisition and towards attending to the social, material and spatially situated relationships through which individual and collective wellbeing are effected.

Looking forward

The case-study chapters begin with Camfield's consideration of what can be learned by mixing qualitative with quantitative methods in developing wellbeing surveys. This opens with a broad review of the limitations of self-reported data, which provides an important frame of reference for subsequent chapters. Camfield then reflects on two of her own experiences of using mixing methods: cognitive de-briefing in which respondents are asked to describe what they were thinking as they responded to a survey and the creation of a taxonomy to guide quantitative analysis, based on open-ended interviews and participatory group activities. She argues that mixing methods in this way brings greater recognition of the value of qualitative approaches to policy. The two contexts in which these pieces of research took place were, respectively, a study of the skills of young entrepreneurs in South Africa and the pathways of poverty and child wellbeing amongst children and their households in rural Ethiopia. With regard to the framework set out above, the studies combine a comprehensive approach to wellbeing with a relational concept of wellbeing. In terms of Figure 1.1, the chapter thus suggests that the combination of multiple baselines linking method and context will lead ultimately to a more robust account of wellbeing. At the same time, each of these lines might perhaps be shown as intermittent, since combining methods makes clear that all data are socially constructed, and so helps to dissolve the notion that there is a strict divide between 'objective' and 'subjective'. Camfield closes with a caution that not all of the tensions between qualitative and quantitative accounts of wellbeing can be resolved through technical solutions, implying that different methods can produce different and non-commensurate accounts of wellbeing. She also suggests that SWB data should be handled cautiously until more is understood about how people interpret the questions they are asked, especially in the Global South.

Chapter 3 addresses the politics of wellbeing methodologies, with Oman's analysis of the UK ONS debate 'Measuring National Well-being: "What Matters to You?"' which took place from November 2010 to April 2011. With regard to the framework in Figure 1.1, the survey reflects comprehensive wellbeing. Oman contrasts the inclusive rhetoric of the debate with the way that qualitative, free-text fields in the survey were largely ignored, resulting in exclusive reliance on quantitative data analysis in the interpretation of results. She points to many ways that politics can inhere in the exigencies of procedures (such as coding too quickly), or routines of practice, such as retro-fitting answers to already established codes and using qualitative statements merely to 'illustrate' points that have been determined through other methods, or that even pre-date the research. Expertise within research teams also has political implications, resulting in some kinds of data and analysis being privileged from the start. The way data were stored for example, which did not allow for the retrieval of individual respondents' answers, indicates that this was not conceived as a fully mixed method project.

Oman argues that the political position of the ONS combined with their strong bias towards quantitative expertise led them systematically either to ignore or misinterpret most of what participants writing in the free-text fields were hoping to convey. Her own discourse analysis of these data demonstrates that the content comprised both political critique and a more relational understanding of wellbeing. In this case, the second point of the triangle in Figure 1.1 (where and with whom: context) is virtually collapsed into the first, as the combination of the institutional position of the ONS (the 'who') and its strong bias towards statistical analysis (the 'how') significantly over-determined the account of wellbeing that the 'debate' could produce.

Chapter 4, by Brangan, explores what qualitative methods can add to quantitative surveys, as she contrasts the universalising constructs of so-called health behaviours with the ways in which people managed food and physical exercise in their everyday lives. The 'where and with whom' this time is a largely black township in Cape Town, South Africa. The main characters in the 'who and how' are Brangan and her research assistant, using ethnography and semi-structured qualitative interviews. In the background are public health professionals who had undertaken a quantitative epidemiological study of 'health behaviour' and non-communicable diseases with the same respondents. Far from being hostile to Brangan's perspective, they were eager to hear about her work and recognised their own was missing something. In some instances the qualitative data help explain some apparent anomalies in the quantitative data. In others, the two forms of data present very different profiles of the individuals involved. The overall model here is personal wellbeing, informed strongly by a public health, bio-medical perspective. Into this, Brangan brings a relational wellbeing perspective. This emphasises how the material and social context significantly construct the 'choices' that people are able to exercise. Like Camfield, Brangan finds that her interviewees' interpretation of questions about life satisfaction inverts the normal expectations. Like Eyber (see below), she finds that religion is of great significance to how people talk and think about wellbeing. In terms of policy implications, the message is clear: understanding people's own perspectives and the interplay of material, relational and subjective dimensions within them is critical to the design of an effective and appropriate health policy design.

White and Ramirez's chapter, Chapter 5, explores the importance of the economic within subjective dimensions of wellbeing. It presents data from Chiawa, Zambia, where men and women villagers were subjects both of a predominantly quantitative survey and of more in-depth, life history interviews. The research as a whole took a comprehensive approach to wellbeing, looking across a range of factors such as health and educational status and provision, livelihoods and subjective dimensions of wellbeing. A new, relational concept of 'inner wellbeing' was produced. In this case two very different approaches of statistical and discourse analysis reinforce each other in emphasising the importance of economic perspectives. Quantitative analysis shows that within inner wellbeing it is the economic domain that is most strongly associated with happiness. Objective economic status also has a significant effect on subjective and inner wellbeing scores. Qualitative analysis shows how economic capacity plays a central role in (male) gender identities and ways that people emphasise reciprocity and the *moral* dimensions of the economy. It also shows how people use economic references as an expressive idiom in speaking of the self. Taken together, therefore, both qualitative and quantitative evidences suggest the need for adjustment in the account of wellbeing, from the psychological subject generally assumed by much wellbeing research, to one that gives greater weight to the economic dimensions of subjectivity.

In Chapter 6, Jha and White present data from the same overall project as Chapter 5, but this time from Chhattisgarh, Central India. The focus is on women and a discussion of close relationships. The authors describe the challenges they encountered in developing a quantitative measure of wellbeing in family relationships and the difference between the high scores given in response to direct survey questions and much less positive qualitative accounts. They relate this to ideologies of the 'happy family' which make people feel they should project a positive image whatever their actual experience. The chapter demonstrates how understandings of wellbeing are place-specific, in that for some women at least, the family household was a place where strength was expressed in staying silent, rather than in speech. This is in contrast to general assumptions that identify wellbeing with self-expression and close relationships with the sharing of intimate thoughts and feelings. In addition to the survey data, the chapter presents in-depth case studies of two unusually empowered women. These develop understandings of wellbeing as process, as they demonstrate how women's management and negotiation of relationships play a significant part in its active construction day by day.

The second section of the case studies is dedicated to qualitative methods. In Chapter 7, Huovinen and Blackmore describe the centrality of relationships to the wellbeing of people in the midst of geographical mobility in Peru. Place emerges as a key theme through which people structure their life stories. The research location is a shantytown in Lima, Peru. Semi-structured interviews through which people narrated their 'mobility stories' are the main research instrument. As in other chapters, gender emerges as a key factor structuring people's responsibilities within, and capacities to maintain, relationships. As with Jha and White, the in-depth interviews provide evidence of the complexity and ambivalence of relationships and the ways they shift over time. In some ways, Huovinen and Blackmore's emphasis on the importance of affect chimes with the psychological subject of dominant wellbeing discourses. Where they differ, however, is in representing relationality as central to their subjects' constitution of self, rather than seeing them as free-standing individuals to whom relationships might be attached. Huovinen and Blackmore also make clear that the experience of affect takes particular cultural forms in different places. They identify in particular two key concepts that are central to the Peruvian elaboration of relational wellbeing in contexts of mobility. The first is 'relational anchoring', which describes how key relationships are built and reworked over distance and time. The second is *pena*, which describes the acute sadness and longing for what is lost. In contrast to Jha and White's findings of Indian women choosing to keep their sorrows to themselves, Huovinen and Blackmore show how, in Peru, people's expression of *pena* may mobilise others to provide support.

Eyber's chapter (Chapter 8) takes as its thematic focus religion in the context of psychosocial interventions addressing personal wellbeing. The location is Angola in 2000, during a period of armed conflict. As with Oman, and to some extent Brangan, the main argument concerns what is missed due to the professional blinkers of the main actors charged with wellbeing, in this case the mental health and psychosocial support workers. Eyber initially shared these blinkers, but her methods of participant observation, semi-structured interviews and focus-group discussions forced her to recognise and see beyond them. In terms of accounts of wellbeing, the key message is that professional investments can prevent (in this case religious) dimensions from being acknowledged. As psychosocial approaches were already positioned as 'less rigorous' than the 'hard sciences', acknowledging religion could have jeopardised workers' hard-won and still somewhat fragile professional status. They were also not sure what to do with religion, if it were acknowledged. The irony is that the religious discourses in many ways mirror those in personal wellbeing, as they emphasise individual responsibility ('many people are sick because of their sins') and the need for personal action for change. With regard to wider policy implications, Eyber makes the interesting suggestion that accounts of wellbeing need to be assessed not for their 'truth' but according to what other accounts they silence or exclude, or what alternatives they enable to flourish.

In Chapter 9, Davies describes how participatory photography enabled villagers in a mine-affected part of Cambodia to reveal many different interconnecting levels of what wellbeing meant to them. This indicates an often forgotten aspect of dominance in research methods: that of the spoken word. Davies' analysis points to the limits of the verbal – people may experience wellbeing, but may not label it as such or analyse it in such abstract terms. It may also be something, quite simply, that is difficult to put into words. Another important dimension of this approach is that it passed the initiative to villagers to set the agenda of discussions, as they chose what to photograph and then sorted through the pictures in advance of the interview to decide which they would talk about and what they wanted to say. The accounts of wellbeing that emerged were multi-relational, interweaving past, present and future, the changing environment and sense of space, family, food and above all, land. This again points to the difficulty of separating objective and subjective, or indeed material, relational and subjective. It also substantiates the argument above that accounts of relational wellbeing must configure a process: it happens in motion, not stasis.

The last two chapters reflect the face of wellbeing as an alternative to development. They report research with indigenous peoples in Mexico and Venezuela, respectively, whose community identities are intertwined with the articulation of a distinctive vision of wellbeing. They thus point to the politicisation of indigenous notions of 'living well together', or *buen vivir*, in Latin America more generally. But they also show that what it means to live well is not a settled cultural script, but a matter of internal contestation. In Chapter 10, Loera-González presents research in two indigenous communities in Mexico. With regard to the 'who and how', he reflects on the importance of his own positionality, and particularly the way he entered the village, in privileging some kinds of voices over others. Echoing other chapters, he emphasises the importance of ethnography and time spent simply being amongst people in enabling him to move beyond his initial presumptions and enabling different narratives to emerge. He emphasises how power is associated with different representations of wellbeing, as a strong narrative of social homogeneity and ethnic solidarity is enunciated by the elders, while younger, more socially marginal men stress economic hardship and their search for a better life in town. But he also makes clear how the politics of wellbeing narratives differ by place. In Mexican society more broadly, it is the narrative of indigenous identity and difference that appears marginal, and the search for a more individualised wellbeing through the market the more authorised form.

The volume concludes with Rodríguez's reflection on her participatory research with the Pemon-Taurepan in Venezuela. Anxieties about the loss of identity triggered processes of community reflection that led ultimately to a reassertion of rights and visions of wellbeing and development. Here again the understanding of wellbeing as process is very strong. It was through the re-construction and recovery of community history that the Pemon-Taurepan were able to produce the book of their *Life Plan*, which expressed their vision of the future. However, this process was also difficult and conflictual: the doubts and hostility of one of the elders were only overcome when the book was finally published. Along with this sense of process, something shifting and twisting and happening in time, goes the awareness of politics. At its simplest, the energy behind producing the *Life Plan* ebbed and flowed according to the political leadership. More significantly perhaps, the *Life Plan* was important to the Pemon-Taurepan both intrinsically – in recovering their sense of identity – and instrumentally – giving them a basis to negotiate with outsiders about property rights and resources. Whereas all the other chapters show the researchers as outsiders, Rodríguez entered at the invitation of the community because they saw she could be of use to them. This chapter thus draws the two base points of the triangle in Figure 1.1 very closely together: the researchers and researched are no longer distinct from one another, as the community is engaged in defining its own project of wellbeing.

Conclusion: Wellbeing as a field of power

As wellbeing becomes a more accepted part of policy discourses, so the need to address wellbeing – for individuals, organisations, businesses and government – becomes ever greater. This may have positive outcomes, with greater attention being paid to promoting the conditions which enable people to thrive. But it may also intensify self-monitoring, with greater pressure to produce and perform happiness or wellbeing as a marker of personal or collective value. To recognise this dilemma is to recognise wellbeing as a field of power.

This introductory chapter has set out four main 'faces' of wellbeing in public policy and four main concepts that underlie these. It has suggested some dimensions of the methodological complexities that attend the study of wellbeing and outlined the chapters to come. It has suggested that the *subject* and what it means to be *subjective* remain radically under-theorised in the literature on subjective dimensions of wellbeing and that relational wellbeing presents an important emerging approach.

Across the different contributions of this book, based in different places and reflecting on different areas of life, there are a number of common messages. The first is that wellbeing should not be seen as a 'real thing' that people may 'have', but that constructions of wellbeing are intrinsically connected to the places in which they are produced, the people who present the account and the methods of data generation and analysis. This suggests the importance of modesty and methodological reflexivity, recognising the strengths and limitations of one's own approach, how the various methods are governed by specific assumptions and being prepared to recognise the value in a quite different perspective. The second is that understandings of wellbeing vary across cultures. The vision of wellbeing as a source of alternative policy and practice needs to be founded not on some comparative ranking against a single measure, but on finding means to listen and discuss that can promote a genuine inter-personal and intercultural dialogue. The third is that the translation of wellbeing into policy is by no means straightforward, but carries a serious risk of co-option by anti-progressive forces and being ransacked of all meaning so it simply becomes a performance to expectations. Underlying all these three points is an appreciation of wellbeing as a field of power.

In closing, I recall the words of Robert Serpell, Professor of Psychology at the University of Zambia, who pointed out to me how culturally specific is the aspiration for universality. For most people it is no problem to accept that their lives are lived in a particular form belonging to a specific context. It is a modern Western intellectual conceit to seek a framework that can comprehend the world.

Notes

1. This work is supported by the Economic and Social Research Council/Department for International Development Joint Scheme for Research on International Development (Poverty Alleviation) grant number RES-167-25-0507 ES/H033769/1.
2. The websites for these indices are as follows: Global Agewatch Index: http://www.helpage.org/global-agewatch/; Happy Planet Index: http://www.happyplanetindex.org/; Legatum Institute: http://www.prosperity.com/; OECD Better Life Index: http://www.wikiprogress.org/; Social Progress Imperative: http://www.socialprogressimperative.org/; data/spi [all accessed 12 July 2015].
3. More information about Gross National Happiness is available at: http://www.grossnationalhappiness.com/articles/ [accessed 12 July 2015].
4. There is no discussion of the political implications of this. The analysis is also very thin. For Egypt and Tunisia for the years leading up to 2011, declines in scores on life satisfaction from the Gallup World Poll are contrasted with rises in GDP. There is no mention, for example, of indices of inequality over the same period.
5. For many years, the most commonly used measure was in fact gross national product (GNP) rather than GDP. Both are measures of national output and income, but GNP also includes the calculation of net income flows in and out of the country. For simplicity I just use the term GDP in this chapter as the most commonly used measure in the wellbeing debates.
6. *Buen vivir* is the Spanish term. Other terms in indigenous languages include *suma qamaña* (Aymara) and *sumac kawsay* (Quechua).
7. The SWLS asks people to respond using a seven-point scale from strongly disagree to strongly agree to the statements: 'In most ways my life is close to my ideal'; 'the conditions of my life are excellent'; 'I am satisfied with my life'; 'so far I have gotten the important things I want in life'; 'if I could live my life over, I would change almost nothing' (Diener *et al.* 1985).
8. The PWI domains are standard of living, personal health, achieving in life, personal relationships, personal safety, community-connectedness, future security and spirituality-religion (International Wellbeing Group 2013).

9. The source of this approach is Cantril's (1965) Self-anchoring Striving Scale.
10. This is reinforced by Gallup's classification of responses into 'thriving', 'struggling' and 'suffering'.
11. Somewhat ironically, they also note, however, that experience sampling 'has never been applied to a representative population sample because it is burdensome' (Stiglitz et al. 2009: 147).
12. Preamble to the Constitution of the World Health Organization as adopted by the International Health Conference, New York, 19–22 June 1946; signed on 22 July 1946 by the representatives of 61 states (Official Records of the World Health Organization, no. 2, p. 100) and entered into force on 7 April 1948.
13. Ryff's domains are self-acceptance, positive relations with others, autonomy, environmental mastery, purpose in life and personal growth.
14. This includes figures such as Jahoda (1958), Maslow (1954), Allport (1961) and Rogers (1961).
15. It can also be reduced to three items per domain, but this is less reliable psychometrically, so not recommended.
16. Responses to this item would be reverse coded, so strong agreement would score as a negative wellbeing.
17. Sahlins (1976: 211) argues that in 'bourgeois society', 'economic symbolism is structurally determining'. Different kinds of society have different 'dominant sites of symbolic production' and in this case it is the economy (in others it might be religion, for example). This means that 'the cultural scheme is variously inflected by a dominant site of symbolic production, which supplies the major idiom of other relations and activities' (Sahlins 1976: 211).
18. Atkinson references this point to Panelli and Tipa (2009).

References

Ahmed, S. (2010) *The Promise of Happiness*. Durham and London: Duke University Press.

Alesinaa, A., Di Tellab, R. and MacCulloch, R. (2004) Inequality and Happiness: Are Europeans and Americans Different? *Journal of Public Economics* 88: 2009–2042.

Alkire, S. and Foster, J. (2011) Counting and Multidimensional Poverty Measurement. *Journal of Public Economics* 95: 476–487.

Allport, G. W. (1961) *Pattern and Growth in Personality*. New York: Holt, Rinehart and Winston.

Angner, E. (2011) The Evolution of Eupathics: The Historical Roots of Subjective Measures of Wellbeing. *International Journal of Wellbeing* 1(1): 4–41.

Artaraz, K. and Calestani, M. (2014) Suma Qamaña in Bolivia Indigenous Understandings of Well-Being and Their Contribution to a Post-Neoliberal Paradigm. *Latin American Perspectives*. Online first. 1–18. DOI: 10.1177/0094582X14547501.

Atkinson, S. (2013) Beyond Components of Wellbeing: The Effects of Relational and Situated Assemblage. *Topoi* 32: 137–144.

Atkinson, S., Fuller, S. and Painter, J. (eds.) (2012) *Wellbeing and Place*. London: Ashgate.

Barker, P. (1998) *The Regeneration Trilogy*. London: Penguin Books.
Berridge, K. and Kringelbach, M. (2011) Building a Neuroscience of Pleasure and Well-Being. *Psychology of Wellbeing: Theory, Research and Practice* 1(3): 1–26.
Biswas-Diener, R. (ed.) (2011) *Positive Psychology and Social Change*. London: Springer.
Brickman, P. and Campbell, D. (1971) Hedonic Relativism and Planning the Good Society. pp. 287–302 in M. H. Appley (ed.) *Adaption Level Theory: A Symposium*. New York: Academic Press.
Calestani, M. (2013) *An Anthropological Journey into Well-Being*. Insights from Bolivia: Springer.
Cantril, H. (1965) *The Pattern of Human Concerns*. New Brunswick, NJ: Rutgers University Press.
Chirkov, V. I., Ryan R. M. and Sheldon, K. M. (eds.) (2011) *Human Autonomy in Cross-Cultural Context: Perspectives on the Psychology of Agency, Freedom and Well-being*. New York: Springer.
Christopher, J. (1999) Situating Psychological Well-Being: Exploring the Cultural Roots of Its Theory and Research. *Journal of Counseling and Development* 77: 141–154.
Clark, D. A. (ed.) (2012) *Adaptation, Poverty and Development: The Dynamics of Subjective Well-Being*. Basingstoke: Palgrave Macmillan.
Collard, D. (2006) Research on Well-Being: Some Advice from Jeremy Bentham. *Philosophy of the Social Sciences* 36(3): 330–354.
Cooper, F. and Packard, R. (eds.) (1997) *International Development and the Social Sciences: Essays on the History and Politics of Knowledge*. London: University of California Press.
Craib, I. (1994) *The Importance of Disappointment*. London: Routledge.
Crush, J. (ed.) (1995) *Power of Development*. London: Routledge.
Deaton, A. (2012) The Financial Crisis and the Well-Being of Americans. *Oxford Economic Papers* 64(1): 1–26.
De la Cadena, M. (2010) Indigenous Cosmopolitics in the Andes: Conceptual Reflections beyond Politics. *Cultural Anthropology* 25(2): 334–370.
Diener, E. (2000) The Science of Happiness and a Proposal for a National Index. *American Psychologist* 55(1): 34–43.
Diener, E., Emmons, R. A., Larsen, R. J. and Griffin, S. (1985) The Satisfaction with Life Scale. *Journal of Personality Assessment* 49: 71–75.
Diener, E., Ng, W., Harter, J. and Arora, R. (2010) Wealth and Happiness across the World: Material Prosperity Predicts Life Evaluation, Whereas Psychosocial Prosperity Predicts Positive Feeling. *Journal of Personality and Social Psychology* 99(1): 52–61.
Diener, E., Scollon, C., Oishi, S., Dzokoto, V. and Suh, M. (2000) Positivity and the Construction of Life Satisfaction Judgments: Global Happiness Is Not the Sum of Its Parts. *Journal of Happiness Studies* 1(2): 159–176.
Easterlin, R. A. (1974) Does Economic Growth Improve the Human Lot? pp. 88–125 in Paul A. David and Melvin W. Reder (eds.) *Nations and Households in Economic Growth: Essays in Honor of Moses Abramovitz*. New York: Academic Press, Inc.
Ehrenreich, B. (2009) *Smile or Die. How Positive Thinking Fooled America and the World*. London: Granta Publications.

Fabricant, N. (2013) Good Living for Whom? Bolivia's Climate Justice Movement and the Limitations of Indigenous Cosmovisions. *Latin American and Caribbean Ethnic Studies* 8(2): 159–178.
Fischer, E. (2014) *Aspiration, Dignity and the Anthropology of Wellbeing*. Stanford: Stanford University Press.
Frey, B. S. and Gallus, J. (2013) Subjective Well-Being and Policy. *Topoi* 32(2) 207–212.
Gallup (n.d.) 'Understanding How Gallup Uses the Cantril Scale.' Available at: http://www.gallup.com/poll/122453/understanding-gallup-uses-cantril-scale.aspx [accessed 23 November 2014].
Gasper, D. (2010) Understanding the Diversity of Conceptions of Well-Being and Quality of Life. *Journal of Socio-Economics* 39(3): 351–360.
Goffman, I. (1959) *The Presentation of Self in Everyday Life*. New York: Anchor Books.
Gough, I. R. and McGregor, J. A. (eds.) (2007) *Wellbeing in Developing Countries: New Approaches and Research Strategies*. Cambridge: Cambridge University Press.
Graham, C. (2011) *The Pursuit of Happiness: An Economy of Wellbeing*. Washington: Brookings Institution Press.
Grossberg, L. (1996) Identity and Cultural Studies – Is That All There Is? pp. 53–60 in S. Hall and P. du Gay (ed.) *Questions of Cultural Identity*. London: Sage.
Held, B. (2002) The Tyranny of the Positive Attitude in America: Observation and Speculation. *Journal of Clinical Psychology* 58(9): 965–992.
International Wellbeing Group (2013) *Personal Wellbeing Index: 5th Edition*. Melbourne: Australian Centre on Quality of Life, Deakin University. Available at: http://www.deakin.edu.au/research/acqol/instruments/wellbeing-index/index.php [accessed 21 November 2014].
Jackson, M. (2011) *Life within Limits: Wellbeing in a World of Want*. Durham, USA: Duke University Press.
Jahoda, M. (1958) *Current Concepts of Positive Mental Health*. New York: Basic Books.
Jimenez, A. (ed.) (2008) *Culture and Well-Being: Anthropological Approaches to Freedom and Political Ethics*. London: Pluto Press.
Kahneman, D. and Deaton, A. (2010) High Income Improves Evaluation of Life But Not Emotional Well-Being. *Proceedings of the National Academy of Sciences of the United States of America* 107(38): 16489–16493.
Larson, R. and Csikszentmihalyi, M. (1983) The Experience Sampling Method. *New Directions for Methodology of Social and Behavioral Science* 15: 41–56.
Layard, R. (2006) *Happiness: Lessons from a New Science*. London: Allen Lane.
Lloyd-Sherlock, P. and Locke, C. (2008) Vulnerable Relations: Lifecourse, Wellbeing and Social Exclusion in Buenos Aires. *Ageing and Society* 28(8) 1117–1201.
Maslow, A. (1954) *Motivation and Personality*. New York: Harper.
Mathews, G. and Izquierdo, C. (2008) *Pursuits of Happiness: Well-Being in Anthropological Perspective*. New York/Oxford: Berghahn books.
McGregor, J. A. (2007) Researching Wellbeing: From Concepts to Methodology. pp. 316–350 in I. R. Gough and J. A. McGregor (eds.) *Wellbeing in Developing Countries: New Approaches and Research Strategies*. Cambridge: Cambridge University Press.

Miller, J. G., Das, R. and Chakravarthy, S. (2011) Culture and the Role of Choice in Agency. *Journal of Personality and Social Psychology* 101(1): 46–61.

NDP Steering Committee and Secretariat (2013) Happiness: Towards a New Development Paradigm. Report of the Kingdom of Bhutan. Available at: http://www.newdevelopmentparadigm.bt/wp-content/uploads/2013/12/NDP_Report_Bhutan_2013.pdf.

Nettle, D. (2005) *Happiness: The Science behind Your Smile*. Oxford: Oxford University Press.

Noll, H. (2011) The Stigliz-Sen-Fitoussi-Report: Old Wine in New Skins? Views from a Social Indicators Perspective. *Social Indicators Research* 102: 111–116.

Nussbaum, M. (2012) Who Is the Happy Warrior? Philosophy, Happiness Research, and Public Policy. *International Review of Economics* 59(4): 335–361.

OECD (2013) *OECD Guidelines on Measuring Subjective Well-Being*. European Union: OECD Publishing.

ONS (2011) Measuring National Well-Being: A Discussion Paper on Domains and Measures. Available at: http://www.ons.gov.uk/ons/rel/wellbeing/measuring-national-well-being/discussion-paper-on-domains-and-measures/measuring-national-well-being---discussion-paper-on-domains-and-measures.html.

ONS (2014) Measures of National Wellbeing. Available at: http://www.neighbourhood.statistics.gov.uk/HTMLDocs/dvc146/wrapper.html [accessed February 6 2015].

Panelli, R. and Tipa, G. (2009) Beyond Foodscapes: Considering Geographies of Indigenous Wellbeing. *Health Place* 15: 455–465.

Radcliffe, S. A. (2011) Development for a Postneoliberal Era? Sumak Kawsay, Living Well and the Limits to Decolonisation in Ecuador. *Geoforum* 43(2012): 240–249.

Ramirez, V. (forthcoming) The Roles of Human Relationships in Wellbeing: The Case of the Oportunidades Social Programme in Mexico. Unpublished PhD thesis, University of Bath.

Rasmussen, D. and Akulukjuk, T. (2009) 'My Father Was Told to Talk to the Environment First before Anything Else:' Arctic Environmental Education in the Language of the Land. pp. 285–298 in M. McKenzie (ed.) *Fields of Green: Restorying Culture, Environment, and Education*. Cresskill, NJ: Hampton Press.

Rogers, C. R. (1961) *On Becoming a Person*. Boston: Houghton Mifflin.

Rothstein, B. (2010) Happiness and the Welfare State. *Social Research* 77(2): 441–468.

Ryan, R. M. and Deci, E. (2001) On Happiness and Human Potentials: A Review of Research on Hedonic and Eudaimonic Well Being. *Annual Review of Psychology* 52: 141–166.

Ryff, C. D. (1989) Happiness Is Everything, or Is It? Explorations on the Meaning of Psychological Well-Being. *Journal of Personality and Social Psychology* 57: 1069–1081.

Ryff, C. D. and Keyes, C. L. M. (1995) The Structure of Psychological Well-Being Revisited. *Journal of Personality and Social Psychology* 69: 719–727.

Sahlins, M. (1976) *Culture and Practical Reason*. Chicago: University of Chicago Press.

Samuelson, P. (1938) A Note on the Pure Theory of Consumers' Behaviour. *Economica* 5 (17): 61–71.

Schwarz, N. (1999) Self-Reports. How the Questions Shape the Answers. *American Psychologist* 54(2): 93–105.
Schwarz, N. and Clore, G. L. (1983) Mood, Misattribution, and Judgements of Well-Being: Informative and Directive Functions of Affective States. *Journal of Personality and Social Psychology* 45: 513–523.
Seligman, M. (2011) *Flourish. A Visionary New Understanding of Happiness and Well-Being*. New York: Simon and Schuster, Inc.
Sen, A. (1983) Poor, Relatively Speaking. *Oxford Economic Papers* 35(2): 153–169.
Sen, A. (1993) Capability and Wellbeing. pp. 30–53 in A. Sen and M. Nussbaum (eds.) *The Quality of Life*. Oxford: Oxford University Press.
Sen, A. (2009) *The Idea of Justice*. London: Allen Lane.
Sointu, E. (2005) The Rise of an Ideal: Tracing Changing Discourses of Wellbeing. *The Sociological Review* 53(2): 255–274.
Stewart, F. (2014) Against Happiness: A Critical Appraisal of the Use of Measures of Happiness for Evaluating Progress in Development. *Journal of Human Development and Capabilities* 15(4): 293–307.
Stiglitz, J., Sen, A. and Fitoussi, J-P. (2009) Report of the Commission on the Measurement of Economic Performance and Social Progress. Available at: http://www.stiglitz-sen-fitoussi.fr/documents/rapport_anglais.pdf.
Tennant, R., Hiller, L., Fishwick, R., Platt, S., Joseph, S., Welch, S., Parkinson, J., Secker, J. and Stewart-Brown, S. (2007) The Warwick–Edinburgh Mental Wellbeing Scale (WEMWBS): Development and UK Validation. *Health and Quality of Life Outcomes* 5(63). DOI: 10.1186/1477-7525-5-63.
Thin, N. (2012) *Social Happiness: Theory into Policy and Practice*. Bristol: The Policy Press.
Thomas, D. (2014) Wellbeing Wales: The Sustainable Wellbeing Framework. pp 161–169 in S. C. White with A. Abeyasekera (ed.) *Wellbeing and Quality of Life Assessment: A Practical Guide*. Rugby: Practical Action Publishing.
Thompson, S., Aked, J., Marks, N. and Cordon, C. (2008) *Five Ways to Wellbeing: The Evidence*. London: New Economics Foundation.
United Nations (2011) Happiness: Towards a Holistic Approach to Development. Sixty-fifth session Agenda item 13. 65/309. Available at: http://www.un.org/ga/search/view_doc.asp?symbol=A/RES/65/309.
Veenhoven, R. (2000) Freedom and Happiness: A Comparative Study in 46 Nations in the Early 1990s. pp 257–288 in E. Diener, E. and E. M. Suh (eds.) *Culture and Subjective Wellbeing*. Cambridge MA: MIT Press.
Watson, D., Clark, L. A. and Tellegen, A. (1988) Development and Validation of Brief Measures of Positive and Negative Affect: The PANAS Scales. *Journal of Personality and Social Psychology* 54(6): 1063–1070.
White, S. C. (2002) Being, Becoming and Relationship: Conceptual Challenges of a Child Rights Approach in Development. *Journal of International Development* 14(8): 1095–1104.
White, S. C. (2010) Analysing Wellbeing: A Framework for Development Policy and Practice. *Development in Practice* 20(2): 158–172.
White, S. C. with Abeyasekera, A. (ed.) (2014) *Wellbeing and Quality of Life Assessment: A Practical Guide*. Rugby: Practical Action Publishing.

Part I
Mixed Methods

2
Enquiries into Wellbeing: How Could Qualitative Data Be Used to Improve the Reliability of Survey Data?

Laura Camfield

Introduction

This chapter makes a methodological contribution to wellbeing approaches by exploring how mixing qualitative and quantitative methods in developing measures of factors contributing to wellbeing can increase researchers' understanding of the strengths and weaknesses of survey data. I argue that mixing methods highlights the subjective nature of 'objective' data, for example, the conscious, unconscious and often contingent influences on the way people respond when asked about their income. It also highlights the fragility of 'subjective' data such as judgements of satisfaction where there is no external referent against which a response can be evaluated. In the first part of the chapter, I look at cognitive interviewing or debriefing, which is not widely used in survey development outside the Global North. Using an example with young entrepreneurs in South Africa, I suggest that given the dominance of survey approaches within applied economic and health research, there may be a role for cognitive debriefing, not least in highlighting the temporal and cultural specificity of this form of measurement. But while cognitive debriefing can capture the conscious and articulable aspects of how people respond to questions (Tourangeau 1984), there are also processes that operate beneath people's awareness. I briefly discuss whether theories from psychology and behavioural economics can be applied in very different settings to help researchers understand these processes.

In the second part of the chapter, I highlight an additional role for qualitative research in the context of measurement. This is to increase the extent to which indicators and measures capture people's knowledge and values. I take as an example a taxonomy developed to understand how households move out of poverty in rural Ethiopia and the impact of this on child wellbeing (Roelen and Camfield 2012). This example enables me to look at how qualitative information from narratives and group discussion can be turned into measures or used to select indicators. I argue that quantifying this information might be a way of making the 'subjective' (or personally meaningful) 'objective' in the sense that it becomes externally visible and thus more amenable to being used in policy. This would at once increase the salience of qualitative data gathered in wellbeing research and potentially extend the capacity of quantitative measures to capture experienced changes in wellbeing. The chapter closes with a brief discussion of challenges for wellbeing research that may not be amenable to technical solutions.

Wellbeing and development

The potential of wellbeing as an alternative measure of development (Stiglitz *et al.* 2009) is limited, at least amongst economists, by a lack of confidence in the subjective measures used to represent it (Bertrand and Mullainathan 2001). For qualitative researchers, a far greater challenge is the incorporation of context to give some meaning to the results of 'global' measures such as satisfaction with life as a whole. How, for example, might global value chains and globalised tastes shape the self-reported wellbeing of children in coffee-growing communities in Southern Ethiopia? These influences are undoubtedly reflected in measures of subjective wellbeing, but how can researchers reliably draw out the extent and nature of their contribution?

Before I talk about the subjective aspects of measurement, I will start with some definitions. In this chapter, I take subjective data to be data that represent people's subjective experiences, for example, happiness, and the judgements they make about those experiences. I see objective data as data that are externally verifiable, which is not usually the case for descriptions of internal states or judgements about the quality of people's lives. Finally, I define self-reported data as data given in response to a question, whether objective (how many years of education do you have?) or subjective (how satisfied are you with the level of education you have received?). To talk of 'objective' data is itself a convention, of course. All these forms of data are subjective in the sense that they are human-made and inevitably influenced by the circumstances in which they were generated. This means that the way that data are generated matters a great deal. For example, in developing countries, households with landlines are likely to be wealthy and located in urban areas. Drawing on our own experiences, we can infer that people willing to answer telephone surveys are likely to be a very particular group (e.g. older and more influenced by norms of cooperation and service). It is therefore very important for the quality of data that responses to the World Values Survey and Afrobarometer are always elicited through face-to-face interviews rather than telephone interviews or self-completed questionnaires. This information tells us something about sampling, response rates and possibly even the nature of what will be reported (De Maio 1984). Psychological studies (reviewed in De Maio 1984) also show that face-to-face interviewing is likely to invoke particular forms of bias. This sensitivity of data to the context in which they are gathered suggests that good practice would not seek to compare data gathered through face-to-face interviews with survey data generated through other methods.

Influences on measurement of wellbeing using self-reported data

In relation to studies of wellbeing in developing countries, given that the pre-eminent research method is the household survey, almost all of the data used are likely to be self-reported. This may present problems including cognitive challenges such as comprehension and recall, issues with survey and research design such as framing effects, translation and the influence of the interviewer and a range of social, cultural and cognitive influences on how people make judgements. These are briefly explained below.

Responding to a survey raises issues of comprehension – do people understand the question? – and recall – will they accurately remember household consumption during the whole of the dry season, or household illness over the past four years? When we ask someone to make a global assessment of their wellbeing in the context of a survey, we present them with a considerable cognitive challenge. Research in psychology and behavioural economics suggests that people are 'cognitive misers' (Fiske and Taylor 1991). Consequently, they will deploy any number of shortcuts or heuristics to come to a judgement without too much intellectual effort. One shortcut is the accessibility of information, which relates to whether information is used frequently, recently, relates to personal or societal values, or to bodily experiences (for example, chronic illness, Schwarz and Strack 1999). The way the survey is designed may also have an influence on the self-reported data. All surveys are vulnerable to 'framing effects', which relate to how questions are asked or ordered (e.g. whether the survey question about satisfaction with life comes before or after the question about recent deaths within the household) and the context of survey administration (e.g. whether respondents are being interviewed on their own by an enumerator of the same gender or in the same room as their husband). For example, Strack et al. (1988) describe how if people are asked about frequency of dating just before evaluating their life satisfaction, their dating performance disproportionately influences their judgement, relative to those who are asked about dating after evaluating their life satisfaction.

Another concern that arises particularly for wellbeing researchers relates to translation and whether literal translations are genuinely comparable in terms of what they mean to respondents (Acquadro et al. 1996). For example, translation of the SF-35 health status measure into Russian found that whereas in the United States 'social activities' (items 6 and 10) means different activities with different people, in Russia it means, 'to participate in political meetings or act like a trade union leader', which is very different (International Quality of Life Assessment, unpublished report). Aside from potential distortion of meaning through translation, the language itself may have a framing effect as it evokes different ways of interacting. For example, Triandis et al. (1965) found systematic differences in the responses of Greek students attending an American school in Greece according to whether they were questioned in English or Greek.

Few qualitative researchers would disagree with the statement that all data, whether narrative or numerical, are co-generated through a particular interaction between a researcher and a respondent. This way of thinking about data is less familiar to survey researchers coming from a positivist research tradition. However, this does not mean that they are not aware of these problems and might describe how respondents answer questions strategically to avoid losing face, or potentially gain access to resources, or use interviewers as a reference group when they make a judgement about the quality of their life. If we accept this then it does not seem surprising that the identity and perceived objectives of the researcher affect the responses given. Nonetheless, psychologists have conducted ingenious experiments to prove this beyond doubt, for example, Strack et al. (1990) showed that respondents reported higher life satisfaction in interviews if the interviewer was of the opposite gender and lower life satisfaction if they believed the interviewer had a severe disability.

Understanding *how* people make the judgements they do also helps us understand why they make them. For example, whether their past experiences or future aspirations become part of the judgement they make about their wellbeing, or whether these are used as a point of contrast to make this judgement against. Elder (1974) noted that North American children who had been adolescents in the Great Depression were more likely to make positive evaluations of their current wellbeing. He suggests that this is because their experience of deprivation at a key stage in their lives had become their standard of comparison, although other literature suggests it may also be an effect of age. While comparisons are an important part of making judgements about wellbeing, they are not only about personal expectations or experiences (Michalos 1985), but may also be about one's own performance relative to others'. This is why, in the increasingly unequal contexts within which most development researchers are working, relative deprivation is becoming as great a research focus as absolute poverty. The interest is due both to the prevalence of inequality, which is often exacerbated by economic growth, and the detrimental effects of negative comparisons with more prosperous others on subjective wellbeing (d'Ambrosio and Frick 2004). For example, Graham and Pettinato (2002) identify a new and visibly less satisfied group of people in Peru – the 'frustrated achievers' – whose social mobility has put them at the bottom of a new economic reference group rather than at the top of their old one.

Another influence on people's judgements is the 'focusing illusion' (Schkade and Kahneman 1998), where respondents focus on a single, visible difference in making judgements about their own wellbeing relative to others'.[1] This may partially explain the observed influence of mood on overall judgements of wellbeing. Temporal biases are also important and Kahneman and Krueger (2006) argue that survey questions on wellbeing ('retrospective evaluations') are not reliable for this reason.[2] One example, which echoes debates about defining chronic poverty, is 'duration neglect' where when respondents evaluate whether an experience was good or bad, they do not appear to take into account how long it lasted. Instead, their memory is 'telescoped' into the best or worst moment and what happened at the end (Redelmeier and Kahneman 1996). The greater memorability of events that were intense, unusual, or recent is a possible source of distortion even with apparently 'objective' retrospective questions in household surveys. Another potential influence on responses is a tendency, identified by Kahneman and Tverskey (1979) and others, to focus on losses rather than gains (perhaps understandably in contexts where even small losses can have devastating consequences, see Mani *et al.* 2013). This makes people less satisfied with their lives when they can imagine things turning out better. Medvec *et al.* (1995), for example, established that silver medallists reported lower subjective wellbeing than bronze medallists, despite being in an objectively better position.

Finally, an important influence on subjective judgements of wellbeing and one of the main reasons why they are not considered credible or sufficient as a measure of wellbeing is adaptation, or the way humans adapt to socio-economic and environmental stimuli and adjust their judgements of these stimuli accordingly. Respondents may adapt upwards – becoming discontented – or downwards – accepting the unacceptable because they see no possibility of change. The capacity to adapt is not necessarily negative – as Nussbaum (2000: 137 in Clark ed. 2012: 9) observes: 'we get used to having the bodies we do have, and even if, as children, we wanted to fly like birds, we simply drop that after a while, and are probably the better for it.' However, it may obscure the difficulties that people are facing or act as an argument against addressing them – if the Global South is full of the 'happy peasant[s]' described by Graham (2009), it becomes easier to argue that the structures that keep them poor do not need to be addressed.

Cognitive debriefing amongst young entrepreneurs in South Africa

The Introduction points to some of the factors researchers may need to take into account in drawing conclusions about wellbeing using data from surveys and measures, or assessing the validity of others' claims. One of the best techniques for understanding what lies behind these data is cognitive debriefing, exemplified by Bowden *et al.*'s (2002) account of the development of the KENQOL measure to study self-reported health in Makueni district in Kenya. Cognitive debriefing aims to capture people's thought processes in responding to questions to identify potential problems. This reduces 'response errors',[3] improves data quality and informs the interpretation of the data (see also Fahmy *et al.* 2011, Pan *et al.* 2008, Willis 1999). The goal is for measures of wellbeing to work equally well during the four cognitive stages required to answer a question: comprehension – what does this question mean; recall – what information do I need to answer it; judgement – how does this information affect my evaluation; and response – given the preceding stages and my understanding of what is expected of me in this situation and what I can expect, how do I respond (Tourangeau 1984). As with pre-testing, the sample for cognitive debriefing should represent socio-economic and cultural diversity within the population. However, there may be a balance between capturing the experiences of people who might struggle to respond to the questions and getting useful data, since the process requires articulacy and meta-cognitive skills (i.e. recalling and interrogating your own thought processes). It also requires considerable skill on the part of the interviewer to ask questions that can be easily understood and develop rapport with the respondent which encourages them to continue participating and reduces concerns that they are being 'examined'. Non-verbal techniques of cognitive debriefing that are considered to work well with less articulate respondents include observing people while responding to the questionnaire, noting signs of difficulty, confusion, hesitation, or annoyance. People may also be asked to either describe how they are responding to the measure as they complete it ('think aloud') or recall what they thought each question was asking and how they chose their answer (retrospective 'verbal probing'). Finally, they are asked whether there were any words they did not understand or found offensive.

One example of why cognitive debriefing might be helpful comes from a comparison of data gathered using the Global Person Generated Index (GPGI) in rural Ethiopia with data from semi-structured interviews with the same individuals (reported in Camfield and Ruta 2007). One 73-year-old man from rural Ethiopia had an overall score for quality of life that was low but positive (63 per cent); however, his description of his current situation was, 'I am living a dead life, and I want to die [...] I am living a life that is horrible and very bad/worst', which suggests a much lower score. He also nominated 'health' as an important life area in his GPGI and rated it 6 out of 6, indicating great satisfaction. This does not seem to correspond to his interview, where he described himself as 'getting physically weak and old'. Mallinson (2002: 19) also observed these discrepancies between how people talked about their health and rated their health status because 'people are responding from different premises to each other and from the surveyor'. A technique such as cognitive debriefing can help resolve some of these by allowing us to explore the premises that people are responding from.

In the remainder of this section, I illustrate the value of cognitive debriefing using seven interviews I collected as part of a study of non-cognitive skills amongst young entrepreneurs in South Africa. I used the

World Bank's STEPS skills measures[4] as the basis for a longer measure of non-cognitive skills which initial qualitative work and consultation had suggested might be important for this group. It was administered to 683 respondents participating in the Awethu entrepreneurship programme in Soweto.[5] Almost all respondents (99 per cent) were black African and a third were female. The majority were educated to at least grade 12 (52 per cent) and fewer than five per cent had lower than grade ten, which may be an artefact of the selection criterion for the programme of fluency in English (this information is relevant given the demanding nature of cognitive interviewing). The seven respondents appeared to find responding to the 50 items easy and gave a good account of their thought processes, both retrospectively (one person) and concurrently (the remainder), using the think-aloud technique illustrated below. Particularly interesting was the way that cognitive debriefing showed how people made the questions personally meaningful. In the quote below, for example, the respondent relates items in a measure of self-esteem specifically to his experience of being a father.

> PULE: 'Are you able to do things as well as most other people?' Almost always. 'Do you feel that you have a lot to be proud of?' Definitely, almost always. One of the things that I am proud of is that I have got two daughters and I have been very involved in their upbringing since day one and they make me feel such like the best daddy in the world.

There were some practical problems relating to the four-point response scale, which was taken from the STEPS study, as respondents perceived a much larger gap between 'never' and 'most of the time' than between 'most of the time' and 'almost always'. This is a common form of wording in Likert scales and therefore a common problem. It suggests that the data generated using these scales cannot be treated as interval (where the gaps between each response option are treated as if they were the same) and analysed with parametric tests,[6] as is conventionally the case within psychology. Some were reluctant to use the extreme ends of the scale, for example, one person playfully refused to say that they were always talkative because they did not talk when they were asleep. Others found it easier to think in binaries (always/never) and harder to use the more qualified response options. Apparently simple questions, such as the main language spoken and occupational status, also proved challenging. The example below shows myself and two respondents discussing the best occupational classification for one of them:

NAUB: Yes, any of the following, shew, I am not a wage employee, I am not a casual worker, I am not unemployed either and I am not a business owner.
LAURA: Do you categorise yourself as not unemployed because you are working on your business?
NAUB: Perhaps, but then again I am involved in another business but then I run operations.
LAURA: Oh right.
NAUB: So I am not the business owner but then I run the operations of the business.
REGINALD: So that could be casual work.
NAUB: So I am not unemployed, I am not a casual worker.
LAURA: You might be a business partner then rather than a business owner.
NAUB: Okay, perhaps a business partner yes, that would be a better suited... [intervenes]
REGINALD: Owner/business partner.
NAUB: Partner, yes.

In responding to items from the personality measure, there were moments when the inherent individualism of some of the questions proved problematic as respondents felt that action often involved others, as in the example of an item addressing locus of control below:

MATHI: Can you do much to change important things in your life, yes I can but then I did not know where to classify it there. I cannot say most of the time because you know changing things in life it does not only take yourself, it takes other people as well so that is why I could not put it in any of those, I cannot say almost always, I cannot say most of the time, I cannot say sometimes and I cannot say never because it involves other people as well.

People also saw patterns within the items that may not have been anticipated by the measure designers, for example, the link between feeling tired and useless:

LAURA: Were there any other examples of possible repetition?
MATHI: You know feeling useless and feeling tired... Sometimes people feel tired because they feel useless you know, let me rather go and sleep, go and relax because they feel useless at that time, there is nothing I can do. Tiredness sometimes is not about what

you have done, the activities that you have done, sometimes it is because of your emotions that you feel strained and you feel like you know I am not worth it, ja so to me they are more or less the same.

Within this sample there was also a high level of self-criticism, or perhaps dissatisfaction relative to high aspirations, which might have reduced their scores relative to other samples. This can be seen in the examples below in relation to satisfaction and success:

> PULE: Are you satisfied with yourself, I am not, I am definitely not satisfied with myself, my family life, my career, I think there is still a lot of improvement that can be done so almost never. At times do you think you are no good at all, definitely not, I know that I always strive to be the best that I can be, so I can say almost never.
> GLEN: Like this one, do you think you have been successful in life, I mean if you talk about the word success, it is a big word. According to me success is to be fulfilled, financially, family wise you understand, so I do not think I am a successful person, according to the way we are now.... [If] that word successful means not yet complete up until I reach my goal then I would say yes I am successful most of the time, according to the way you want me to answer.
> LAURA: Could you phrase it differently then to make it better?
> GLEN: Do you think you have been successful in life, ja do you think are you heading towards your goals or you have achieved your goals because for me successful, to be successful I mean you are complete like in every aspect of life.

Glen's responses highlight the multiplicity of possible responses to these questions and the role of convention, or 'the way you want me to answer' in deciding which is the most appropriate (many of the respondents understood the principles behind scale construction, for example, the importance of repetition). Nonetheless, Glen seems to have a different conception of success to the one encoded in the question as he sees it as a state of completion where there is nothing more to be attained rather than an on-going process or something you can have more or less of. A similar observation, also in South Africa, is made by Brangan (this volume).

Many of the sample were born-again Christians and this influenced their responses in relation to pride, satisfaction and also the perceived need to set a good example:

PROFESSOR: Okay 'do you think about how the things you do will affect others?' Yes, I always think about that. I always think especially on my line of duty because I preach, I preach something else and then I cannot be seen doing something else.

Finally, respondents showed a great deal of patience both with my questions and the measure itself, which may be because many of them had responded to similar measures or even administered them, which might not be the case in a more typical sample.

MATHI: All these questions are okay because like we are saying, another person will answer the very same, the very two questions that we are talking about, another person will say almost never to 2.2 and to the other one says almost always, and then as a person who is looking at them then you wonder what kind of a person is this... if you ask one question in three different ways it will tell you whether this person is telling the truth or if this person is not telling the truth.

Some of the problems identified through this process are technical, however, the majority cannot be resolved by tweaking the wording of items (Fahmy *et al.* 2011), but require an understanding of 'higher order normative contexts' (White 2010: 162) where the measures are being administered. Structured research methods such as surveys are often perceived as easier to use than open-ended methods, but if researchers do not understand the context they are working in, or recognise the specificity of the measures they are using, they are likely to generate data that have the appearance of rigour, but may not be meaningful. To some extent this can be addressed by thorough piloting, or by developing a survey for a particular context, as described in White (Chapter 1, this volume). However, less structured methods offer the opportunity to probe, to adapt the language of the questions, to change the direction of questioning, or even abandon direct questions altogether if that approach is not working. While this is considered beneficial in initial 'exploratory' research, arguably all research is exploratory to some extent so this fundamental openness to unexpected information should not be lost, even within a quantitative hypothetico-deductive research design.

Developing a taxonomy of household and child poverty

There are other ways of addressing the accuracy of measures of wellbeing. Assessments of poverty, for example, may be strengthened by creating indices that represent valued stages or outcomes in particular types of communities, which may also represent pathways out of poverty, using content from open-ended interviews or focus groups. Roelen and Camfield (2012) describe the creation of a taxonomy of households in rural Ethiopia in relation to the level of child wellbeing they were able to support. The taxonomy reflected local understandings of which households or children were poor and why. This was then applied to three rounds of Young Lives[7] survey data, to show how the wellbeing of children in these households changed over time, in relation to broader changes in poverty and social mobility in rural Ethiopia. The taxonomy was based on qualitative data collected from children and adults in four of the 13 Young Lives rural sites in 2007, 2008 and 2009. The data were generated through interviews and group activities which were semi-structured or entirely open-ended and conducted separately with children and adults during the three fieldwork periods (2007–2009).

The taxonomy consisted of four categories, ultra-poor, poor, near-poor and non-poor, which were then applied to the quantitative survey data to group children and their households. We adopted the 'stages of progress' method developed by Krishna (2006) to translate the qualitative information on what children and adults associate with poverty or a good standard of living into a taxonomy of child poverty. For example, ultra-poverty was represented by child malnourishment, not being enrolled in school, having no animals, no land used for agriculture and unreliable credit. However, this process was not straightforward. One fundamental problem, illustrated by Table 2.1, was the difficulty of capturing the relational and symbolic understandings of wellbeing through circumscribed and more individually focused survey variables. A 'simple' material indicator like ownership of oxen, for example, might be seen to be of great significance in symbolic/relational terms. This is shown by the statement: 'if an individual buys a pair of oxen then he is considered as [...] equal to others since he is able to farm [his] own land independently.' The importance of clothing, similarly, went far beyond its material or practical dimension, to encompass issues of self-esteem and social participation: 'they are well clothed and hence are proud to mix with the community in places where the community meets.'

Such limitations are inherent to questionnaire survey data; they simply cannot convey the social and symbolic richness of qualitative methods. The bias towards materiality in the survey also meant that two of the indicators perceived as most important – food and clothing – either

Table 2.1 Focus-group data to inform taxonomy and selection of indicators

Indicator	Importance	Illustrative quotes from interviews and group activities	Mapped to quantitative?
Food (frequency, quantity, variety, quality)	Mentioned first in all sites	'They eat only shiro sauce all the time but we eat a variety of sauces every time' (children, Aseb)	Yes (*During the previous 24-hour period, did the child consume: number of meals?*), but this could not capture variety or quality
Clothing	Mentioned first or second in almost all sites	'They are well clothed and hence are proud to mix with the community in places where the community meets' (female household heads, Tana)	No. Mentioned in round 2 and 3 only, and then as an indicator of the propensity to feel shame, e.g. *I am ashamed of my clothes*
Animals (poultry, sheep, goats, cattle)	Mentioned in almost all sites, usually ranked third, fourth or fifth	'Those who are wealthy, they milk the cows, they herd goats and sheep which they have never had before. Yes they have improved their life' (women, Tana)	Yes (*Has anyone in the household owned any of the following animals at any time in the last 12 months?*)
Oxen	Mentioned in the majority of sites, usually as the threshold between poor and non-poor	'If an individual buys a pair of oxen then he is considered as [...] equal to others since he is able to farm his own land independently' (mixed adults, Leki)	Yes (*Has anyone in the household owned any livestock in the last 12 months?*)
Land	Mentioned in the majority of sites	'The criteria give more weight to having land than oxen. This is because cattle are mortal, but land is fixed' (male household heads, Tana)	Yes (*In the last 12 months, has anyone in your household owned, borrowed or rented any land?*)
Access to medical treatment	Mentioned in the majority of sites	'People prefer to go to holy water because they don't have money for medical expenses' (children, Aseb)	No. Only asked in response to severe illness, so the number of respondents was small
Daily labour	Mentioned in at least a third of sites	'The demand for daily labour in our village is too low and periodic [there is money only] in big cities like Addis Ababa, where there is continuous demand for daily labour work' (mixed adults, Galafi)	No, as the activity codes are not sufficiently differentiated (e.g. casual work may not be equivalent to daily labour)

Table 2.1 (Continued)

Indicator	Importance	Illustrative quotes from interviews and group activities	Mapped to quantitative?
Irrigation	Mentioned in at least a third of sites	'Irrigated land helps the household to produce different kinds of cash crops including onions, tomatoes, etc. The income obtained from the sale of the vegetables helps the owners to expand the irrigated land by renting land from the poor' (children, Leku)	Yes (*In the last 12 months, have you irrigated any of the land?*)
Having a corrugated iron roof	Mentioned in at least a third of sites	'They eat as they like and have covered their house with corrugated sheets of iron' (women, Tana)	Yes (*Observe and record main roof material*)
School performance	Mentioned in at least a third of sites	'School performance of our children is getting better [now we have more money]. For example, my daughter stood third in her class. Our children are being awarded for their ranks' (mixed adults, Galafi)	No. Mentioned in round 3 only as education became a stronger focus as the project progressed
Uniforms and school materials	Mentioned in at least a third of sites	'If they go without wearing their uniforms, they will be chased out of school. Due to fear of that, they miss school days' (children, Negele)	No. Mentioned in round 2 and 3 only
Connections to govt.	Mentioned in at least a third of sites	'Those who have nothing, even a single hen to dig the compound, let alone an ox, are excluded [from the Productive Safety Net Scheme]. It is those government elites and local elites. They include their relatives until the quota is full' (men, Tana)	Partially (*Is any member of your household an active member of an organization, group or informal association?*)
Children not doing paid labour	Mentioned in at least a third of sites	'Being poor is thinking about daily labour in class because daily labour is the work of the poor' (children, Leku)	Yes (*Have you [the child] done anything in the last 12 months to earn money for yourself and/or your family?*)

Source: Adapted from Roelen and Camfield (2012).

could not be mapped to the dataset, or could only be mapped in a limited way. For example, concerns about the variety and quantity of food were reduced to frequency of meals. Those about being able to dress appropriately were proxied by the amount of money spent on clothing for men, women and children within the household, regardless of the size of the household. The variables also focused on quantity rather than quality so it was possible to find out how frequently a person ate each day, but not whether the food they ate was good quality, varied and satisfying.

Table 2.1 gives some further examples of issues that arose in the qualitative data and how these were translated into indicators for quantitative analysis.

We faced two other problems in creating and using the taxonomy. First, Krishna's method was developed to be participatory and community-based with the development of the taxonomy and the classification of households to be undertaken at the community level and informed by other information about these households. Our partial use of the method created a potential inconsistency between the poverty classifications identified by children and adults and the extent to which these various classes actually represent a particular pathway out of poverty that can be observed in the quantitative survey data. For example, while the ownership of draught animals may be defined as a distinct stage and a considerable improvement in living conditions and seen as following on from progress made in malnourishment or school enrolment, the survey results showed that some children suffer malnourishment despite having draught animals in the household. In other words, children and households identify a linear process of progress in interviews and focus groups, perhaps indicating the ways in which data are constructed through and shaped by a particular instrument such as a timeline or the normative and performative context of a focus group (White, Chapter 1 of this volume). However, the quantitative survey findings point towards a more iterative process, presumably involving a number of trade-offs. The question of whether the taxonomy worked in identifying key stages in the advancement of child wellbeing cannot really be answered at this stage as we would need to confirm it with further rounds of quantitative data. However, even though 'types' will never perfectly match empirical examples, it proved a good way of selecting cases to exemplify particular trajectories (Camfield and Roelen 2013). We found that combining qualitative and quantitative data on particular children and their households revealed some lacunae, but also considerable convergence in that the quantitative data and the life history data collected from parents agreed about the direction in which households were moving.

Conclusion

The aim of the chapter was to demonstrate how qualitative approaches and psychological understandings of how people respond to measures can be used to improve the accuracy of survey data, and how translating some qualitative data into quantitative indicators may increase recognition of the value of qualitative research, especially in a policy context. In Introduction, I discussed the potential of qualitative methods to blur what is often presented as a rigid divide between subjective and objective data by demonstrating the constructed nature of all measures. I showed how simple techniques such as cognitive debriefing can highlight technical problems and point towards differences between how people understand the questions and the assumptions on which the measures are premised. I described some of the unconscious factors that influence the way people respond to measures and the practices of researchers, for example, an orientation towards unusual or striking examples. Finally, I showed how qualitative and quantitative methods can work together in creating taxonomies or measures.

In conclusion, I would like to make a somewhat different point: that not all of the challenges of translating expansive visions of wellbeing into simple measures are amenable to technical solutions. Understanding that one respondent's reference group is the people in her neighbourhood and another person's is his or her brother who works in Dubai can only partially explain differences in reported wellbeing. There are also other cognitive and contextual factors that shape people's responses, for example, how questions are phrased and what constitutes a 'good' answer in particular contexts. Greater attention and reflection on the methods used to study wellbeing, facilitated by volumes such as this, demonstrate the complexity of subjective wellbeing data and the danger of treating them as a transparent measure of the state of the world. Macro-level data offer great potential to address questions such as why wellbeing changes over the life course, what factors support people's wellbeing, whether experiencing wellbeing is a resource in and of itself and how and why understandings of wellbeing differ and change over time. However, these data have micro-foundations and we do not yet know enough about how subjective wellbeing measures work in developing countries to understand the potential dangers in relying too heavily on them. If measures are not completely accurate, this can to some extent be smoothed over through the use of large samples. However, if these inaccuracies only occur with particular types of respondent (e.g. people with low education), they may be reinforcing the entrenched inequality that much wellbeing research seeks to challenge.

Notes

1. In the Schkade and Kahneman example, respondents focused on the difference in climate in predicting whether people would be happier in one locale or another.
2. The alternative they propose is asking someone to make multiple judgements of their wellbeing over the course of one day, which are then aggregated. This requires a personal digital assistant and as far as I'm aware has not been trialled outside the Global North.
3. For example, in response to lack of clarity as to the purpose or order of the questions, or the correct use of the response scales.
4. Available at: http://siteresources.worldbank.org/EXTHDOFFICE/Resources/5485726-1281723119684/STEP_Skills_Measurement_Brochure_Jan_2012.pdf, downloaded 12/01/14.
5. Available at: http://awethuproject.co.za/.
6. Parametric statistical techniques are the most commonly used method of analysis but can be misleading with small and heterogeneous samples as they assume a normal or even distribution which isn't 'skewed' to one side or the other.
7. Young Lives is a longitudinal study of children growing up in poverty in four developing countries. Available at: www.younglives.org.uk.

References

Acquadro, C., Jambon, B., Ellis, D. and Marquis, P. (1996) Language and Translation Issues. pp. 575–585 in B. Spilker (ed.) *Quality of Life and Pharmacoeconomics in Clinical Trials.* 2nd ed. Philadelphia: Lippincott-Raven.

Bertrand, M. and S. Mullainathan (2001) Do People Mean What They Say? Implications for Subjective Survey Data. *The American Economic Review* 92(2): 67–72.

Bowden, A., Fox-Rushby J. A., Nyandieka L. and Wanjau J. (2002) Methods for Pre-Testing and Piloting Survey Questions: Illustrations from the KENQOL Survey of Health-Related Quality of Life. *Health Policy Planning* 17(3): 322–330.

Camfield, L. and Roelen, K. (2013) Household Trajectories in Rural Ethiopia – What Can a Mixed Method Approach Tell Us about the Impact of Poverty on Children? *Social Indicators Research* 113(2): 729–749.

Camfield, L. and Ruta, D. (2007) 'Translation Is Not Enough': Using the Global Person Generated Index (GPGI) to Assess Individual Quality of Life in Bangladesh, Thailand, and Ethiopia. *Quality of Life Research* 16(6): 1039–1051.

Clark, D. A. (ed.) (2012) *Adaptation, Poverty and Development: The Dynamics of Subjective Well-Being.* Basingstoke: Palgrave Macmillan.

D'Ambrosio, C. and Frick, J. R. (2004) Subjective Well-Being and Relative Deprivation: An Empirical Link. *Social Indicators Research* 81(3): 497–519.

De Maio, T. J. (1984) Social Desirability and Survey Measurement: A Review. pp. 257–281 in C. G. Turner and E. Martia (eds.) *Surveying Subjective Phenomena.* Vol. 2. New York: Russell Sage Foundation.

Elder, G. H. (1974) *Children of the Great Depression.* Chicago: University Press.

Fahmy, E., Pemberton, S. and Sutton, E. (2011) Cognitive Testing of the UK Poverty and Social Exclusion Survey. Poverty and Social Exclusion in the UK Working Paper – Methods Series No. 17.

Fiske, S. T. and Taylor, S. E. (1991) *Social Cognition.* 2nd ed. New York: McGraw-Hill.

Graham, C. (2009) *Happiness around the World: The Paradox of Happy Peasants and Miserable Millionaires.* Oxford: Oxford University Press.

Graham, C. and Pettinato, S. (2002) *Happiness and Hardship: Opportunity and Insecurity in New Market Economies.* Washington, DC: Brookings Institution Press.

Kahneman, D. and Krueger, A. (2006) Developments in the Measurement of Subjective Well-Being. *Journal of Economic Perspectives* 20(1): 3–24.

Kahneman, D. and Tverskey. A (1979) Prospect Theory: An Analysis of Decision under Risk. *Econometrica* 47(2): 263–292.

Krishna, A. (2006) Subjective Assessments, Participatory Methods and Poverty Dynamics: The Stages of Progress Method. Paper presented at the *Workshop on Concepts and Methods for Analyzing Poverty Dynamics and Chronic Poverty.* 23–25 October. University of Manchester, UK.

Mallinson, S. (2002) Listening to Respondents: A Qualitative Assessment of the Short-Form 36 Health Status Questionnaire. *Social Science and Medicine* 54(1): 11–21.

Mani, A., Mullainathan, S., Shafir, E. and Zhao, J. (2013) Poverty Impedes Cognitive Function. *Science*, 341(6149): 976–980.

Medvec, V. H., Madey, S. F. and Gilovich, T. (1995) When Less Is More: Counterfactual Thinking and Satisfaction among Olympic Medalists. *Journal of Personality and Social Psychology* 69(4): 603–610.

Michalos, A. C. (1985) Multiple Discrepancies Theory. *Social Indicators Research*, 16: 347–413.

Pan, Y., Landreth, A., Schoua-Glusberg, A., Hinsdale- Shouse, M. and Park, H. (2008) Cognitive Interviewing in Non-English Languages: A Cross-Cultural Perspective. Special Invited Paper for the *International Conference on Survey Methods in Multinational, Multiregional and Multicultural Contexts.* 25–29 June. Berlin, Germany.

Redelmeier, D. A. and Kahneman, D. (1996) Patients' Memories of Painful Medical Treatments: Realtime and Retrospective Evaluations of Two Minimally Invasive Procedures. *Pain* 66(1): 3–8.

Roelen, K. and Camfield, L. (2012) A Mixed-Method Taxonomy of Child Poverty – The Case of Ethiopia. *Applied Research in Quality of Life* 8(3): 319–337.

Schkade, D. A. and Kahneman, D. (1998) Does Living in California Make People Happy? A Focusing Illusion in Judgments of Life Satisfaction. *Psychological Science* 9(5): 340–346.

Schwarz, N. and Strack, F. (1999) Reports of Subjective Well-Being: Judgmental Processes and Their Methodological Implications. pp. 61–84 in D. Kahneman,

E. Diener and N. Schwarz (eds.) *Well-Being: The Foundations of Hedonic Psychology*. New York: Russell Sage Foundation Press.

Stiglitz, J. E., Sen, A. and Fitoussi, J-P. (2009) Report of the Commission on the Measurement of Economic Performance and Social Progress. CMEPSP. Available at: www.stiglitz-sen-fitoussi.fr

Strack, F., Martin, L. L. and Schwarz, N. (1988) Priming and Communication: Social Determinants of Information Use in Judgments of Life Satisfaction. *European Journal of Social Psychology* 18(5): 429–442.

Strack, F., Schwarz, N., Chassein, B., Kern, D. and Wagner, D. (1990). The Salience of Comparison Standards and the Activation of Social Norms: Consequences for Judgments of Happiness and their Communication. *British Journal of Social Psychology* 29: 303–314.

Tourangeau, R. (1984) Cognitive Science and Survey Methods: A Cognitive Perspective. pp. 73–100 in T. B. Jabine, M. L. Straf, J. M. Tanur and R. Tourangeau (eds.) *Cognitive Aspects of Survey Methodology: Building a Bridge between Disciplines*. Washington, DC: National Academy Press.

Triandis, H. C., Davis, E. E., Vassilou, V. and Nassiakou, M. (1965) Some Methodological Problems Concerning Research on Negotiations between Monolinguals. *Technical Report 28*. Urbana: Department of Psychology: University of Illinois.

White, S. C. (2010) Analysing Wellbeing: A Framework for Development Practice. *Development in Practice* 20(2): 158–172.

Willis, G. (1999) Cognitive Interviewing: A 'How To' Guide. Reducing Survey Error through Research on the Cognitive and Decision Processes in *Surveys Short Course* presented at the 1999 Meeting of the American Statistical Association (8–12 August 1999).

3
Measuring National Wellbeing: What Matters to You? What Matters to Whom?

Susan Oman

Introduction

The Office for National Statistics' (ONS) Measuring National Well-Being: 'What Matters to You?' debate ran between November 2010 and April 2011. The five-month debate took place across various platforms: an online questionnaire and forum, social media, postal submissions, a telephone line and 175 live events. The latter varied from workshops and focus groups with 'people from all walks of life', including some groups thought 'hard-to-reach',[1] to large-scale public events with hundreds in attendance (Evans 2011: 5). In creating the debate, the ONS presented a space in which to listen to, discuss, collect and collate descriptions of what was important to individuals and communities in order to understand 'what matters' for the nation[2] (Cameron 2010, Matheson 2011, Self *et al.* 2012). More than 30,000 responses describe what mattered to participants about wellbeing, which the ONS has indicated formed the basis of the UK's national wellbeing domains and measures (Self *et al.* 2013: 2).

The national debate was part of ONS' on-going Measuring National Well-Being (MNW) programme, called 'Measuring What Matters'. The debate and wider programme were officially launched in November 2010 and were symptomatic of a broader international research agenda surrounding wellbeing as an alternative measure of progress. A year earlier, the Sarkozy Commission's Report by the Commission on the Measurement of Economic Performance and Social Progress[3] recommended, with some influence, that individual national statistics offices measure wellbeing (Stiglitz et al. 2009). In the UK, the ONS had committed to investigating national wellbeing in 2007 (Allin 2007), a point obscured in the 2010 launch, as David Cameron stated he had 'tasked the ONS to look at how the nation is doing', in order that 'we really know what matters to people' (Cameron 2010). The new prime minister's eagerness to align himself to the wellbeing agenda suggests that political points were to be won in doing so. This demands closer attention to the motives driving such a large-scale consultation, most prominently, 'what mattered to *whom?*' in 'What Matters to You?'

This chapter looks at the debate as an indicator of how wellbeing knowledge is constructed (White, Chapter 1, this volume) and problematises the way in which methods are treated as 'reliable tools for describing and so enacting social reality' (Law 2009: 242, discussed at length in Law et al. 2011, 2013). Based on accounts in published ONS reports, I describe the ONS' approaches to working with the debate's various qualitative data. ONS debate outputs do not fully account for these approaches, especially how these data were analysed. As a result, I infer some possibilities based on usual practice from outside the ONS in consideration of what might have led to an apparent marginalisation of the debate's qualitative data from the MNW programme's evidence base.

Using discourse analysis, I re-examine the wellbeing debate as a case of knowledge produced through social science technologies (methods, approaches and systems) which creates politically performative 'representations' (Law 2009: 239). This analysis points to choices made in the MNW programme which discounted valuable opportunities for qualitative analysis of thousands of narratives of the meaning of wellbeing in favour of dominant quantitative technologies. Policymakers and statisticians are more conversant in quantitative approaches, as they are 'tasked' to manage, create, read and describe them, which might indicate that the programme defaulted to the most familiar, rather than most apposite approaches. Whatever the reason, the outcome is that those 'tasked' to understand wellbeing produced a knowledge base which reinforced the significance of pre-existing statistical measures, and the importance new subjective wellbeing (SWB) measures, referred to as 'the work of the ONS' (ONS 2011).

I outline how incomplete approaches to knowledge production are problematic when attempting to construct a wellbeing evidence base. I present my own secondary analysis of data found in free-text fields which the ONS labelled 'Other' to highlight some of the ethical, practical and political issues which result from a selective or discriminatory approach to data forms. Referring to prior work on 'the art of listening'

(Back 2007, Fromm 1994, Gunarantam 2012), I return to these survey data in order to 'listen' to how debate participants describe wellbeing in their own words, arguing these 'Other' forms and descriptions present opportunities for a more complete understanding of wellbeing, which better represents the concerns of the British public.

I compare my analysis of free-text fields with default shortcuts taken to create a quantitative evidence base, and argue that these offer alternate realities of how wellbeing is constructed, based on the respondents' descriptions on the one hand and those of 'knowledge producers' on the other. In so doing, I argue that survey data have potentially 'richer' qualities than the indicators to which they are usually reduced and that the failure to analyse them appropriately marginalised various 'qualities of life' which people saw as critical to their expressions of wellbeing.

The matters of the debate

In the five-month MNW debate, the ONS reached 7,249 people at 175 events 'in a range of formats including workshops, focus groups, seminars, round table discussions and informal chats'. According to the Findings from the National Well-Being Debate report (Evans 2011), they sought the advice of various experts, establishing a National Statistician's Advisory Forum and a Technical Advisory Group. In addition, there were online debate channels via blogs, websites and forums, as well as postcards and a dedicated telephone line, which generated an additional 34,000 responses (Evans 2011: 5).

> ONS conducted the national debate in order to engage with experts on wellbeing who would provide an insight into what to measure and how to measure it, and interested members of the public who not only know best about what matters to them but would also be affected by any policies that would result from this work.
>
> (Evans 2011: 4)

The debate also comprised a public 'consultation paper', which asked the nation five main questions with three sub-questions and an 'Any Other Comments' field. On 23 February 2011, the ONS amended the questions and the choices available to tick by way of response. The ONS refers to the two different versions of the consultation as Questionnaire 1 (10 November 2010–22 February 2011) and Questionnaire 2 (23 February 2011–15 April 2011), which are summarised in Tables 3.3 and 3.4. The consultation received more than 7,900 responses and these

Table 3.1 Question 1: What things in life matter to you? From Questionnaire 1

What things in life matter to you?	
What things in life matter to you? Please choose all that apply	Percentages*
Health	89
Having good connections with friends and relatives	89
Job satisfaction and economic security	86
Present and future conditions of the environment	73
Education and training	69
Personal and cultural activities, including caring and volunteering	68
Income and wealth	62
Ability to have a say on local and national issues	59
Crime	56
Other	28

Note: *Percentages will not add up to 100 per cent as this is a multi-code question.
Source: Evans (2011: 4).

questionnaires are the foundation of the evidence base, as it is predominantly referred to in subsequent ONS reports and presentations; and as such, they form the focus of this chapter.

Table 3.1 indicates how people answered the first of the nine questions from the first questionnaire. It lists the nine tick-box response options available, together with a field labelled 'Other', which was '[e]xtra space available to write in other things that were important' (Evans 2011: 7) using free text. This table also explains the response rate for each tick box and the 'Other' field.

Free-text fields, often signposted 'Other', are generally used in order to enable participants to describe 'what matters to them' in relation to the posed question, but outside the closed parameters of tick-box options. This additional possibility is understood to encourage retention of respondents, who are often deterred from completing the survey in full if their chosen response is not represented by a suitable tick box. The inclusion of these fields also offers potentially richer data for survey designers, enabling richer understanding when analysed than tick boxes alone.

Table 3.2 outlines the ways in which question one was amended from 'What things in life matter to you? Please choose all that apply' in the first questionnaire, to 'What things in life matter *most* to you?

Table 3.2 A summary of question 1: What things in life matter most to you? From Questionnaire 2

'What things in life matter most to you? Please choose all that apply' Tick-box title	Response Percentage	Comparison to Questionnaire 1
Income and wealth	45	Same
Job satisfaction	73	Split
Economic security	68	Split
Ability to have a say on local and national issues	47	Same
Having good connections with friends and relatives	85	Same
Having a good relationship with a spouse or partner	72	Added
Present and future conditions of the environment	66	Same
Crime	30	Same
Health	83	Same
Education and training	56	Same
Personal and cultural activities*, including volunteering	56	Split
Cultural activities	46	Split
Unpaid caring, such as for children or other family members	41	Added
Spirituality or religion	29	Added
Other – please specify	16	

Note: *This should read 'Personal activities, including volunteering', but an oversight in the report does not correctly label this field.
Source: Adapted from table in Evans (2011: 10).

Please choose all that apply' (my italics) in the second. In addition to a slightly different wording of the question, the tick-box options were also amended. Some were split and new ones were added, which changed the response percentages; and notably for this chapter, also seems to have reduced free-text use by 12 per cent in question one of the second questionnaire. The methodological benefits of this are not acknowledged in the Findings from the Debate report, and the changes in questions are not highlighted. Furthermore, an error in the reporting of the field, 'Personal and cultural activities, including volunteering' might indicate a lack of attention to certain details when summarising the debate for the report.

Tables 3.3 and 3.4[4] represent how these adaptations may have affected the ways in which people interacted with the survey. For example, one

Table 3.3 A summary of Questionnaire 1 from the ONS MNW debate consultation: Tick-box responses compared to 'Other' free-text field responses

Question	Tick-box responses	'Other' free-text field
Q1. What things in life matter to you? Please choose all that apply.	Highest response: Health, 4,780 Having good connections with friends and relatives, 4,783	Other, 1,533
Q3. Of the things that matter to you, which should be reflected in measures of national well-being? Please tick all that apply.	Highest response: Health, 2,031	Other, 774
Q5. Which of the following sets of information do you think help measure national well-being and how life in the UK is changing over time? Please tick all that apply.	Highest response: Life satisfaction, 523	Other, 649
Q7. Which of the following ways would be best, to give a picture of national well-being? Please tick one option.	Answered question unknown	Unknown
Q8. How would you use measures of national well-being? Please tick all that apply.	Highest response: To help understand the longer-term implications of our current activities, 285	Other, 401
Q9. We welcome any other comments you have regarding the measurement of national well-being.	Free text, 1,864	
TOTAL 'Other' responses		5,221*

Note: *This number would be considerably higher, but I was not permitted access to a figure for question 4.
Source: Adapted from data kindly provided by the ONS.

might interpret that as the questions and the tick boxes were refined in Questionnaire 2, people felt more encouraged to respond using a tick box and felt the need to respond in free-text less.

Despite this refinement, there remained a large proportion of respondents across the two questionnaires who wanted to respond in free text and take the opportunity to use their own words to describe their sense

Table 3.4 A summary of Questionnaire 2 from the ONS MNW debate consultation: Tick-box responses compared to 'Other' free-text field responses

Question	Tick-box responses	'Other' free-text field
Q1. What things in life matter most to you? Please choose all that apply.	Highest response: Health, 1,839 Having good connections with friends and relatives, 1,885	Other, 346
Q3. Of the things that matter to you, which should be reflected in measures of national well-being? Please choose all that apply.	Highest response: Health, 989 Same as my response to the previous question, 1,047	Other, 168
Q5. Which of the following sets of information do you think help measure national well-being and how life in the UK is changing over time? Please choose all that apply.	Highest response: Life Satisfaction, 1,576 Health Statistics, 1,583	Other, 190
Q7. Which of the following ways would be best to give a picture of national well-being? Please choose one option only.	Highest response: Small selection of indicators, 658 Small set of indicators, 555	Other, 100
Q8. How would you use measures of national well-being? Please choose all that apply.	Highest response: To help understand the longer-term implications of our current activities, 1,532	Other, 145
Q9. We welcome any other comments you have regarding the measurement of national well-being.	Free text, 616	
TOTAL 'Other' responses		1,565

Source: Adapted from data kindly provided by the ONS.

of wellbeing.[5] In response to the question 'What things in life matter to you?' in the first iteration of the survey, for example, from the 5,401[6] who answered the question, most used tick boxes, while 1,533 people chose to describe the 'things in life [that] matter' in their own words. Question three in Questionnaire 1 has a 25 per cent higher response rate using free text than the highest tick-box response, 'quality of life', for example; and rather than using the predefined answers, 40 per cent more people used their own words to respond to the question, 'How would you use measures of national well-being?' In addition, there was a space called 'Any Other Comments' which 2,480 people participated in, many writing at length about the things that matter to them.

When the debate has been cited to corroborate certain decisions regarding the ONS' wellbeing programme and measures,[7] the 'evidence' comprises responses placed in the tick boxes which are aggregated and then recited as statistics. I will not outline these in detail here, as most of the ONS' outputs refer to these percentages, but will turn to the under-represented 6,787 answers offered by debate questionnaire respondents using their own words in *free* text. I argue these fields are of methodological significance to what is claimed to be the evidence base. I also maintain they are of political significance in a large-scale research event designed to understand 'What Matters to You?' across the nation. Furthermore, they are of practical interest, proposing an insight into alternative approaches to working with survey data and understanding wellbeing.

Finding out the 'Findings from the Debate'

The debate was profiled as an exercise which engaged a variety of different people 'from different walks of life' (Evans 2011: 5) and this 'participatory spirit' has been congratulated when compared to initiatives in other national wellbeing programmes (Kroll 2011: 7). The tens of thousands of responses would have generated a high volume of different types of qualitative data, thereby presenting an opportunity to investigate 'what matters' beyond what is knowable through quantitative practices which are widely regarded as dominating evidence-based policy, especially for wellbeing (e.g. Camfield and Palmer-Jones 2013).

While numerous ONS reports on the MNW programme summarise analysis of quantitative elements of the debate, only the Findings from the Debate report refers to analysis of the vast and varied qualitative responses described above. This report describes the events as:

> an invaluable process [that] reinforced the fact that well-being is multifaceted and can be affected by a lot of things. This was illustrated well at an event with a voluntary group in London that provides assistance to elderly people. They highlighted the connection between social connections, fuel poverty and car parking; for an elderly person

74 *Measuring National Wellbeing in UK*

> living alone, the lengths of their visitors' stay was determined by how long they were allowed to park when they came to visit and how warm the house they were visiting was.
>
> (Evans 2011: 6)

This account presents the only real description of a finding from an event, which is here used to illustratively reinforce something which was already considered as 'known', that wellbeing is multifaceted. Although other observations are bullet-pointed and tabulated, these are apparently descriptive, rather than offering analysis, and there is no indication that these responses found their way into what is called the evidence base.

According to the Findings from the Debate report, the 2,480 'Any Other Comments' fields (Q9) were analysed by an external consultant, offering the following observation:

> [participants] used this question as an opportunity to express what they understood by the term well-being, providing rich personal accounts of what aspects of well-being were important to their individual sense of well-being and noting particular interventions or actions that could be used to enhance well-being.
>
> (Evans 2011: 18–19)

With regard to the 'rich personal accounts of what aspects of well-being were important', only 'key messages' were chosen and summarised in brief. It is not explained how these 'key messages' were distilled and they do not account for the various 'aspects of well-being [that] were important to [participants'] individual sense of well-being [or the] particular interventions or actions that could be used to enhance well-being'. As such, this represents a missed opportunity to understand 'what matters' to all the people who took part.

What is notable for this chapter is there is no indication as to the methodological approach to qualitative analysis. In fact, the methodological approach to data *collection* is often confused, with one page saying that the events included focus groups (Evans 2011: 5) and another categorically stating the events were not focus groups (Evans 2011: 19).

The use of qualitative data in other reports from the MNW programme might offer some indication as to how qualitative descriptions might have a role in the final evidence base. For example, the following is cited from a free-text field from one of the two survey questionnaires:

I would hate for someone to be worrying about whether they will have something to eat or a roof over their head. Also doing other things including recreation activities improves your mental wellbeing which in turn affects your general well-being but you can only do those things if you are in a good financial position.

(Self *et al.* 2012: 15)

The ONS chose this quote to illustrate 'personal finance' in its Life in the UK report (Self *et al.* 2012). Yet beyond basic needs of shelter and food, recreation activities were considered most important to wellbeing for this respondent, or in other words, access to qualities of life.[8] While the implication is that this participant saw 'a good financial position' as 'key', it is only because that facilitates access to qualities which impact positively on different modes of wellbeing. Furthermore, that the wellbeing of others is the primary concern of this account is not addressed in the ONS' interpretation. This respondent's view of wellbeing clearly exceeds 'personal finance', reflecting rather a personal concern for *social* welfare. These aspects of wellbeing are not represented in the measures, suggesting that however the fields were analysed, the intended meaning of the descriptions within them failed to make it into the 'evidence base'.

Large qualitative datasets such as those produced by the MNW consultation free text are typically analysed by way of thematically 'back-coding' into an existing coding frame (NatCen and CLS 2003: 7). A predetermined coding frame of this nature is likely to correspond to the tick box options, as outlined in Tables 3.1 and 3.2. If this approach was used, it would have most likely involved forcing free-text descriptions in fields called 'Other' (as in none of the above) to fit the tick-box response options which the participant decided were insufficient or inappropriate representations of what they wanted to say.

In order for the citation from the Life and the UK report to 'best represent personal finance', it seems analysis may have fallen into one of the commonly observed 'coding traps'[9]; either coding too much too quickly (Seidman 2013: 134–136) or being 'too close' to the aims of data collection to analyse them objectively (Richards 2005). This again suggests that analysis of the free-text fields would have probably involved 'retrofitting' them to tick-box codes which met predetermined priorities. In other words, the debate would probably serve to reiterate the relevance of specific existing objective measures of societal 'progress' as suitable measures of wellbeing, rather than being a more open exercise in improving wellbeing knowledge, which would have allowed for recognition of miscellaneous matters, such as, in this case, a social concern for others.

Working with a limited coding frame means that the themes which might be coded from the above citation, such as social justice, equality or the importance of everyday activities, for example, would fail to appear in the 'evidence base', as there would be no code to enable their representation. Interestingly, a more detailed tabulation towards the end of the Evans report (2011) summarises themes from 'the wider debate: other responses' (i.e. not the events or any of the free-text fields previously described). This acknowledges the importance of 'freedom, equality and fairness' and the importance of spare time, but is at the end of the report with other tables which function as appendices, clearly downplaying the importance of these wellbeing attributes (Evans 2011: 24).

The 2012 Life in the UK report reflected on the first iteration of the measures and the previous two years of the MNW programme. The report's press release explained that,

> national well-being is about 'measuring what matters' – bringing together relevant economic, social and environmental statistics to show how the country is doing overall and how people's lives are affected by their circumstances.
>
> (ONS 2012b)

While approaches to data generation in the debate were open and varied, the ONS seems to have been less prepared to utilise mixed approaches to evidence and evaluation, perhaps reverting to more familiar territory when it came to data analysis. Rather than listening to 'how people's lives are affected by their circumstances', the Office FOR National Statistics seems to, as a matter of resource, habit or expertise, have defaulted to collating an index of statistics it deems relevant and justifies by way of 'useful' selective citations from the qualitative data. It is not even clear whether the 'key messages' outlined in the Findings from the Debate report were included as evidence. If this signposts that statistics were always the predominant, perhaps only way to describe wellbeing in the context of the MNW programme, one might question what the real motivations were behind efforts to create an inclusive debate in the context of the wider project.

Without explicit reference to how the consultation's free-text fields or the rest of the qualitative data were analysed, it is difficult to be conclusive with regard to how different forms of data formed its final evidence base. The lack of attention to the qualitative components in debate outputs (beyond the Evans 2011 report) may indicate why it is overlooked by those citing the debate. However, perhaps later reports overlook the qualitative data, unless using it illustratively, as with the personal finance quotation above, because Evans (2011) does not summarise these data in a way which presents them as evidence. It seems these data were largely omitted from reporting mechanisms, owing to habituated practices which rely on the easily quantifiable. It is likely that these practices also failed to recognise the importance of quantifying the less easily quantifiable for those (policymakers and advisors) accustomed to working with statistics. This raises questions regarding the missing evidence and consequently, the utility and comprehensiveness of the evidence base behind the indicators of UK wellbeing.

The methodological issues suggest the political

As outlined above, the published MNW evidence indicates it is likely that only matters pertaining to expedient and existing statistics were destined to become a tool for policy-making. Given the general lack of emphasis on qualitative work across the ONS,[10] perhaps it was inevitable that less importance was placed on the qualitative data than necessary in the task to analyse the debate in a way that made it a complete and usable evidence base. The next question might be whether this *mattered* for the ONS.

In this respect, the debate seems to be less about understanding what matters to *us*, personally, socially, or even as a nation, and more about an imperative to compete internationally,[11] as David Cameron's speech to launch the MNW programme suggests:

> We often talk about the importance of science and research; this is a little bit, if you like, of science and research that is being looked at the world over and I would rather we were in the vanguard of doing this rather than just meekly following on behind. I think there is an opportunity on that front as well.
>
> (Cameron 2010)

Minutes from the Technical Advisory Group (ONS 2011) outline the importance placed on 'the work of the ONS' in the MNW programme fitting into 'international consensus', rather than qualitative work to evaluate the questions asked. 'The government's "happiness tsar"' (Jeffries

2008), Lord Layard, reiterates the status of this work as the aim of the programme, with his concerns that the 'UK is less likely to set international agenda if introducing unnecessary changes' (ONS 2011). Therefore, the 'participatory spirit' alluded to through inclusion of 'people from all walks of life' might be more about including the measures themselves, as described below:

> The measures we intend to develop will be used to compare the UK against other countries. As such it was important that views were collected from a cross section of the population that was as representative of the UK as possible.
>
> (Evans 2011: 5)

Inclusion of public opinion could be read as 'a little bit, if you like, of science and research' tokenism to reinforce the importance and assure inclusion of the 'the work of the ONS' in international consensus when 'evidence-making' for policy is traditionally disinclined towards 'tools which allow for "bottom up" concept development' (Scott et al. 2009: 132).

As a project, the debate offered various 'opportunities [for] innovative ways of developing and using qualitative data investigatively', as advocated by Mason (2007) in respect of approaches to secondary data. Furthermore, as a project driven by the ONS, all modes of inquiry might have carried similar influence to that credited to well-established social surveys, such as the census. By the same token, if methods and knowledge production are 'fully of the world that they are also active in constructing' (Law et al. 2011: 5), a more diverse approach to knowledge-making and representation gives the prospect of a more accurate and representative description of 'national wellbeing', rather than a rearticulation of the status quo.

Law outlines the importance of a 'performative understanding of methodological practice' (2009: 3), explaining that 'knowledge producers' create realities in which their 'knowledges' can flourish. The UK's ONS' very purpose is to generate statistical realities which perform as an evidence base to inform policy-making and media dissemination for 'everyday' international and domestic consumption. In considering how social science performs certain realities, Law highlights how the technologies (methods, approaches and systems) of social science create contexts and narratives in which they can reproduce themselves methodologically, affecting society, politics and culture in the same way as other sciences and technology do.[12]

Therefore, the 'knowledges' produced through analysis of the wellbeing debate by those 'tasked' to measure wellbeing would be inclined to reinforce and legitimate a reality in which measurement is not only plausible, but advisable. Conceivably, then, the debate was imagined in order for survey methodologies to continue to reproduce themselves in a world where international wellbeing measures are an alternative to gross domestic product (GDP) and a new competitive incentive to be 'at the vanguard' of this new 'science and research'. This political context assured that the 'efficiency' and ease of familiar quantitative methodologies and descriptions predominated the efficacy of less familiar qualitative ones.

The politics of method outlined in Law's descriptions of knowledge production and social science offer an interesting alternative answer to the question 'What Matters to You?', or perhaps, even another question seeking different answers. From this perspective, it is imaginable that 'measuring what matters to the nation' will only transpire if the nation answered in agreement with, and using easy to interpret (mainly quantitative) responses to the underlying research question, 'What matters to *us*?' (as wellbeing measurers).

Free text versus forced choices and the participant-author

As previously stated, despite the prevalence of free-text fields in surveys, there is little discussion or guidance on how they might be analysed, or even used (Garcia *et al.* 2004), and concerns regarding 'efficiency...in survey methodology' often justify their omission or minimal attention in analysis (O'Cathain and Thomas 2004: 1). Survey design is evolving, however, and these fields are gaining recognition (Scott *et al.* 2009) as 'a valuable data source, suitable for content, thematic and narrative analysis' (Rich *et al.* 2013: 11). My analysis of the wellbeing debate and its free-text responses (outlined in the following section) suggest this is a 'valuable data source' that is largely unexplored and certainly under-represented.

Whatever the political or practical motives (or oversights) behind omissions from the MNW 'evidence base', 'efficient' analytical shortcuts would ordinarily rely on value judgements of what and who to include without close and careful reading. When trying to understand something as complex as national wellbeing, it is necessary to engage with each respondent and each description in its entirety, rather than simply coding sections to themes of predetermined relevance. In order for interpretation and representation to be 'inclusive', all responses demand attention, as everyone's opinion on their wellbeing is relevant in a debate asking the nation what matters. However, this does not seem common practice when approaching responses to open-ended questions in surveys and may be the reason for oversights in respect of the ONS' national debate.

The free text reveals incongruities in language and meaning and highlights the limits of some of the ONS' knowledge practices to communicate and gather data. Free-text fields present solutions by way of an 'Other' option to a survey respondent, offering a dialogic space between the survey's author and respondent, or 'participant-author', while also exposing differences between 'everyday' and technocratic understandings of something as complex as wellbeing. Terminology and frames of reference used in the questions and tick-box response options were often too specific to the survey-authors' knowledge and practices, as described in comments such as the following, 'Do you really expect people to understand what these options mean?' (Case 12, Q7).

Some free-text field respondents, or 'participant-authors', also seemed unfamiliar with certain nuances of language on occasion. For example, question seven asked, 'Which of the following ways would be best to give a picture of national well-being? Please choose one option only!' One participant wrote, 'Some sort of graph as a picture is required' (Case 62).[13] This 'participant-author's' literal interpretation of the question suggests the metaphor 'painting a picture' is unfamiliar. It indicates cultural differences between the 'survey-author' and 'participant-author' and the importance of incorporating diversity into methods requiring interpretation of questions and answers.

A large number of respondents to the wellbeing debate elected to use the 'Other' field, stating that they 'found the scope of choices limiting' (Case 26, Q9) with 'too many forced-choices an[d] assumptions' (Case 49, Q9). Some even found the tick boxes alienating, and as I have, questioned the reasoning and methods behind the debate:

> These [tick-boxes] are all relevant to government and public bodies. Is this inevitable?
>
> (Case 136, Q8)

This participant-author suggests that making the debate,

> more interesting to the individual, and thus the means of increasing the credibility of the exercise, is to establish consensual measures.
>
> (Case 136, Q8)

The free-text field as a place of inclusion is not simply practical in that it improves the perceived experience of participation, or methodological in that it improves the outcomes of participation, but is ethical in that it includes the opinions and experiences of those who do not identify with generalised and predicted assumptions typical of survey practices. Consequently, these fields offer a public political space in which those taking part are able to author their own wellbeing and voice 'what matters' in a way appropriate to them. It is therefore imperative that these voices are heard.

Some of the 'Other' field responses in the consultation contained extensive contributions, which demonstrated the eagerness of the participant-author to talk about 'what matters' to them and influence the debate's outcomes. A participant's response often conveyed the sense that they were really trying to tell something of the world, their world, or how they see the world, even if this was within imposed and alien frames, such as a government survey.

Methodological alternatives and the art of listening

While free-text fields may not offer the 'rich descriptions' typical of, for example, a biographical one-to-one interview, some contain quite extensive testimony describing people's lived experiences and multiple concerns related to the meaning of wellbeing. This is evident in the response below:

> All citizen [sic] should feel valued and respected. I used to work as a specialist nurse, I was well-respected, ran a busy department, managed a multi-million pound budget and a group of staff and earned a very good salary. Due to sudden, serious ill-health I had to finish work early and found this very hard to accept. Now I have had my DLA [Disability Living Allowance] stopped and will soon have my incapacity benefit stopped as I have been getting it for more than a year and do not qualify for means-tested benefits. So after working extremely hard for 32 years including at least 10 hours of unpaid overtime every week and paying my taxes I will now get precisely nothing. So much for making work pay. Those of us who have worked and paid NI but have a working partner (who only earns a low wage, less than he did 20 years ago thanks to [the redundancies]) get nothing, but those who haven't worked will still get their benefits. In case you haven't guessed my well-being is rapidly deteriorating, contributed to by the stress of losing the little income I still had and

worrying how I am going to manage with nothing. My condition is made worse by stress, maybe I will worry myself into an early grave and the government might be happy then.

(Case 73, Q9)[14]

Were this narrative to be analysed using the customary methods described in this chapter's Finding out the 'Findings from the Debate' section, retrofitting this description to codes from the 'forced choices' of the tick boxes would impose detrimental limitations on representing this account. Even with a multivariate coding representing family, health and finance, for example, such a coding practice would deny the shame that this nurse describes, going from feeling 'well-respected' to the implication that she no longer feels valued. In fact, a resounding theme of this narrative is how government systems can disempower and deplete individual wellbeing.

If a predetermined coding frame was used, it was perhaps unlikely that either the frame or the analysis would have had the capacity to criticise government policy. Yet, if methods of analysis do not incorporate research participants' experiences of wellbeing, or their opinions on what contributes to, or depletes it, research is open to criticism for reinforcing the interests of research designers. This tension highlights the important role for an analyst independent of the research framework. Not only can independent researchers see new potential for data to ask different questions and answer different problems (Savage 2007), but they can also distance themselves from the context of the data's creation. In short, they have better claims to impartiality.

In the light of this, I sought an alternative methodology to approach analysis of these fields which foregrounded the descriptions and narratives found within the free-text fields called 'Other'. This 'investigative epistemology' (Mason 2007) and how it was 'performed' as Law (2009) might say, is corroborated methodologically by the content of the free-text fields themselves. Participants wanted to be listened to:

> Your [sic] talking to people about their lives, not selling them a product. Empathy and understanding with how you word your surveys will make people actually give a damn and 'want' to take part as they believe (rightly or wrongly) that they will be listened too [sic] and their opinion might just count for something.
>
> (Case 6)

Recalling 'the art of listening' (Back 2007, Fromm 1994, Gunarantam 2012) and therefore consciously avoiding pre-set ideas regarding what the themes 'would' or 'should' be, or how they should be labelled, I 'listened' to the participants' descriptions and allowed themes to make themselves apparent. In other words, I enacted the 'participant-author's' account into analytic description, rather than back-coding into what the 'survey-author' might have labelled in the survey design. Approaching the qualitative data in this way, the voice of the participant-author could be heard, thereby gaining a hand in the production of knowledge, rather than this remaining in the hands of traditional 'knowledge producers'.

As one might expect when listening to 'Other' narratives, they were diverse in content and their analysis highlighted a large number (75) of themes (Table 3.5). This approach often required numerous codes for any one particular narrative. Consequently, multi-coding was necessary in my secondary analysis of these free-text fields, as the meaning of the narrative would shift if coding was too generalised, and retaining the integral meaning and complexity of the whole narrative was paramount to the project.

While this method presented 'coding traps' of its own for secondary analysis, large numbers of codes are common when analysing text relating to wellbeing. For example, Janet Scott *et al.*'s (2009: 128) analysis of British Household Panel Survey free-text fields on quality of life created 77 codes despite the clear analytical questions posed by the research team. I propose that this reflects the complexity and diversity of meanings of wellbeing, which 'efficient' shortcuts in analysis would overlook, but which are of paramount importance in a project designed to listen to voices of 'various walks of life' in a national debate on wellbeing.

The matter of understanding of wellbeing and 'Other'?

In returning to the 6,787 debate responses which were voiced in free text, I present a second chance for these voices to be heard, while this secondary data analysis contributes to the evidence base of national wellbeing and highlights the significant differences in emphasis across response registers with regard to 'what matters most' (see Tables 3.3 and 3.4). Eighty-nine per cent of respondents to the first questionnaire ticked 'health' in response to 'What things in life matter to you? Please choose all that apply.' This is unsurprising, given that 'health and wellbeing' is a common discursive construction and health is undoubtedly important to wellbeing. What is perhaps unexpected, however, is that 11 per cent of people didn't tick 'health' at all, and even more perplexing is that changing the emphasis of the question to 'What things in life matter *most* to you? Please choose all that apply' (my italics) and adding five extra tick-box response registers reduced the

Table 3.5 A summary of categories from secondary thematic analysis of free-text field usage. Codes are listed in the right-hand column, with their thematic cluster to the left. Given the large number of codes, these two columns have been split into two for ease of presentation

Cluster	Code	Cluster	Code
Financial	Business/industry	Governance	Access to services
	Expanding economy		Freedom
	GDP		Government
	Lower tax		Politics
	Stability		Targets
Definitions of/synonyms for wellbeing	Well paid	Measurement	As alternative to GDP
	Satisfied/content		Comparisons
	Fairness/social justice		Empirical evidence
	Happiness		How to/is it possible?
	Health/care		Problem of labels and categories
	Life satisfaction		Longitudinal
	Meaning in life		Problems with aggregation
	Essence of wellbeing		Quants vs quals
	Equality		Social Indicators
	Mobility		Subjective perceptions of WB
	Behavioural		Theory
	Cognitive		Waste of public funds
	Context/circumstance		Who is being measured?
	Emotional	Social aspects (inc. responsibility)	Alone time
	Potential/aspiration		Community
	Psychological		Cultural difference
	Resilience		Family
	Purpose for living		Friends
	Security	The 'story' of wellbeing	Cameron
	Happiness of others		Media
	Social definitions		Previous research
Environmental	Sustainability	What we do – personal activities	Access to services
	Overpopulation		Commute/transport
	Protection of 'nature' or 'the planet'		Quality of/access to 'natural environment'
	vs GDP		Job
Cultural identity	Faith		Physical activity
	Religion		Everyday
	Morality/values		Role in society
	Ethnicity/religious groups		Routine
	Spiritual		Spare time
			Unemployment

response rate to 83 per cent for health, especially as a lower percentage of people used free text in the second questionnaire. Cursory analysis might suggest that when presented with more dimensions of wellbeing, health becomes less important, but this seems unlikely. Even more remarkably, secondary analysis of the free-text fields identified that only nine per cent describe health in response to the same question. These counter-intuitive outcomes present further reason to investigate the different response registers and reiterate that there are methodological complications with the consultation that have been overlooked.

This discrepancy between tick-box and free-text priorities might indicate that most of the 11 per cent who did not tick health, did not tick anything and exclusively used the free-text field. Owing to limitations in the way the data were stored, it is not possible to know how participants used the different response registers available. We are unable to compare who ticked health and also ticked family, for example, or indeed how many ticked every single box. It is also not possible to compare the proportion who only used tick boxes, how many exclusively wrote in the 'Other' field, or what percentage used both response registers. While this poses problems for re-analysis, the way that the data were stored serves to reiterate the point that this was not a fully conceived mixed method project, despite the multiple approaches to collecting the data.

Table 3.6 outlines my analysis of the top-14 free-text response themes. It demonstrates that the most import theme was 'spare time and leisure' with 40 per cent of people describing the importance of where and how it is spent. This was corroborated by brief acknowledgements at the end of the Evans report and the quotation to illustrate 'personal finance' in the 2012 Self *et al.* report (both described above). When asked 'What things in life matter to you?' in Questionnaire 1, 68 per cent ticked 'Personal and cultural activities, including caring and volunteering'. This response register was split over two fields in Questionnaire 2, where 56 per cent ticked 'Personal Activities, including volunteering' (which was misreported in the Evans report) and 46 per cent ticked 'Cultural activities'. This might suggest that if free-text field analysis finds 40 per cent of responses choose to describe how they spend their spare time, it is of less importance. Yet, in Questionnaire 1, the tick boxes represent domains comparable to 'Spare time' as only the sixth most important contributor to wellbeing, when compared to 'Health' (89 per cent), 'Having good connections with friends and relatives' (89 per cent), 'Job satisfaction and economic security' (86.4 per cent), 'Present and future conditions of the environment' (73 per cent) and 'Education and training' (69 per cent).

Table 3.6 A summary of themes coded from secondary thematic analysis of free-text field usage from question 1, Questionnaire 2. 'What things in life matter most to you? Please choose all that apply.' See Table 3.2 for the tick-box responses

Free-text preferences, my own analysis	%
1. Spare time	40
2. Quality of natural environment	19
3. Family	11
4. Security	10
5. Protect planet/nature	10
6. Freedom power	9
7. Access to 'leisure' possibilities	9
8. Health/care	9
9. Equality	8
10. Happiness/WB of others	8
11. Government	8
12. Fairness/social justice	7
13. Access services	7
14. Politics	7

As far as possible given the limitations of the way the data were stored, my concern in this chapter is to bring out the difference in emphasis across the two fields of qualitative and quantitative responses. Not only did the methods of asking the debate's questions (survey, focus group or telephone line) change the results, but the way of answering (free text or tick box) altered the preferential outcomes also. Therefore, to analyse only one response register provides a very partial account of what matters to people.

The following excerpt is one of many which was coded as 'spare time', as well as 'access to leisure services':

> Having access to good local services at minimal cost that enrich cultural and physical life e.g. libraries, parks....
>
> (Case 114)

As Evans also acknowledged, the qualitative responses offer much potential for holistic insight into policy decisions and predictions (2011: 6). In respect of the importance of spare time, how and where it is spent, this offers a vital perspective on the value of investment in recreation and other services, or the importance of reserving public space from private development. While these aspects of wellbeing are acknowledged by academic (Haworth 2010: 7, Jeffres *et al.* 2009, Lovell *et al.* 2014) and sector-specific research (Fujiwara 2013, Galloway 2008, Hicks *et al.* 2011, O'Brien 2010), they have been largely neglected in literature with claims to informing policy (e.g. Bok 2010, Dolan *et al.* 2011, Hicks *et al.* 2013, O'Donnell 2013, Stoll *et al.* 2012). Furthermore, despite their prevalence in 40 per cent of 'Other' responses to what matters, the proposed domains and measures (Beaumont 2011) only account for satisfaction with amount of leisure time, a different and very partial indicator of wellbeing as an evaluator of policy decisions (see Oman 2012, 2013 for further discussion).

In her policy analysis, Karen Scott (2014: 4) describes 'a bundle of entities which can be described as "wellbeing" and another set of entities which fall outside these descriptions and are therefore "other"'. The ex-nurse, cited above (Case 73), used the free-text field to describe how certain policies are detrimental to her wellbeing, which could be interpreted as describing how she is alienated (and thus 'othered') by dominant wellbeing forms and frameworks. Positive articulations of wellbeing were also prevalent in these 'Other' fields, which might also proffer suggestions or recommendations for the beginnings of improved means of policy appraisal. Cost–benefit analysis and market valuations of non-market goods are currently stipulated by HM Treasury's *The Green Book* as the focus of public policy evaluation (2003, updated 2011). However, if wellbeing is measured by the amount of leisure time, rather than the value of services that contribute to leisure time, for example, we cannot understand the values of what matters to wellbeing and the role of government to facilitate access to these. I argue that it is only through recognition of 'Other' forms and descriptions that we can make steps towards a more complete and representative understanding of wellbeing as well as how to make policy which betters the wellbeing of all, no matter how multifaceted.

Many of these 'Other' narratives were as equally complex as Case 73 above, and so 'efficient' analytical approaches seem unlikely to be able to respect the 'rich description' of wellbeing present. Aggregating 'shortcut' analyses to represent the nation thereby corrupts the evidence base, making evidence-based policy-making to institute positive social change more problematic and less possible. While the debate was constructed to understand the nation, ignoring the intricate qualities of life and wellbeing outlined in the qualitative data leave the project vulnerable to misinterpretation and thus misrepresentation in the evidence base which policymakers draw upon. If those analysing the debate did not listen to 'how people's lives are affected' (Self *et al.* 2012), as articulated in the qualitative data, the evidence base will be limited and the wellbeing measures that are developed as a result will be flawed in their capacity to assess policy outcomes.

Conclusion

The question of wellbeing is a 'whole life' question, cutting across many 'domains' in everyday lived experience. 'The social survey has historically been able to capture and describe various realities, including seemingly mundane descriptions of everyday material conditions to aid policymaking'[15] (ONS 2001: 9). Free-text fields offer an opportunity for valuable description and are common in social survey design (e.g. Scott *et al.* 2009), yet detailed analysis of them remains atypical as survey practitioners 'naively rely on numerical survey responses without considering the interpretive value of descriptive comments' (York *et al.* 2012: 103).

The discrepancy between tick-box and free-text priorities from the debate consultation illuminates the importance of understanding the qualitative possibilities of social surveys, rather than dismissing them, in what Sarah White calls the 'construction of wellbeing knowledge' (see Chapter 1, this volume). Understanding the complexity of wellbeing thereby obliges analysis, which accommodates multiple approaches and perspectives in order 'to translate knowing into telling' (White 1987: 1) and telling into knowing. In the case of 'knowledge producers' (Law 2009), *telling* narratives of 'wellbeing', methods of interpretation and translation should also be communicated to assure the inclusion of everyday ways of knowing and narratives of wellbeing expressed as qualities of life, as found in spaces such as the free-text fields called 'Other'. This is all the more urgent if we are to make the most of knowledge in an era of big data, where analysis is driven even more by efficiency.

Analysis of the wider debate situates the intellectual issues raised by different practical engagements and highlights the potential these methodologies offer to 'understand the world'. The ONS' implied promise to listen to declarations of 'what matters most' to people who participated in the debate and its statement to look for 'what lies beneath' norms in the first major report on the MNW programme (Self *et al.* 2012) rests on epistemologically dubious ground, owing to its approach. Despite the credible breadth of participation, the interpretive interventions necessary to understand and utilise the data excluded these descriptions from outputs by nature of their form, if not their content. Thus the evidence base referred to as the wellbeing debate painted a partial picture of 'what matters' for national wellbeing, seemingly happy with what it calls a 'snapshot of life in the UK' (ONS 2012a).

No method or mode of representation is without politics, although appeals to science obscure this. My analysis of the free-text fields resulted from pre-existing knowledge of data and contexts following discourse analysis of wellbeing-related policy documents, speeches and meetings. I have described these realities and 'performed' an alternative analytical method based upon 'the art of listening' to address the gap between the participant-author, survey-author and analyst through close reading of (or listening to) the participant-author's described realities. Deconstructing the ONS' debate, its creation, direction, interpretation and dissemination may imply I intend an alternative 'truer' representation of wellbeing. Instead, this chapter is an attempt to present the potential of alternative realities as contributions to knowledge, rather than an ultimate truth.

It is important to reflect the ultimate and unique epistemological privilege of the 'Other' narrator as participant-author, rather than the researcher (survey-author or analyst) in a democratic project, as suggested by the creation of a national debate. Acknowledging the performativity of methodologies recognises the political potential of the performativity of other actors as authors, rather than being limited to habituated practices which 'feel [like] solid and reliable' realities of knowledge-making and representation (Law 2009: 242).

This chapter suggests that habitual methodological practices forgot, even ignored thousands of 'Other' narratives which are unique contributions to understanding qualities of life, including what matters and what lies beneath or outside of 'norms'. Furthermore, as Law (2009) suggested when describing the social survey, the thousands of wellbeing realities described in the free-text fields and other methods of response may have been marginalised to create a reality of wellbeing measurement as *the norm*. In dismissing the significance of free-text field analysis, the content of these fields is under-represented, excluded even, from concepts of wellbeing. Thus qualities of life that emerge from different social and cultural contexts are sidelined, as are the arguably already marginalised 'voices' of participant-authors who identified with 'Other', rather than with the predefined labels of the tick-box options.

The latter approach discounts the degree of national engagement in a debate on its own wellbeing and ignores the opportunities free-text fields offer to survey-authors for reflecting upon and improving on their own methodological practices. Without inclusive and reflexive engagement, social science remains limited to 'imagin[ing] the nation' (Savage and Burrows 2007) rather than engaging with it.

This chapter's analyses of the MNW debate have highlighted the potential practical and intellectual contributions of qualitative methodologies to tendentious quantitative practices in a project to understand wellbeing. Questions of 'what matters' in these contexts thus extend beyond the debate across social science and evidence-making practices for policy. I argue that the question 'what matters' together with the significance of answers to 'why it matters' appears to have been marginalised, disadvantaging attempts to evolve from 'imagining the nation' to 'understanding the world'. Furthermore, I argue that were this the case, then the debate creates a reality in which wellbeing measures flourish, rather than being an exercise primarily concerned with listening to descriptions of human flourishing and wellbeing, yet it is only through this shift that evidence-based policy-making can address wellbeing inequalities.

Notes

1. These groups included parents, including vulnerable mothers; youth affected by mental health; gypsy travellers; religious groups; and hospital patients and carers. For a full description of the live events, see Evans (2011).
2. 'The nation' was not specified, which was problematic for some respondents, especially those from Scotland, Wales and Northern Ireland. There were also other concerns relating to the concept of nation in relation to migration and who belongs to 'nation', which were voiced in debate responses.
3. In 2008, the French president, Nicolas Sarkozy, established the Commission on the Measurement of Economic Performance and Social Progress, chaired by the economists Joseph Stiglitz, Amartya Sen and Jean-Paul Fitoussi. This commission, along with the Organisation for Economic Co-operation and Development (OECD) 'Beyond GDP' international conference, was incredibly influential on the international imperative to measure wellbeing (see Bache and Reardon 2013 and Scott 2012).
4. These are summary tables. Questions two, four and six in the case of each questionnaire request a top three for questions one, three and five, respectively. They have been omitted from the tables for clarity of presentation, as they do not contribute understanding to the use of fields in this chapter.
5. Ideally, this chapter would outline the number of respondents who chose to use the free-text field, instead of or as well as the tick-box options, but according to email correspondence from the ONS, the debate data were not stored in such a way as to make this level of analysis possible. It is important to acknowledge that the 89 per cent of respondents who ticked 'health' may have done so by default, with little need to expand upon its meaning or outline why in a free-text field. This might go some way to explain its lack of prevalence in the free-text fields. It does not, however, ameliorate the methodological issues with ignoring differences across response registers.
6. There are issues with some of the ONS figures, which makes exacting analyses of the responses even more difficult. For example, '5,401 people answered this question and almost nine out of ten people told us that health (89 per cent) was most important' (Evans 2011: 8).

7. As witnessed in various All Party Parliamentary Group meetings, workshops, symposia, roundtables and other events I have seen representatives of the programme speak at.
8. Sen's capability theory is a useful and popular approach to wellbeing datasets. It suggests that a framework which accounts for equality in what people are able to do is more valuable than a model based on the availability of resources ([1985] 1999). While many of the narratives from the ONS' debate lend themselves to Sen's capability framework (various, including 1985), it is not the approach used in this analysis.
9. While most who talk of 'coding traps' refer to the dangers of using software, these traps are found in coding practices which do not rely on software.
10. A qualitative methods unit was formed within the social survey methodology unit in 1996 – mainly to do cognitive question testing and to advise on qualitative projects carried out by the social survey.
11. There are a number of discussions surrounding how the wellbeing agenda addresses competition; on the one hand, it pretends to flatten competition, while on the other, it reinforces it. See OECD (2014) and concepts such as 'sustainable competitiveness' (Global Economic Forum [GEF] 2013).
12. Science, technology and society (STS), also referred to as science and technology studies, is the study of how social, political and cultural values affect scientific research and technological innovation, and how these, in turn, affect society, politics and culture.
13. For the reasons outlined above, it is not possible to confirm whether this participant only responded via the free-text field, or whether they ticked one of the following boxes as well: 'Economic measures only; Single measure of overall life satisfaction/happiness; Small selection of indicators; Large set of indicators; Single index of national well-being (lot of information combined into a single number).' However, I would suggest his response indicates that these terms did not correspond to his idea of what giving a picture meant.
14. There are numerous narratives which refer to very personal and localised governance issues relating to disability, public-sector work and pit closures. While electing to use a single quote from almost two-and-a-half thousand is problematic in terms of representing the narrative content, this quote is used to illustrate a point regarding problems with dominant coding practices, rather than to represent the debate as a whole.
15. For example, surveys in the mid-1940s discovered almost one in ten households did not have the number of cups deemed necessary for essential use and 'the shortage of scrubbing brushes seems to have been extensively felt' (ONS 2011: 9).

References

Allin, P. (2007) Measuring Societal Wellbeing. *Economic and Labour Market Review. Office for National Statistics* 1(10): 46–52.

Bache, I. and Reardon, L. (2013) An Idea Whose Time Has Come? Explaining the Rise of Well-Being in British Politics. *Political Studies* 61(4): 898–914.

Back, L. (2007) *The Art of Listening*. Oxford: Berg.

Beaumont, J. (2011) *Measuring National Well-Being: A Discussion Paper on Domains and Measures*. Newport: Office for National Statistics.

Bok, D. (2010) *The Politics of Happiness: What Government Can Learn from the New Research on Well-Being.* Princeton and Oxford: Princeton University Press.
Cameron, D. (2010) *Prime Minister's Speech on Wellbeing on 25 November 2010.* Available at: https://www.gov.uk/government/speeches/pm-speech-on-wellbeing [accessed 15 March 2013].
Camfield, L. and Palmer-Jones, R. (2013) Improving the Quality of Development Research: What Could Archiving Qualitative Data for Reanalysis and Revisiting Research Sites Contribute? *Progress in Development Studies* 13(4): 323–338.
Dolan, P., Layard, R. and Metcalfe, R. (2011) *Measuring Subjective Well-Being for Public Policy.* Newport: Office for National Statistics.
Evans, J. (2011) *Findings from the National Well-Being Debate.* Available at: http://www.ons.gov.uk/ons/guide-method/user-guidance/well-being/publications/findings-from-the-national-well-being-debate.pdf [accessed 1 May 2012].
Fromm, E. (1994) *The Art of Listening.* New York: Continuum.
Fujiwara, D. (2013) *Museums and Happiness: The Value of Participating in Museums and the Arts.* Suffolk: The Happy Museum.
Galloway, S. (2008) *The Evidence Base for Arts and Culture Policy.* Edinburgh: Scottish Arts Council.
Garcia, J., Evans, J. and Reshaw, M. (2004) 'Is There Anything Else You Would Like to Tell Us' – Methodological Issues in the Use of Free-Text Comments from Postal Surveys. *Quality & Quantity* 38: 113–125.
Global Economic Forum (2013) *Global Competitive Report.* Available at: http://www3.weforum.org/docs/WEF_GlobalCompetitivenessReport_2013-14.pdf [accessed 1 February 2014].
Gunarantam, Y. (2012) Learning to Be Affected: Social Suffering and Total Pain at Life's Borders. *The Sociological Review,* 60(S1): 108–123. Available at: http://onlinelibrary.wiley.com/DOI: 10.1111/j.1467-954X.2012.02119.x [accessed 13 May 2013].
Haworth, J. (2010) *Life, Work, Leisure, and Enjoyment: The Role of Social Institutions.* ESRC. Available at: http://www.wellbeing-esrc.com/downloads/LifeWorkLeisure&Enjoyment.pdf [accessed 13 March 2012].
Hicks, D., Creaser, C., Greenwood, H., Spezi, V., White, S. and Frude, N. (2011) *Public Library Activity in the Areas of Health and Well-Being. Final Report.* Birmingham: Museums, Libraries and Archives Council.
Hicks, S., Tinker, L. and Allin, P. (2013) Measuring Subjective Well-Being and Its Potential Role in Policy: Perspectives from the UK Office for National Statistics. *Social Indicators Research* 114(1): 73–86.
HM Treasury (2003, updated 2011) *The Green Book: Appraisal and Evaluation in Central Government.* London.
Jeffres, L. W., Bracken, C. C., Jian, G. and Casey, M. F. (2009) The Impact of Third Places on Community Quality of Life. *Applied Research in Quality of Life* 4(4): 333–345.
Jeffries, S. (2008) Will This Man Make You Happy? *The Guardian,* Tuesday 24 June 2008. Available at: http://www.theguardian.com/lifeandstyle/2008/jun/24/healthandwellbeing.schools [accessed 12 June 2012].
Kroll, C. (2011) *Measuring Progress and Well-Being: Achievements and Challenges of a New Global Movement.* Berlin: Friedrich-Ebert-Stiftung.
Law, J. (2009) Seeing Like a Survey. *Cultural Sociology* 3(2): 239–256.

Law, J., Ruppert, E. and Savage, M. (2011) The Double Social Life of Methods CRESC Working Paper 095. Available at: http://www.cresc.ac.uk/sites/default/files/The%20Double%20Social%20Life%20of%20Methods%20CRESC%20Working%20Paper%2095.pdf [accessed 15 August 2012].

Law, J., Ruppert, E. and Savage, M. (eds.) (2013, July) Special Issue on the Social Life of Methods. *Theory, Culture and Society.* 30(4): 3–21.

Lovell, R., Husk, K., Bethel, A. and Garside, R. (2014) What Are the Health and Well-Being Impacts of Community Gardening for Adults and Children: A Mixed Method Systematic Review Protocol. *Environmental Evidence* 3: 20.

Mason, J. (2007) Re-Using Qualitative Data: On the Merits of an Investigative Epistemology. *Sociological Research Online* 12(3). Available at: http://www.socresonline.org.uk /12/3/3.html. DOI: 10.5153/sro.1507 [accessed 12 December 2013].

Matheson, J. (2011) *National Statistician's Reflections on the National Debate on Measuring National Well-Being.* Newport: Office of National Statistics.

NatCen and CLS (2003) *Millennium Cohort Study, First Survey: Code Book and Edit Instructions.* Centre for Longitudinal Studies, Bedford Group for Lifecourse and Statistical Studies and Institute of Education, University of London.

O'Brien, D. (2010) *Measuring the Value of Culture: A Report to the Department for Culture Media and Sport.* London: DCMS.

O'Cathain, A. and Thomas, K. (2004) 'Any Other Comments?' Open Questions on Questionnaires – A Bane or a Bonus to Research? *BMC Medical Research Methodology* 4(25). Available at: http://www.biomedcentral.com/1471-2288/4/25 [accessed 13 December 2013].

O'Donnell, G. (2013) Using Well-Being as a Guide to Policy. pp. 96–111 in J. F. Helliwell, R. Layard and J. Sachs (eds.) *World Happiness Report 2013.* New York: UN Sustainable Development Solutions Network.

Oman, S. (2012) Measuring National Wellbeing: The Public Debate That Was Never Ours. *Arts Professional* (257): 8, September 2012.

Oman, S. (2013) A 'Snapshot of Life'? What's Missing from this Picture? Two Years of Measuring National Well Being. *Arts Professional*, February 2013.

OECD (2014) *Competition.* Available at: http://www.oecd.org/daf/competition/ [accessed 1 March 2014].

Office for National Statistics (2011) *Measuring National Well-Being Technical Advisory Group.* Friday 4 February 2011. Minutes available at: http://www.ons.gov.uk/ons/guide-method/user-guidance/well-being/measuring-national-well-being-technical-advisory-group/Notes-from-the-meeting-on-4-february-2011.pdf [accessed 15 March 2014].

Office for National Statistics (2012a) *Measuring What Matters – Understanding the Nation's Well-Being.* Available at: www.ons.gov.uk/wellbeing [accessed 1 September 2012].

Office for National Statistics (2012b) *ONS Sheds More Light on Life in the UK News Release.* Available at: http://www.ons.gov.uk/ons/dcp29904_287921.pdf [accessed 30 November 2012].

Office of National Statistics (2001) *60 Years of Social Survey: 1941–2001.* Norwich: HMSO.

Rich, J. L., Chojenta, C. and Loxton, D. (2013) Quality, Rigour and Usefulness of Free-Text Comments Collected by a Large Population Based Longitudinal Study – ALSWH. *PLoS ONE* 8(7). Available at: http://www.plosone.org/

article/info%3Adoi%2F10.1371%2Fjournal.pone.0068832 [accessed 1 December 2013].
Richards, L. (2005) *Handling Qualitative Data: A Practical Guide*. London: Sage.
Savage, M. (2007) Changing Social Class Identities in Post-War Britain: Perspectives from Mass-Observation. *Sociological Research Online* 12(3): 6. Available at: http://www.socresonline.org.uk/12/3/6.html. DOI: 10.5153/sro.1459.
Savage, M. and Burrows, R. (2007) The Coming Crisis of Empirical Sociology. *Sociology* 41: 885.
Scott, K. (2012) *Measuring Wellbeing. Towards Sustainability*. London: Routledge.
Scott, K. (2014) Happiness on Your Doorstep: Disputing the Boundaries of Wellbeing and Localism. *The Geographical Journal* 181(2): 129–137.
Scott, J., Nolan, J. and Plagnol, A. (2009) Panel Data and Open-Ended Questions: Understanding Perceptions of Quality of Life. *21st Century Society* 4(2): 123–135.
Seidman, I. (2013) *Interviewing as Qualitative Research: A Guide for Researchers in Education and the Social Sciences*. 4th ed. New York: Teachers' College Press.
Self, A., Thomas, J. and Randall, C. (2012) *Measuring National Well-Being: Life in the UK, 2012*. Newport: Office for National Statistics.
Self, A., Thomas, J. and Randall, C. (2013) *Measuring National Well-Being – Review of Domains and Measures, 2013*. Newport: Office for National Statistics.
Sen, A. (1999) *Commodities and Capabilities*. 2nd ed. Delhi New York: Oxford University Press.
Stiglitz, J. E., Sen A. and Fitoussi, J. P. (2009) *Report by the Commission on the Measurement of Economic Performance and Social Progress*. OECD. Available at: http://www.stigliz-sen-fitoussi.fr/ [accessed 3 April 2012].
Stoll, L., Michaelson, J. and Seaford, C. (2012) *Well-Being Evidence for Policy: A Review*. London: New Economics Foundation.
White, H. (1987) *The Content of the Form: Narrative Discourse and Historical Representation*. London: John Hopkins University Press.
York, G. S., Churchman, R., Woodard, B., Wainright, C. and Rau-Foster, M. (2012) Free-Text Comments: Understanding the Value in Family Member Descriptions of Hospice Caregiver Relationships. *American Journal of Hospice and Palliative Medicine* 29: 98.

4
Staying Well in a South African Township: Stories from Public Health and Sociology

Emer Brangan

Introduction

The current approach to preventing noncommunicable diseases[1] (NCDs) in low- and middle-income countries draws heavily on the disciplines of public health and biomedicine, which unsurprisingly construct health as a dominant normative goal and a central component of wellbeing. The research which this chapter draws on was driven by my sense that something important was missing from much policy on NCD prevention: a broader understanding of how health and the so-called health behaviours[2] implicated in causing NCDs were related to wellbeing, particularly in very challenging environments such as a South African township. It seemed to me that one of the reasons that such an understanding was lacking was the approach to knowledge which was being taken: the discourse around public health policy on prevention was 'expert' driven; the vast majority of the research on which policy was based was quantitative and had been carried out in high-income countries; and the 'public' were often cast as a group to be manipulated in order to change their behaviour, rather than as stakeholders with knowledge, values and reasons which warranted respectful attention. In order to explore this, I carried out qualitative research alongside a quantitative epidemiological study which was already underway in a township in South Africa. This chapter presents some of the stories which the combined data told and considers the implications of the different disciplinary approaches for the ideas about health and wellbeing which emerged.

Methods

This chapter draws on research using a case study design carried out in the township of Langa in South Africa – a low-income urban area with high rates of unemployment and crime (City of Cape Town 2012, Gie 2009) and multiple health burdens (Groenewald *et al.* 2012). The primary data generated included semi-structured interviews with 40 residents[3] of Langa (20 female and 20 male) with an average age of 49 years. These interviews[4] explored the respondent's life history and satisfaction, health, daily routine, physical activity, and views of local challenges and how to address them. After a discussion about the respondent's life more generally and their satisfaction with it, specific questions about health were asked, followed by questions about physical activity and other so-called health behaviours. This was done in an attempt to reduce the extent to which these topics would be taken as cues indicating what we thought was important (e.g. along the lines of 'physical activity is important for health which is important for wellbeing'). Nevertheless, our association with the epidemiological study in which the respondents were already involved is likely to have been one of the many things which influenced how people answered our questions (see White, Introduction to this volume).

Interviews were carried out in the first language of the respondent, usually Xhosa, and were transcribed into English. They took place during visits to respondents' homes by the author and a local female researcher[5] whose mother tongue was Xhosa and who was a resident of a nearby township. Triangulation and further context were provided by eight interviews with key informants working in the fields of health, physical activity and policy in Langa; field notes and photographs generated during observation in Langa; and secondary data on Langa such as unemployment and crime rates.

Secondary data on respondents was comprised of a set of questionnaires completed approximately ten months earlier by respondents for the Prospective Urban and Rural Epidemiological (PURE) study. These questionnaires sought to capture quantitative information about respondents' health, using closed questions about a range of disabilities, symptoms, diagnoses, injuries, risk factors and stresses. In addition, physical measurements – such as weight, height, blood pressure, electrocardiogram (ECG), spirometry, blood and urine samples – were taken by PURE.

In this chapter, I focus on a selection of the stories about staying well told by the combined quantitative and qualitative data for each respondent.

Stories

Nombeko

Nombeko's small front room appears to function as both a living room and a kitchen. It is furnished with a sofa, a TV and an armchair cushioned with uncovered foam. An old fridge stands beside a small table covered with a plastic Coca Cola design tablecloth – the external landscape of the township is awash with the drink company's logo and now I see that it has invaded homes as well. Another Coca Cola cloth covers a table on the other side of the room where an electric hotplate stands on bricks. A frying pan sits on the shelf under the TV and there is a kettle in the glass-fronted cupboard beneath this.

The smell of cooking is in the air. There are two kids on the sofa – one is very little and is struggling somewhat as he eats pasta with a big spoon from a Blossom margarine tub. A baby is crying in the background. Flies buzz. Fifty-five-year-old grandmother of three, Nombeko, wears earrings, black trousers, a white tunic and white, laced shoes. Her outfit is reminiscent of a healthcare uniform. She seems energetic and animated, and uses her hands a lot as she talks. She had a variety of jobs in the past but gives her current occupation as 'home-based carer'. She did not complete the final two years of secondary school when she was younger (her first child was born when she was 16), but she is studying to pass them now. She is also on a training course for the unpaid social work which she is doing in the township via a local non-governmental organisation (NGO):

> I go door to door looking for children whose CD4 count[6] is less than 200. I am looking for children that are sick and who are not getting support from the government. I am also responsible for making sure that they take their treatment. I am in the children's forum. I am also looking after children who are abused by their mothers.

Nombeko had five sons of her own, of whom three are still living. One had learning difficulties and suffered from epilepsy, but he 'just disappeared', aged 29, eight years earlier. More recently she lost her third-born to tuberculosis (TB), just when she thought he was starting to recover.

The epidemiological questionnaires give the impression of a woman with many health problems. Diagnoses of diabetes, high blood pressure, heart failure and asthma are recorded, along with a history of stroke and TB, and there is a long list of medications she is taking. In the section on disabilities, 'yes' is ticked for every option except for 'trouble speaking and being understood'. This implies that she has problems with her sight, hearing, walking about, bending down, picking things up and grasping/handling things. Nombeko brings up the same diagnoses in her interview (although she does not mention heart failure, and does mention having arthritis, which was not one of the tick boxes available on the questionnaire), but they do not seem to dominate her life. She does not mention any disabilities, nor is any impairment apparent during our interaction with her. When asked how her health is, she says that she has 'no problem' in the summer, but that winter is more difficult. She talks about lots of charitable and domestic work which she carries out on a daily basis, thus it appears that functionally she is doing well.

Nombeko was unusual amongst female respondents in reporting that she smoked (five cigarettes a day according to her questionnaire) and drank alcohol (spirits and beer, quantities not clear).

Yes I smoke and I am craving as we speak! [Laughter]

However, unlike the majority of the women we interviewed, Nombeko was not overweight as defined by the World Health Organization (WHO)[7] when she was weighed at the time she completed the questionnaires. She did not speak about her diet during her interview but she walked a lot for exercise, saying that she has to exercise because she had a stroke, and that it is good for her asthma. However she also enjoyed it for its own sake:

> Nombeko: Even now you saw me sweating, walking very fast; I cannot walk slowly, I have to walk fast.
> Int: Really; so do you see yourself as an active person?
> Nombeko: Yes because I love exercising; I am able to walk from here, Langa, and go to Bellville [approximately eight miles].
> Int: You walk to Bellville!?

Her description of her walking is in stark contrast to the tick in the box on her questionnaire stating that she had trouble walking about and another tick stating that she needed to use a cane/walker. Ten months had passed since the questionnaire had been completed, and so it may have been that her physical capacity had been different then, but she did not mention any such changes during her interview. In addition, a physical activity questionnaire for her had been completed on the same day as the questionnaire with the questions about disability, and this reported a lot of walking as well as high levels of domestic physical activity. Might other factors have influenced the difficulties she reported at that time? It had not been long since the death of her son, and in her questionnaires she had reported 'permanent stress' and that she had experienced symptoms of depression. Nombeko did feel that the losses she had experienced had affected her health:

> My health changed ever since my children passed on.

In her interview however, she came across as a very optimistic person. Keeping busy and active was one of the strategies she used to stay positive amidst such challenging circumstances:

> Yes, exercising is very good and you should not stress yourself by thinking too much. You see now I am concentrating on this because I know that I must do this work. I forget about other things, you see.

A general life satisfaction question was asked within the context of the interview and Nombeko's response to this helped to illustrate the importance of caution in interpreting the option on the response scale chosen by respondents:

> Nombeko: I am not satisfied with life because I am still going on, getting skills.
> Int: You are not satisfied?
> Nombeko: No I still want to further my studies and become whatever I want to be.

Nombeko's response seems to imply that she associates being satisfied with being content to stay where you are; perhaps giving up a little. Her dissatisfaction seems somehow positive. She radiated pride in the things she had achieved and was confident that she would continue to progress (see also Camfield, this volume).

The questionnaire items on crime and safety in Langa raised further questions for me: Nombeko's walking was done despite the almost universal agreement amongst questionnaire respondents, including Nombeko, with the statements 'the crime rate in my neighbourhood makes it unsafe to go on walks during the day' and 'at night'. However, like several other respondents, a few questions later in the same questionnaire she reported that she was satisfied with safety from the threat of crime in her neighbourhood. This apparent contradiction in the questionnaire data was confusing: how could people whose main form of local transport was walking be satisfied in this situation? The structured questionnaire data did not offer anything further which I was able to use to make sense of this. The stories which people told in their interviews however did: respondents had developed strategies to help them stay safe in their neighbourhood, despite the threat from crime. Limitation of movement in Langa was one such strategy, but others included careful consideration of what you carried with you, and how you carried it, what times you moved, where to and who with. Another strategy was to be known by perpetrators of crime, as this made it less likely that you would be chosen as a target. Another respondent explained why walking for exercise was not a problem:

> No, people who want to be active do it because when you are active and they see that you are exercising, they know that you don't have money and a cell phone on you; so what are they going to take? But the minute you are carrying a handbag or whatever, obviously they think that there is money in the bag, you know what I am trying to say.
>
> (Cebisa, 57-year-old female)

The qualitative data thus provided useful explanatory information for those interested in using the quantitative data on perceptions of safety to inform policy on physical activity. Physical activity was possible on the streets of Langa, but it was constrained by safety concerns. Other qualitative data were also of relevance here – such as the finding that obvious purposeful exercise, such as that described by Cebisa above, was often seen as socially inappropriate for older adults, particularly women. Such exercise also had a higher opportunity cost than, for example, getting exercise by walking to places you needed to get to such as shops, work or visiting people – when you would be more likely to be carrying things with you and the threat from crime increased.

Xolile

Like Nombeko, 47-year-old Xolile ticked a box on the negative side of the scale for the life satisfaction question, however his outlook on life was very different. Also like Nombeko, Xolile was unemployed and his main concern at the time we spoke to him was where his next meal would come from.

> Int: How do you spend your days during the week and on weekends?
> Xolile: I just stand here and wait for someone who might call me and ask me to do something for him... or go to Athlone [nearby suburb] but even there, when you get there you are greeted by a 'no vacancy'

sign so it does not help. It is a waste of time to go there in the first place because sometimes I go there and when I come back I hear that someone was looking for me. I then feel sad because I wasted time going there while I could have done the small job here so that I can get even if it is R10 [less than £1 sterling] so that I can eat.

He has limited family to provide support – his mother died when he was 13 (he does not mention his father), and this meant that he had to leave school to help support himself and his grandmother. He managed to find casual work as a general labourer for a shop and then as a window cleaner, but the contracts were temporary: 'that is the last job I had. I did not get a job again.' Now his only surviving adult relative is an aunt. He lives behind her house in one of the 'backyard shacks' which are common in the township and she can sometimes help him out with food. He is conscious however of being a burden:

Some days I go for two days without eating because there is nowhere else to go to. Where can I go? I am ashamed because maybe my aunt gave me four bread slices and I ate that, I am ashamed to go and ask her again. I would rather to go to sleep with an empty stomach.

Xolile has a 12-year-old son from a past relationship who lives with his mother and she receives a child support grant of R200 per month. Xolile wants to be able to provide more for the boy but finds himself frustrated:

To add to that my son needs a tracksuit for school; like now I am stressing about that, I need to get the tracksuit. I have to try and get money for that because the only thing that is helping him out is the grant and it is too little. I am really struggling.

We sit in the living area of the main house to talk. Xolile is thin – measurements taken ten months earlier put his Body Mass Index (BMI) at 17.3, which is considered underweight. He is wearing clothes which are flecked with paint, a baseball cap and a beard. Occupants of the main house are around and about, answering the phone, talking and watching TV. Xolile sits on a sofa facing us. The embroidery pattern of the cushions is protected by a clear plastic cover. He is bent forward at the waist and uses few gestures as he talks. When I arrived, I gave him my contact details card and throughout the conversation he holds this in one hand.

Xolile's questionnaires for the epidemiological study reported no disabilities, symptoms, diagnoses, injuries or medications, although physical measurements indicated that he might have high blood pressure.

However, at the time of his interview ten months later he rated his health as very bad. He said he was weak, which was not usual for him, and he did not know what was happening. He wondered if he might have high blood pressure, but said he had not been given results of the measurements taken for the research. He mentioned that he had had TB in the past (this was not recorded in his questionnaire) and wondered whether this might be coming back. He had not been to see a doctor.

When asked what he did to protect or improve his health, he said that he was not doing anything, and seemed to base this solely on the fact that he was not taking any treatment or medication. He did not mention health in connection with any of the so-called health behaviours which are the focus of WHO policy on NCD prevention. Xolile's emphasis was different. Food was about survival – he was not in a position to choose what he ate:

> I eat everything that is in front of me... It does not matter what kind of food it is; sometimes I get leftovers from next door. I eat everything that was left over from what they were eating; rather than throwing it away, they give it to me and that is how I survive. I eat anything so that there can at least be something in my stomach; like now I do not know what I am going to eat since the soup kitchens are no longer running.

He does not think much of the idea of taking part in sport – there were various costs associated with sport which adults in his position could ill afford:

> You need to have money; you don't just go in, you have to pay. Even if you have money, that is not going to help you with anything because the only thing you do there is to play and at the end of the day you go to sleep hungry. Playing is just a waste of time because you have to have something to eat; how can you play with an empty stomach?
>
> (Xolile speaking about the local sports centre)

A former soccer player, he thinks he is now well past the age at which it would be sensible to play this anyway, but other types of physical activity are okay:

> Xolile: Soccer... now?! No I cannot do that; the age limit for soccer is 25 years.

Int: You can just play to keep yourself active.
Xolile: No I cannot.
Int: So how do you keep yourself active?
Xolile: I keep myself active by doing all the hard work in the township like when someone wants their grass to be cut short; that is how I use my energy. I like that, I like working.

He also walks a lot because transport costs money which he does not have, thus he may well be meeting the WHO guidelines on physical activity (WHO 2010), but staying healthy was not his motivation for this. Xolile has smoked cigarettes since he was 20, as well as some cannabis. He also reported in his epidemiology study questionnaires that he drinks alcohol regularly, although not large amounts. Like many other respondents he sees links between unemployment, alcohol and drug use, and crime in the township:

> There is a lot of crime here. There is a lot of crime because our sons are on drugs. They say they are on drugs so that they can make the day go faster; that is what they say.

Unemployment was a terrible burden for many of the respondents. Xolile's interview, and the questions about stress levels and symptoms of depression in the questionnaires he completed ten months previously, gave clear indications of his distress. He was asked about his life satisfaction during the interview:

> I am not satisfied at all because I am struggling too much now that I do not have people. It is worse than before... if I do not have something, there is nowhere else to turn to. People in the township do not help each other; even if you cry out to someone, the person will tell you to go and fend for yourself. You go looking for stuff and you return with nothing and then you end up regretting the fact that you even went to look for something in the first place because you still return with an empty stomach. Sometimes you get to maybe clean a garden; I sometimes ask the people to please let me clean their gardens. I ask the people because it is hard... I am really struggling; there is nothing that satisfies me with my life. It is very bad.

Behind him a lunch of sandwiches with brown bread is being prepared for the children of the house, but not for Xolile. The 'thank you' parcel of stationary, tea, biscuits and fruit juice which we give him at the end of the interview seems pitifully inadequate.

Nkosazana

We come into Nkosazana's well-kept home through the kitchen, pass a bedroom on the right and sit together in the living room. There are two sofas and an armchair here, surrounding a coffee table. A dining table and matching chairs are pushed against the wall in the area between us and the kitchen, opposite a sideboard. A trophy stands on this sideboard – it turns out later that Nkosazana won this when she was younger and a bit of a netball star. Girls from the township still come to ask her for advice about the game. The wooden floor is brightened up with a rug. The message 'The Lord is our Shepherd' is framed and hanging on one of the whitewashed walls. A radio is on in the background.

Nkosazana is a slim, well-looking 40-year-old woman. She was born in this house, one of a large family, several of whom live here now with their children and grandchildren. Nkosazana had her first child at 15 while still at school. She has since worked as a cleaner and tea lady, but lost her job before her fourth child was born. She gives her occupation now as 'unemployed', but she spends her days caring for her elderly mother, her brother's child and her sister's grandchild. She is called away by her mother at one point during the interview, and comes back with her baby nephew, who she proceeds to feed from a bottle. Later, contented, he sits on my knee.

After feeling unwell for some time, Nkosazana found out on Valentine's Day 1999 that she was HIV positive. She was very open about her HIV status – it was almost the first thing she told us when we arrived. For the majority of respondents, the question about HIV on the epidemiological questionnaire was not answered and many people also responded 'no' to the question about whether they knew people with HIV.[8] The stigma associated with the illness had wounded Nkosazana deeply:

> Nkosazana: You know what? When you are sick, people laugh at you, people laugh at you when you are sick. In my street...
> Int: Was there no one there for you?
> Nokosazana: My family was there, my family was next to me but that day I remember I had friends but from that day I never had friends again.

Nkosazana brought her family together to tell them about the results of her HIV test and found them supportive:

> They are looking after me and they don't want me to struggle for anything. They are doing everything for me... they love me and they show me love.

When asked about her health right at the start of the interview, Nkosazana responded:

> Int: How can you rate your health; how would you say your health is now?
> Nkosazana: It is very bad.
> Int: How bad is it?
> Nkosazana: It is very bad, I am always sick.

But later in the interview, having spent some time talking about her situation, she was asked a similar question and said:

> Int: So health-wise, how satisfied are you?
> Nkosazana: It is OK.
> Int: So there is nothing that is bothering you?
> Nkosazana: No there is nothing that is bothering me despite the fact that I have swollen feet.

This was the first interview. I had intended the health question to be asked at this second point. However, I had confused my colleague with the layout of the paperwork I had given her, and so, in this interview only, the questions about general life satisfaction and self-rated health were asked twice.

The difference in responses indicates once again how cautious we need to be in interpreting responses to such questions – the answer may be strongly influenced by very short-term context. When we arrived, Nkosazana had started by telling us about problems she was having with her feet. She was quite bothered about this and had not had a response from the doctor which satisfied her. Later, after sitting talking about her life for a while, and reflecting on how she had managed to deal with her illness, and the love and support she had received from her family, she seemed calmer and more at peace with things. There was a similar change in her response to the general life satisfaction question asked at the same two points, going from 'I am extremely not satisfied because of what I see in my past life' to 'sister, my life is alright.'

However, Nkosazana did feel that her health problems had limited both her own and her children's possibilities in life, saying 'my health is pulling me back':

> It feels like if I hadn't fallen sick, my children would be far. Neliswa and Mibono are not studying. They are not studying just because they passed grade 12[9] and now they are not studying. Mibono is studying computers here in Roma; it was his aim to go and study. He passed his grade 12 very well; I was supposed to take him further but I am not working and I don't have money so I said: my child, go and study computers rather than doing nothing. My firstborn, Neliswa, is not doing anything.

The previous year, Nkosazana had found a job with the municipality but 'I could not stay because of my feet.' This lack of employment could have very harmful effects on self-esteem:

> I see myself as useless; people say that I am useless because I am... if I was HIV negative I would be a good person. A person that works; I used to work, my sister.

But Nkosazana had been able to draw on the strength which came from her relationship with her family to get through very tough times in the past, such as the health crisis which had led to her HIV diagnosis:

> I stayed in hospital the whole year, the whole year!... But I told myself when I was in hospital that I will never die, my children are very young. I will never, never! I got well.

Nkosazana had never smoked or drunk alcohol but told us that 'most of my peers here drink', and she saw this as a preventing them from involving themselves in other activities. Asked about what could be done to help people keep themselves healthy she responded:

> In my area what is finishing young people are drugs, there is a lot of drugs.

She thought that providing young people with training, and creating jobs, was the way to reduce the level of drug abuse in Langa. Nkosazana spoke to me about the terrible burden of unemployment in the township. She told me that there was nothing to do; people just walked up and down the street to fill in the time. She worried about her children – two of the four had finished their education but had not found work and were just sitting at home. The third one would finish grade 12 shortly and she fully expected him to do exactly the same.

Nombeko's poor health as a consequence of HIV had frustrated her and left her in a very different position from what she believed would otherwise have been possible – affecting her social relationships, her ability to find and keep work, and, linked to this, her ability to provide for her children. She felt that as a result her children's prospects were now similarly blighted. Although unemployment was a pervasive barrier to wellbeing in Langa, Nombeko believed that with better health she would have been able to support her children in further education and that they would have been better placed to overcome this. Her own wellbeing in the face of these frustrations was built on her position within her family – living with four generations in the house of her birth, caring for the young and the old amongst them and having them next to her in her most difficult times.

Malusi

We could not find Malusi at first, but when we enquired locally, someone was kind enough to fetch him for us so that we could walk together back to his home. We come round the back of the house and go in through a blue door whose paint is flaking. Inside the door is a bed with an elderly man in it. He seems a little startled at first, but then he says that we can sit on the side of his bed.[10] The room is small and crowded with possessions. Malusi clears some stuff off a chair for himself. The slim 39-year-old is dressed in a blue V-neck jumper, green tracksuit bottoms and battered-looking, white New Balance trainers. He has short hair and a beard, and his face is very expressive as he speaks. He occasionally consults with the older man before answering a question. Malusi is unusual amongst our respondents in that he does not have children. From what he tells us, the household has fallen on hard times of late and the house itself is sinking into disrepair.

The reason that we, and, judging by the fridge and the stack of armchairs in the corner, most of the furniture are crammed into this room is that the house has been colonised by bees. Malusi believes that this has happened because the ancestors are angry and that this is also why the household is not doing well and cannot get jobs.

Malusi's questionnaires, completed eight months earlier, report no disabilities, diagnoses, or symptoms. During his interview, he rated his health as good. He said that as an adolescent he had a calling to be a traditional healer, but that his family, and practitioners of Western medicine, did not recognise this, mistaking his condition for a nervous ailment. It was only when he went to the Eastern Cape[11] that a different opinion on the source of his illness was offered.[12] However, he ended up dropping out of school and getting 'piece jobs' instead.

Sport is Malusi's passion in life and he wishes he could get a job as a sports coach but he thinks his lack of education and family connections mean that this will not happen.

> I grew up playing football, cricket, swimming and roller-skating, and riding bicycles... God gave me sports as a talent; it is just that I did not go to school. I am supposed to be teaching and coaching in the two community halls, my sister, or in the stadium.

Asked what he does to stay healthy, he talks about his exercise, but he feels he needs the right food to be able to do this, so has not been for ten days now because food is short:

> Like, my sister, the only thing that is helping my health is that I like exercising; the only thing that is keeping me from doing that is what I was telling you about, that we do not have food. I like exercising, I grew up doing that; when I do not go to the gym I can feel that there is something that I did not do. My body is used to that and when I do not do it I feel pains in my body.

Food is a big problem. Malusi suddenly gets up and goes into the next room. He comes back with a yellow plastic pot and an empty orange squash bottle and shows them to us:

> We always ate good food in this house and we were always happy; you can now open that fridge, there is nothing; there isn't even sugar and there is no mealie-meal.[13] We used to put sugar in this. With the one rand that I had, I bought a sweet-aid and ate the bread that I came back with yesterday, from Pinelands [nearby affluent suburb]. So there is no sugar now and there is no bread, but a black person can hang on.

Malusi came back to the theme of food repeatedly, seeing the right kind of food as essential for fuelling and building the body:

> I like eating porridge in the morning and also have bread and egg. Later in the day I make mashed potatoes, after that I have fruits and then in the evening I eat rice, cabbages and chicken; that is when there is some money. When there is no money, the body also gets slow because the immune system is not getting the nutrition. It takes time to build your body when you eat dry bread and tea, especially when you eat that late in the evening. That is what is happening here in this house, my uncle also knows that. When I am eating those foods, my body gets built and I exercise more but it is a different situation when I do not have money. I get lazy because what is the use of exercising when there is nothing to eat. Do you understand my sister? I really love sports. I was telling my uncle that it becomes hard when there is no sugar and no mealie-meal in the house because in the mornings I have to go and run and then come back, take a shower and make some porridge. It becomes hard because I am draining myself by going to the gym, while not eating healthy food.

Despite his love of sport and his interest in a healthy diet, Malusi has been smoking since a young age – about five cigarettes a day. He also drinks beer, but says he never drinks a lot in one go. He spoke negatively at times about those in his community who drank:

> Other people don't like keeping their bodies in a good condition; they like being down, smoking and drinking and as a result, they get old before their time.

However, later in the interview he displayed more understanding of the stresses which may drive people to drinking and using drugs:

> There are things that are finishing people and those things have been here for a long time and we cannot stop them. I am talking about things like drugs and alcohol, when we got here, those things were already here. People get tempted; there are home situations that drive you to that. Sometimes you feel like you cannot handle the stress and decide to kill the pain with a drug or alcohol, not knowing that you are making the situation worse. I don't know if I am making sense?

Many respondents linked several of the other commonly mentioned challenges for people in Langa to the unemployment situation. In particular, drug and alcohol abuse, and the crime that went alongside, were seen to be strongly connected to unemployment:

> So you end up committing a crime because you see that all your friends are working and you ask yourself why you are not working. You see my sister; you end up telling yourself that it is better to be a criminal and do wrong things.

Malusi feels that his own problems are caused by his inability to get a job:

> The only thing that is frustrating me in my life is being unemployed. I do not like begging my sister.

His pride prevents him from asking his neighbours for help – he feels better about going to a nearby 'white' community:

> I have to go to Pinelands around 4pm to try and get the sugar; I am definitely sure that I will get it from the whites. If you ask someone from here for some sugar, he will give it to you but after that he will make fun of your situation. You know our situation, how we are living.

Malusi shared the views of several other respondents – mostly women – that how well you were doing was influenced by your attitude and how you responded to your circumstances. He believed that his ability to reflect on his life had saved him from ending up in a worse situation:

> I am not satisfied with the things that I wanted for my life because downfalls have happened in my life. If I had decided not to give thought to everything that has happened I would be in jail or dead as we speak.

Spiritual powers – Malusi maintained Christian and traditional beliefs alongside each other – had the ability to bring about real change:

> There is only one person who can change a person's life and a person's condition; it is the person with power, the one who is up there. When you want to change your life, you ask the ancestors and also ask God.

But you also needed to be proactive: 'If you just sit here in the township, you will not get anything.' Like Nombeko, Malusi relied on keeping active to stay well in difficult times:

> At the same time, keeping myself active helps me to forget the things that happened to me. When I am not exercising, everything becomes too much for my brain but when I am exercising, it becomes easier. So exercising helps me with that, and it also protects my body.

Mandisa

We go outside to the backyard of Mandisa's house as people are watching a film inside. The kitchen and living room are both small. Young men are gathered in the former and several teenagers in the latter. We bring out plastic chairs for my colleague and 69-year-old Mandisa to use, and I sit on the steps. The yard is surfaced with uneven bricks and sand. There are wooden buildings along one side and rusty corrugated iron sheets extending from the back of the neighbouring house make a fence on the other side. A hockey stick and cricket bat are propped against a wall. Mandisa is very breathless and very heavy. She is wearing a dress, a head scarf and flip-flops. My poor colleague ends up sitting in the hot sun, which will move round and catch Mandisa too if we stay here for long.

Twelve people live in this house, including seven of Mandisa's grandchildren and two toddlers she takes care of who I think are her great grandchildren. She, along with many other respondents, feels that a shortage of housing is a major problem in Langa:

> They have to build houses for us because we are staying with children in our yards, you understand? Look at these old sons that we have staying with us, they are old but there are not places.

Some of the respondents were themselves these grown up 'children' and expressed their frustrations that they were still living with their parents. The shortage of housing caused conflict within families, with adult siblings forced to share, or compete for, space.

Mandisa was now a pensioner, but had been employed for most of her adult life, firstly as a domestic and then in the laundry of an old-aged home.

Mandisa had never smoked or drunk alcohol. When it came to food she liked to eat porridge, oats and vegetables, but did not see her diet as being connected to her health. In fact she said she was not doing anything to protect her health. She had been devastated eight years earlier when she was diagnosed with asthma and had to give up her job:

> They told me that I am suffering from asthma because of the chemicals; the doctor said that they must give me a light job. There is no light job in an old-aged home. You make beds, wash the walls, wash the dishes and I said I could not manage... and then the law was against them, they could not let a person like that work. And then I stopped working. I didn't want to sit around and I was wondering why I got asthma at such an age, my children were young,[14] what was I going to do?... They were sleeping on the floor, the house is small and there was no fresh air, I would sit outside and weep.

While the view that people must be proactive to improve things for themselves arose many times across the interviews, 'acceptance' was also sometimes seen as being good – for example in circumstances where there was little an individual could do. Coming to terms with her situation had been important in reducing Mandisa's distress.

> The child used to tell me that there is nothing that I am crying for because God knows what He is going to do. He said it doesn't matter what the situation is, I have to accept it. And I ended up accepting the situation and I stopped stressing myself.

Her religious beliefs had played a role in this acceptance:

> I am satisfied because you cannot change where God has placed you. There is nothing that you can do, you just have to accept it because He is the one who will free you and put you in a better place. It doesn't help to walk up high... our hearts want to but we are not able to do that so we have to accept it.

But Mandisa was also a believer in being proactive. 'Just sitting' was not an option:

> Int: Do you see yourself as an active person?
> Mandisa: Yes I force myself because I hate sitting around because nothing becomes right. So I force myself because I get tired because of my chest. There is nothing wrong with my body, it's the chest. I get tired and I struggle to breathe and I also feel that my body is tired and I decide to relax. I sit down and then start again later.

Int: Do you think that being active has something that it does to your health?
Mandisa: Yes because what can you become if you are always sitting around? You cannot sit around; it has something that it does.
Int: OK.
Mandisa: Yes it does something, you have to be strong.

Discussion

The research which this chapter draws on (Brangan 2012) was intended to be exploratory, to be open to different forms and sources of knowledge, and to consider health and 'health behaviours' in the broader context of the person and society. My varied sources of data allowed me to compare findings with each other – which at times helped to contextualise things, or clarify uncertainties, and at other times highlighted tensions and contradictions between different sources of evidence which I needed to seek to explain. Eisenhardt argues that case studies can be used to build theory, because 'creative insight often arises from juxtaposition of contradictory or paradoxical evidence', with the process of reconciling these accounts forcing the researcher to a new 'gestalt' (Eisenhardt 1989: 546 in Fernandez 2005; cited in Berg 2007). While it can be challenging to be confronted with apparent contradictions within your data, in the context of this volume, it is also something to be celebrated in how it promotes methodological reflexivity, and directs attention to the way in which how, and by whom, wellbeing research is undertaken relates to the accounts of wellbeing which are produced (White, Introduction to this volume).

The epidemiological questionnaires sought to collect specific information about aspects of individuals' health, health risk factors and so-called health behaviours in the context of a longitudinal multi-country study which planned to recruit many thousands of participants. I was interested in accounts of wellbeing in Langa and how health and 'health behaviours' were related to wellbeing in these accounts. The pooled data indicated that 27 of the 40 respondents had at least one long-term health issue – from high blood pressure, to HIV, to disability caused by traumatic injury. Yet when people were asked directly during interviews about challenges in Langa generally, health did not really come up. People spoke about unemployment, housing, crime and the abuse of alcohol and other drugs. It was different when it came to questions about respondents' own situations – there was no doubt that poor health was having a major impact on many respondents' wellbeing. The stories above include examples of this, but the other issues which were raised by many respondents as challenges in Langa generally also appear prominently and in interlinked ways in individual stories.

This chapter thus illustrates part of the landscape which any initiative seeking to address health problems in low-income communities must navigate. While NCDs are clearly a major problem within Langa, they are set amidst, and contribute to, other challenges and priorities. It was apparent that the 'health behaviours' targeted in NCD prevention policy were all influenced by the major social problems afflicting the township. Due to low and uncertain incomes, concerns about access to food were raised by many people during their interviews. While under-nutrition in terms of long-term energy intake was clearly not a problem for the vast majority of respondents, many of whom were overweight as defined by the WHO, short-term availability of food, and quality and choice when it came to food, undoubtedly were. Several people spoke about not eating the food which they wanted to eat, or felt that they should be eating to be healthy, but instead were eating whatever they could come by. Eating was rarely seen as a 'health behaviour' – it could be about comfort and pleasure, but often it was about staving off hunger from day to day and surviving. Malusi's and Xolile's stories graphically illustrate this.

Smoking was common, particularly amongst men. Misuse of alcohol was seen as widespread amongst both men and women in Langa, and as something which people often fell into because they had nothing else in their lives – no work, no prospect of further education, no hope. Nkosazana and Malusi were amongst those who spoke about this. Staying positive was thus one crucial way of avoiding situations and activities which would be likely to undermine your wellbeing, and, as one component of this, your physical health. Nombeko was one of several women who spoke about the importance of staying positive. While this often required a proactive approach, there were times when it was important to learn to accept something about your situation, and several respondents drew on their religious beliefs to help them to do this. Mandisa's story illustrates this, while Malusi also ascribed a substantial degree of control over his life situation to spiritual powers.

Being physically active could be one way of staying positive. It could help by providing an alternative to 'thinking too much', and could also help as action – by earning (work) or saving (e.g. transport) money; producing a well-maintained home; supporting physical health; and by generating positive feelings and a sense of achievement, such as described by Nombeko and Malusi. For many respondents, such as

Mandisa and Nkosazana, physical activity was substantially limited by existing health problems however, and this in turn affected their employment prospects. Physical activity could also have costs, as Xolile pointed out – pain, fatigue and hunger; harm to health from overdoing it, especially if you were old or ill; financial costs of participation, or loss of time which would be better spent looking for work; exposure to risk from crime while out and about; and social harm from being seen as behaving inappropriately for your age or gender.

Life in Langa was difficult, but many respondents came across as believing that there was a choice in how you responded and who you were revealed to be by that. Healthy food, exercise, avoidance of tobacco, drugs or too much alcohol: these things were generally seen as good, but not always readily achievable. Policy initiatives which seek to directly tackle these 'health behaviours' without taking account of their socially embedded nature are unlikely to succeed. Those interested in promoting health and preventing NCDs need to look upstream and beyond the sphere of health to consider how to create conditions conducive to the broader wellbeing within which health will more easily flourish.

This is a challenging prospect, but it is an important long-term goal. When working further downstream, one way to start taking steps in the direction of this goal can be to use qualitative methods to allow people such as the respondents in Langa to contribute their knowledge. Strategies used by respondents to stay well despite the context included knowing how to avoid hazards, knowing when acceptance was your best option, staying busy and involved, and being able to maintain a positive, hopeful attitude, while looking out for opportunities to improve your situation. Downstream policy initiatives which build on the knowledge and values of members of the targeted population, as well of those of the 'experts', will be more likely to contribute to supporting wellbeing and protecting health in the shorter term.

Acknowledgements

This research was funded by an Economic and Social Research Council studentship. I wish to thank Kholiswa Mphiti for guiding me in Langa and for her extensive contribution to generating interview data; James Copestake and Sarah White at the University of Bath for their advice throughout the research; the Prospective Urban and Rural Epidemiological (PURE) study group at the School of Public Health, University of the Western Cape (Principal Investigator Prof Thandi Puoane); and most of all, the respondents in Langa for sharing their ideas and experiences with me.

Notes

1. These include illnesses such as stroke, diabetes, heart disease, cancer and chronic respiratory disease (WHO 2008).
2. According to the WHO, 'health behaviours' to be tackled in order to reduce NCD risks include unhealthy diets, physical inactivity, smoking and the harmful use of alcohol (WHO 2008).
3. Respondents were a subsample, stratified by age and gender, of 500 residents of Langa participating at that time in the PURE study. Please see Teo et al. (2009) for further details of PURE and Brangan (2012) for further details of methods for this study.
4. All names etc. have been changed to preserve anonymity. In interview extracts 'Int:' indicates the interviewer.
5. Kholiswa Mphiti.
6. An indicator used in the management of HIV/AIDS.
7. A body mass index (BMI) of greater than 25 kg/m^2 (WHO 2013).
8. This is extremely unlikely to be the case given the high prevalence of HIV infection in the area (City of Cape Town 2011).
9. Final year of secondary school system in South Africa.
10. Malusi later referred to this man as his uncle.
11. Province of South Africa which incorporates the former 'Xhosa homelands' of Transkei and Ciskei.
12. Local sources informed me that a Xhosa traditional healer is believed to be 'called' through an illness with a particular set of symptoms and which is resistant to conventional treatment.
13. Ground maize.
14. Her own children were no longer young by then, but several of her grandchildren were living with her.

References

Berg, B. L. (2007) *Qualitative Research Methods for the Social Sciences*. Boston: Pearson International Edition.

Brangan, E. (2012) *Physical Activity, Noncommunicable Disease and Wellbeing in Urban South Africa*. PhD Thesis, University of Bath. Available at: http://opus.bath.ac.uk/33115/1/UnivBath_PhD_2012_E_Brangan.pdf

City of Cape Town (2011) City Health HIV, AIDS, STI and TB Plan 2012/2013: Annex I of the City 2012–2017 5 Year Plan. Available at: http://www.capetown.gov.za/en/IDP/Documents/Statutory%20compliance%20plans%20201213/AnnexureI_HIV_Aids_STI_TB_Plan_2012_2013.pdf [accessed 26 February 2014].

City of Cape Town (2012) City of Cape Town – Census 2001 – Langa. Available at: http://www.capetown.gov.za/en/stats/2001census/Documents/Langa.htm [accessed 16 August 2012].

Eisenhardt, K. (1989) Building Theories from Case Study Research. *Academy of Management Review* 14(4): 532–550.

Fernandez, W. (2005) The Grounded Theory Method and Case Study Data in IS Research: Issues and Design. pp. 43–59 in D. N. Hart and S. D. Gregor (eds.) *Information Systems Foundations: Constructing and Criticising*. Canberra: The Australian National University E Press.

Gie, J. (2009) *Crime in Cape Town: 2001–2008*. Cape Town: Strategic Development Information and GIS Department.

Groenewald, P., Bradshaw, D., Msemburi, W., Neetheling, I., Matzopoulos, R., Naledi, T., Daniels, J. and Dombo, N. (2012) *Western Cape Mortality Profile 2009*. Cape Town: South African Medical Research Council.

Teo, K., Chow, C. K., Vaz, M., Rangarajan, S. and Yusuf, S. (2009) The Prospective Urban Rural Epidemiology (PURE) Study: Examining the Impact of Societal Influences on Chronic Noncommunicable Diseases in Low-, Middle-, and High-Income Countries. *American Heart Journal* 158(1): 1–8.

WHO (2008) *2008–2013 Action Plan for the Global Strategy for the Prevention and Control of Noncommunicable Disease*. Geneva: World Health Organization.

WHO (2010) *Global Recommendations on Physical Activity for Health*. Geneva: World Health Organization.

WHO (2013) Obesity and Overweight Fact sheet No. 311. Available at: http://www.who.int/mediacentre/factsheets/fs311/en/ [accessed 2 April 2014].

5
Economics and Subjectivities of Wellbeing in Rural Zambia[1]

Sarah C. White and Viviana Ramirez

Introduction

As described in Chapter 1, the call to go 'beyond economics' is central to the wellbeing agenda. One dimension of this is to go 'beyond GDP' (Gross Domestic Product) in measuring national progress. Another is the extended debate on the theme of 'does money make us happy?' which has animated the new field of 'happiness economics' (Graham 2011). While the tenor of that debate is strongly positivist, defining itself in terms of 'what we know',[2] it can also be read against the grain as a discourse on Western cultures of wellbeing, using statistics to debate the relative importance of income, wealth, inequality, human rights, health, employment and family relationships to 'good lives' and 'good societies'. Continuing the well-worn pattern of 'modernity' seeking to know itself in contrast to 'tradition' (Grossberg 1996), this questioning about wellbeing has also looked to 'other cultures' for inspiration, as less materialist, more spiritual, more holistic. *Buen vivir* and allied approaches have inspired significant mobilisation for cultural and political rights in Latin America. However, their celebration in the West also indicates the particular place of indigenous worldviews as a cultural mirror for self-questioning Western modernity. But this is only one side of the picture. The contradictory dynamic within Western modernity is to generalise its own patterns of thought as universal (Mazrui 2001). For current discourses of wellbeing and their preoccupation with subjective experience and 'happiness', informed by the psychological and affective 'turn' across the social sciences (e.g. Craib 1994, Kahneman 2012, Moore 2007), this means the export of a psychological subject, projected onto the peoples of the world.

This chapter presents mixed method research in Chiawa rural Zambia in which people resisted the attempt to render them psychological subjects and instead foregrounded the economic in their representations of self. It begins with a brief discussion of the key terms, economics and subjectivity. It then describes the research design, location and methods. The following sections present a number of different vantage points which demonstrate the centrality of the economic to wellbeing. These begin with the emphasis people place on material sufficiency in their accounts of what wellbeing means to them. This is followed by statistical analysis, first of the relationship between subjective economic confidence and overall happiness, and second of the relationship between measures of objective economic status and subjective dimensions of wellbeing. This leads into further questioning of the form of association between economics and subjectivities, with qualitative data suggesting a more internal relationship of co-constitution than the external causative relationship usually envisaged by quantitative methods. Three snapshots are presented: the role of economic capacity in forging (male) gender identities; the emphasis on reciprocity and a *moral* economy; and the use of economics as an expressive idiom in speaking of the self.

Economics and subjectivities

The definition of the economy and the economic is a matter of major debate. Within economic anthropology, the main divisions concern those who identify the economy in substantive terms, involving the social organisation of, for example, production, consumption and exchange, and those who see it in terms of a logic of decision-making, the 'rational... choice to allocate scarce resources to different possible ends' (Wilk and Cliggett 2007: 35). Amongst economists there is a further difference between those who accept that social norms, institutions and obligations influence behaviour and those who believe that these motivations are merely incidental to the 'rational', maximising motivation. In this chapter, we adopt the first, descriptive approach, classifying as 'economic' any reference to work, production, wealth or assets, income, consumption, material provisioning and exchange of goods or services. While Chiawa operates within a market economy, norms of reciprocity have a powerful influence on behaviour and provide an important idiom for social exchange. Individual decisions are made at the interface of moral intuitions, social obligations and calculations of self-interest, sometimes, as shown below, quite explicitly so.

The emphasis on the subjective in contemporary constructions of wellbeing is paradoxically marked by a widespread failure to theorise subjectivity. Where such theorisation does appear, it is amongst the critics, rather than the advocates (e.g. Ahmed 2010). The mainstream subjective wellbeing (SWB) literature is extraordinarily naïve, assuming that people *know* their own thoughts and feelings, that they can abstract and generalise from these to assign an overall number and that they are ready to give an accurate report to strangers. There is some admission that society and culture may have some effect on scores (e.g. Diener and Suh eds. 2000, Graham 2011). However, the *subject* who is the author of these results remains unexplored, an abstracted point of cognition and affect such that even the individual's state of health is represented as an external factor whose correlation with happiness is a matter to be investigated (e.g. Graham 2011: 67).

The slimness and simplicity of the subject in the SWB literature is in marked contrast to the breadth and multiplicity emphasised in the literature on identity and subjectivity in feminist, sociological and cultural studies. The focus on subjectivities grew out of work on identity, which had built a critique of any claims that identity (often in the context of gender and/or ethnicity) could be seen as naturally given or unitary (e.g. Hall and du Gay 1996). This led to talk of people identifying themselves through a process of identification(s) which are always multiple and relational, rather than fixed identities, complete in and of themselves. The notion of subjectivity combines an understanding of people becoming subjects *of* their lives, with the recognition that they are subject *to* powers and circumstances that are not of their choosing. The stress on multiple subjectivities recognises that there are many different ways in which people identify and experience themselves. But these 'ways' are not random; they are reflective of a particular place and history. Mama (1995: 89) provides a powerful statement of this, as she describes subjectivity as:

> constituted, socially and historically, out of collective experience. I theorise subjectivity not as a static or fixed entity but as a dynamic process during which individuals take up and change positions in discourses. I further propose that these discursive positions can be located in the collective history of the social group in question.

This renders the subject social, rather than psychological; fluid and complex, rather than stable and unitary. Like the psychological subject it is somewhat disembodied, discursive rather than corporeal. It does, nevertheless, provide a basis for exploring the range of ways in which people represent themselves, which we begin to explore in the later sections of the chapter. First, however, we explain the concept of wellbeing used in this study, the methods of research and introduce the location in which it took place.

Methodology and research design

The inner wellbeing approach

Inner wellbeing (IWB) is a psychosocial approach which explores what people think and feel they can be and do. In some ways, therefore, it has conceptual affinities with Sen's capability approach (see Chapter 1) although its methods are quite distinct. In the categories established in Chapter 1, its underlying model is relational wellbeing. It was developed through primary research in two rural communities, one in central India (Sarguja district, Chhattisgarh state) and one in Chiawa, Zambia, 2010–2013. Unease with the fact that standard approaches to SWB had been developed in such different contexts to those of our research, coupled with the wish to explore in a more substantive manner how people were thinking and feeling about their lives, led us to develop our own concept and methods of assessment.

IWB comprises seven domains: economic confidence; agency and participation; social connections; close relationships; physical and mental health; competence and self-worth; and values and meaning. These bring together dimensions identified as important in the psychological wellbeing literature (e.g. autonomy, competence and relatedness, Ryan and Deci 2000) and in the literature on empowerment and social development (e.g. Rowlands 1997). For example, one of the items in the social connections domain is, 'Do you know the kind of people who can help you get things done?' This reflects the fact that in many societies in the Global South, people's access to key resources depends on personal brokerage (e.g. Devine 2002) and the importance of social capital more broadly (Putnam and Leonardi 1994). Two previous research projects were particularly influential in developing the IWB approach. The first was Wellbeing in Developing Countries (WeD), which identified three interlinked dimensions of wellbeing: the material – what people have or do not have; the relational – how people relate to one another; and the subjective – what people think or feel (Gough and McGregor eds. 2007, White 2010). The second was the Colombo-based Psycho-social Assessment of Development and Humanitarian Intervention (PADHI) and their 'social justice approach to wellbeing' (PADHI 2009). This provided five of the seven domains in the IWB model. To these were added two more (on close relationships and values and meaning) which had

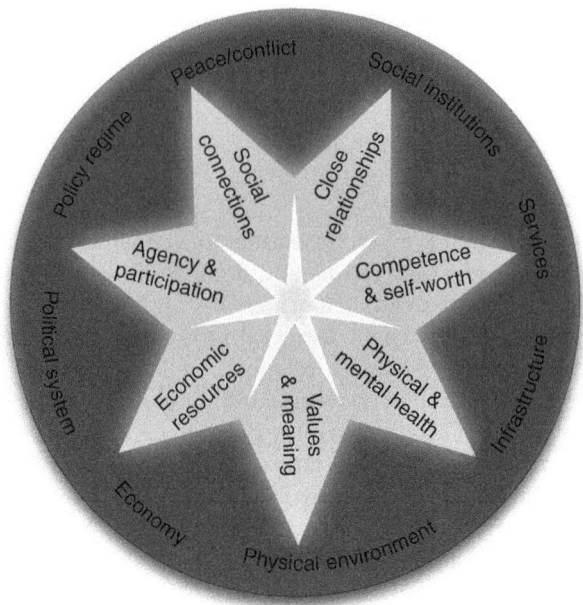

Figure 5.1 Inner wellbeing

been shown to be important in WeD and in a project on religion and wellbeing, respectively (Devine and White 2013).

Each of the domains is assessed through five questions for which answers are provided corresponding to a five-point scale. These items, and the domains themselves, were forged through an extensive process of reflection, grounding and piloting and statistical testing. The IWB model is represented by the star in Figure 5.1. The circle which encompasses the star indicates the broader environment within which people experience wellbeing. Although we had to 'fix' IWB as a set score for the purpose of assessment, we do not view it as something stable that people 'have'. Rather we see the experience of wellbeing as something that happens in interaction, between the domains, between people, and between people and the broader environment (see also White and Jha 2014, White *et al.* 2014).

Methods

The research on which this paper is based took place in two rounds of four months' fieldwork in Chiawa, Zambia, August–November, 2010 and 2012. The main instrument was a survey, which combined objective (self-report) questions about livelihoods, education, health and social support with subjective questions about satisfaction and IWB. We talked to husbands and wives (interviewed separately) and women heading households. In almost all cases, these women had previously been married and were single as a result of widowhood, desertion or divorce. Respondents were asked in all cases to speak as individuals, so for example their main source of livelihood should reflect their own activity, not the main income to the household as a whole. The field research was led by the project research officer (Shreya Jha) who was supported by a team of three local peer researchers who acted as interpreters and undertook much of the survey work themselves. The project director (Sarah White) visited for shorter times, including all piloting at the beginning of each fieldwork period.

For statistical analysis we draw only on the second fieldwork period. This involved surveys with 370 people, including 52 women heading households. Three hundred and fifty-eight of these respondents were also interviewed in 2010. In the qualitative analysis, we draw on data from both fieldwork periods, comprising notes from 54 survey interviews and verbatim transcripts of 40 open-ended life history interviews and one focus-group discussion.

Surveys were conducted in Goba, Nyanja or the English language. If an international member of the research team was present, they were translated into English simultaneously, otherwise they were undertaken solely in the language in which the interviewee was most comfortable. Responses were recorded on a survey form in English and inputted into Excel, then translated for analysis into SPSS. Qualitative interviews and the focus-group discussion were either in English or translated simultaneously. We have coded and analysed qualitative data by hand and using the NVivo qualitative data-analysis software. All direct quotes are identified by type of respondent (MM = married man; MW = married woman; SW = single woman) with the respondent number. Where we quote at length from a particular individual, we give him or her a fictive name.

Chiawa

Chiawa lies in Kafue district of Lusaka province. To the south and southeast, Chiawa is flanked by two major rivers, the Kafue and the Zambezi; to the north, by the Zambezi escarpment. To the southeast it borders Zimbabwe and to the east the Lower Zambezi National Park. Chiawa was declared a Game Management Area in 1991.

Most of the population of 10,929 (Central Statistical Office 2010) live in villages along the line of the rivers. Local amenities are basic: a primary health centre, an agricultural extension office, a community development office, schools and churches. There is no public transport, so most people have to walk, cycle or rely on private pick-ups and small lorries which run along the main route providing transport to work or the ferry in the mornings and evenings. Chiawa has four primary schools and one (primary) community school plus two high schools. A single police station has very limited resources and a traditional court was not operational during our research. Most other official business requires people to travel to the district capital of Kafue, and for hospital care, to the nearest town of Chirundu. In both cases this has meant crossing the river by ferry. The other significant government presence is the Zambia Wildlife Authority. Governance of Chiawa is in the hands of the Chieftainess, who appoints the headmen who lead each village.

Major economic activity is concentrated in large plantations or safari lodges which occupy most of the best land along the river. Farming remains a mainstay of village livelihoods, often in combination with other activities. In 2012, 25 per cent of respondents stated farming as their main source of survival. The main implement remains the hoe and mechanised irrigation is rare – only 23 households report having a water pump. Shockingly, although 70 per cent of people reported planting maize in 2012, only half of them (37 per cent) managed to harvest any. This reflects the extremely precarious nature of local livelihoods, hit that year through a combination of drought and crop damage from wild animals. Asked for how many months they were able to eat their own maize, only 29 per cent answered 10–12 months, 34 per cent saying four–six months and 30 per cent three months or less. Almost 30 per cent of our respondents had gone hungry over the past 12 months, including 22 per cent of married men, 32 per cent of married women and 43 per cent of single women.

After farming, three other activities tie for next place as the most common source of survival, each being reported by nine per cent of respondents. The first is safari lodge employment, which involved 22 per cent of men but no women. The next, petty trading, has a markedly different gender profile, involving 21 per cent of women heading households, 12 per cent of married women and only one per cent of married men. Many of these enterprises are extremely marginal. The third is piecework, which comprises various kinds of casual labour, and shows no significant difference by gender/marital status. Four per cent overall report commercial farm work as their mainstay. This was proportionately more common amongst women heading households (ten per cent).

Chiawa stands on the brink of change. Despite being only 70 miles from Lusaka, it has been relatively isolated with poor quality roads and a daytime-only ferry across the Kafue River. In 2014, however, a new bridge was completed and a new road is also being built. While the improved transport infrastructure has been eagerly awaited, it also carries dangers. Economic development so far has provided some benefit in the shape of jobs, but has also threatened local lives and livelihoods through the growing number of wild animals since it was declared a Game Management Area, and privatisation of the customary land on which local people depend. This has resulted in sporadic social and political protest over the past 20 years, but with little sign of positive action to protect local people's tenure. The fear is that the new road and bridge could raise local land values and accelerate dispossession, pushing local people out of agriculture and into increasingly marginal and precarious activities.

Findings

Economic sufficiency is a major preoccupation

Given the harsh conditions and material scarcity of village life in Chiawa, it is not surprising that economic sufficiency is the first thing that people mention when you ask about wellbeing. The following comment is typical:

> Most essential thing I want to say is that one must be able to have sufficient food for him and also his family.
>
> (MM 13)

Many emphasised the importance of land and farming as the basis of their livelihood. For some this was everything. An elderly man put it like this:

> Wellbeing is all about if you have everything that you want, you are able to farm and harvest whatever is supposed to be harvested and also when things go according to plan and then even other people will also say 'I think he is wellbeing.'
>
> (MM 28)

For others, though, farming was the basis around which other activities might take place. A schoolteacher talked about his hopes for retirement:

> Yes just buy a plot of a farm and just locate myself there. I can do some other things, but meanwhile I have the farm.
>
> (MM 107)

A married woman in her 30s, whose husband had worked in a safari lodge, explained:

> I think that is not only the money that makes a better life because even when you are in the home you don't fight and we are able maybe to farm, get a good harvest, get enough food even without money that would still be a good life.
>
> (MW 54)

In fact, when asked about almost anything, the economic continually intruded. We had real difficulty finding questions for the self-worth domain in particular, as items that are commonly used in wellbeing surveys to gauge self-worth or levels of social trust were interpreted by respondents in economic terms. Asked if they had achieved what they had hoped to in life, people would speak about their limited means; asked if neighbours were helpful, people would say that they did not have the means to help; asked about harmony in the home, they would say how could there be harmony when they were worried about survival?

The most obvious interpretation of this is Maslow's (1954) 'hierarchy of needs' in which he saw physical and material needs as having to be met before social or psychological needs came into play. In contrast to this, however, it was not that people did not talk about other parts of their lives, including what Maslow classified as his highest category of 'self-actualization needs'. Rather, the way they talked about them was more embodied, such that the material was intrinsically interwoven within these other dimensions.

Economics and inner wellbeing: Statistical analysis

In this section, we present our quantitative analysis of the relationship between economic status and subjective dimensions of wellbeing within our sample. Fierce debates regarding the Easterlin paradox notwithstanding (see Chapter 1), there is now quite widespread agreement amongst economists about the general patterns of relationship between economic status and SWB. Confirming Easterlin's (1974) initial observations, most agree that there is little change in happiness scores within a country as GDP rises over time (Graham 2011: 16). Graham (2011: 17) shows that those in the Organisation for Economic Co-operation and Development (OECD) countries tend to report higher scores, but amongst countries with lower GDP, there is no discernible relationship between GDP and SWB. Stevenson and Wolfers (2008) argue against this that there is a consistent relationship across countries between GDP and SWB. Within countries the picture is clearer. Most studies find that wealthier people report themselves as happier than do poorer people and there is a 'basic needs' threshold. For very poor people, the relationship between income and SWB is much stronger than it is for wealthier people (Graham 2011:17). In economists' terms, the marginal utility of income is seen to fall as incomes rise. Where income is seen to continue to have an effect on SWB amongst wealthier people, it seems to be relative income that matters (the level of my income compared with others around me) rather than the amount of income in absolute terms (e.g. McBride 2001).

Differences in findings reflect at least to some degree the use of different datasets, different techniques of analysis and different measures of wellbeing (Graham 2011). Stevenson and Wolfers (2008), for example, employ the Gallup World Poll measure of life satisfaction, which is widely found to be the measure which correlates most strongly with income (Kahneman and Deaton 2010). It is also now recognised that life-satisfaction measures in general correlate more closely with income compared to measures of emotion or affect (Diener et al. 2010, Graham 2011). The way that SWB and happiness are used interchangeably, with either term being used to refer to empirical measures of life satisfaction or affect or a combination of the two, makes it difficult to get clarity.

In order to test the significance of economic dimensions in the quantitative analysis of our dataset, we needed first to ensure that we had statistically robust measures for our wellbeing domains. This involved a procedure called factor analysis (FA) which tests whether people's responses to the items which we have assigned to each domain in fact behave in the systematic way we would expect them to, to show that they all correspond to the same underlying factor (or domain). The analysis validated six domains, with economic confidence emerging as the strongest, first factor. The analysis validated four items for the economic confidence and social connections domains and three items for agency and participation, health, competence and self-worth, and values and

Table 5.1 Items from factor analysis that measured six domains of inner wellbeing

Economic confidence
1. How well would you say you are managing economically at present?
2. If guests come, do you feel you can look after them in the proper way?
3. Do you feel that people around you have got ahead of you?
4. How well could you manage if something bad were to happen (e.g. illness in the family)?

Agency and participation
1. If there is a village meeting, do you have an opportunity to voice your opinion?
2. If official decisions are made that affect you badly, do you feel that you have power to change them?
3. Do you feel that you are heard? (Beyond family)

Social connections
1. Do you know the kind of people who can help you get things done?
2. When do you get to hear about events in the community?
3. Do you feel there are people beyond your immediate family who you'll be able to count on even through bad times?
4. What proportion of people in the community are helpful (to you)?

Health
1. Do you ever have trouble sleeping?
2. How often do you feel too weak for what you need to do?
3. Do you suffer from tension?

Competence and self-worth
1. How far do you feel you are able to help other people?
2. To what extent do you have faith in yourself?
3. To what extent do you tend to doubt the decisions that you have made?

Values and meaning
1. To what extent do you feel that life has been fair for you?
2. How far would you say you feel peace in your heart at the end of the day?
3. To what extent do you feel that life has been good to you?

meaning.[3] These items were thus used in calculating our domain scores.[4] They are shown in Table 5.1. We were not able to validate the close relationships domain. This reflects the difficulty we found in designing items which could track the quality of close relationships in a reliable way, given the strong social pressure to project family harmony (see also Jha and White, this volume). While we recognise the importance of close relationships to wellbeing, we have therefore had to exclude this domain from further analysis in this chapter.

Having produced reliable measures for the six domains, we then wanted to test the relationships between these and our single happiness question ('Taking all things together, how happy would you say you are these days?'), which is a standard SWB measure. The way quantitative analyses such as correlations and regressions are generally used would envisage the relationship between the IWB model and SWB either in terms of determinants (IWB causes SWB, or SWB causes IWB) or components (IWB domains comprise elements of SWB). Our view is that these two approaches reflect distinct concepts and measures of wellbeing, but they are not entirely different. We therefore would expect some overlap between them and are interested in exploring the extent of this.[5]

The mean scores for the happiness item and the six inner domains are given in Table 5.2. These show that people scored happiness above average (3.5, when 3.0 would be the mid-point). The only other scores above the mid-point are those for health and self-worth.

We next wanted to assess the overlap between the IWB domains and the global happiness question through correlation analysis. This simply explores the strength of the association between the two measures of wellbeing, without any view as to whether there is a causal relationship between them, or if so, in what direction. Table 5.3 presents the coefficients. As expected, the results show that all IWB domains have a positive and significant linear association with happiness. The significance is strong at $p < 0.01$.[6] The domains with the highest correlation are economic confidence (0.341) and values and meaning (0.313). This level of correlation is usually considered moderate. In contrast, the

Table 5.2 Descriptive statistics: Happiness and inner wellbeing

	Mean	Std. Dev
SWB		
Happiness	3.50	0.932
IWB		
Economic confidence	2.82	0.686
Agency and participation	2.65	0.770
Social connections	2.67	0.720
Physical and mental health	3.09	0.732
Competence and self-worth	3.26	0.689
Values and meaning	2.96	0.709

Table 5.3 Pearson's correlation: Inner wellbeing and happiness

IWB	Happiness
Economic confidence	0.341**
Agency and participation	0.187**
Social connections	0.174**
Physical and mental health	0.176**
Competence and self-worth	0.210**
Values and meaning	0.313**

Note: **p-value < 0.01.

correlations with the domains of agency, social connections and health are low to moderate.

We then wished to assess the relative effect of the different domains on happiness, when all of the domains were taken into account together. We therefore undertook linear regression analysis with happiness as the dependent variable and the IWB domains as the independent variables. As before, it is important to be clear that we do not envisage IWB domains as either determinants or components of SWB. Rather, we simply wanted to assess whether the degree of overlap for some domains and global happiness is greater than for other domains, when all the domains together are taken into account. As Table 5.4 shows, when all of the IWB domains are entered into the analysis together, the domain of economic confidence remains the most strongly related with happiness, closely followed by values and meaning. The domain of health also shows a statistically significant relationship with happiness. In other words, in this sample, greater overall happiness is most strongly related

Table 5.4 Linear regression analysis of happiness over inner wellbeing

	Happiness
Constant	1.068**
Economic confidence	0.292**
Agency and participation	0.041
Social connections	0.019
Physical and mental health	0.137*
Competence and self-worth	0.101
Values and meaning	0.235**
R-squared	0.176

Note: **p-value < 0.01, *p-value < 0.05.

with economic confidence, followed by the sense of values and meaning and physical and mental health. Relationships between happiness and the other domains were not significant. The R-squared score indicates that IWB helps to explain 18 per cent of the variability of the happiness of participants.

Having considered the relationship between happiness and the way people felt about their economic positions, we then wanted to explore whether there was any association between IWB and their 'objective' economic status. We constructed two indicators of economic status. The first, to give a proxy for income, combined a fivefold categorisation of people's main source of livelihood with the amount of maize they harvested.[7] Maize is the staple crop in Chiawa, and using it in this way to moderate the category of main source of livelihood enabled us to distinguish, for example, between very poor and more wealthy farmers who would otherwise have appeared in the same category. The second indicator, to give a proxy for wealth, was formed through principal components analysis (PCA) on the variables of housing, source of electricity, type of cooking fuel and assets (farm animals, transport, technology).[8]

Having produced these proxies for wealth and income, we undertook similar analyses as before. First, we tested for correlations between the measures of economic status and the IWB domains. The results are presented in Table 5.5. This shows that almost all of the domains have positive and significant correlations with both economic status indicators. The one exception is a lack of relationship between wealth and health. The size of the correlations ranges from moderate to low.

Finally, we wished to explore the relationship between objective economic status, IWB and happiness, after controlling for other personal characteristics of participants such as age, gender, marital status and

Table 5.5 Correlation of economic status indicators and IWB domains

	Livelihood	Wealth
Economic confidence	0.255**	0.418**
Agency and participation	0.267**	0.271**
Social connections	0.202**	0.302**
Physical and mental health	0.188**	0.080
Competence and self-worth	0.230**	0.240**
Values and meaning	0.225**	0.305**

Note: **$p < 0.01$.

Table 5.6 Regressions of IWB domains over economic status and control variables

	Economic	Agency	Social	Health	Self-worth	Values	Happiness
Wealth	0.142**	0.107**	0.099**	−0.014	0.085**	0.128**	0.105**
Livelihood	0.058†	0.075†	0.045	0.075†	0.081*	0.077*	0.076
Controls							
Male	−0.024	0.061	0.023	0.113	0.126	−0.077	−0.035
Age	−0.007*	0.014**	−0.001	−0.011**	0.006	0.004	−0.004
Years of education	0.019†	0.033*	0.027*	0.017	0.009	0.031*	0.033*
Unmarried	−0.368**	−0.159	−0.158	−0.249*	−0.039	0.088	−0.100
Remarried	−0.125	−0.176†	−0.102	−0.065	−0.012	0.065	0.010
Household size	0.012	0.012	0.011	0.003	0.018	0.004	0.006
Constant	2.423**	1.343**	2.117**	3.259**	2.355**	2.035**	2.939**
R-squared	0.269	0.178	0.126	0.102	0.114	0.131	0.095

Note: **p-value < 0.01, *p-value < 0.05, †p-value < 0.1.

years of education. Table 5.6 presents the results. This shows that the livelihood variable loses much of its significance once the control factors are introduced, while the significance of wealth remains. This could suggest that personal characteristics such as age, education and marital status are driving much of the variability captured by the livelihood variable. The most significant finding is, however, that the influence of economic status on people's IWB goes beyond their economic confidence, significantly predicting their wellbeing outcomes in almost all domains such as their sense of agency and participation, competence and self-worth, values and meaning, and the perceived quality of their social connections. As with the two previous tables, the domain of health is the only one not significantly associated with wealth, though it does show marginal significance ($p < 0.1$) with livelihood. Overall, the R-square values show that happiness is the subjective variable least explained by this model, at under ten per cent. This is in line with the wider findings discussed above.

Dwarfing the effect of all other variables is the fact of being a woman heading a household alone. This is captured in the dummy variable Unmarried. Because of the way we constructed our sample of married couples and single women, this variable mainly reflects the gendered effect of being a single, divorced or widowed woman.[9] For economic confidence, this is significant at $p < 0.01$, with a coefficient of −0.368. The next highest effect is again negative, and again for single women, in relation to health (−0.249 at $p < 0.05$). No other coefficient is above 0.2 and most cluster around 0.1 or below. This result does not undermine the significance of economic factors, but demonstrates how they can be compounded by other social dimensions. Results not reported here showed that single women were significantly poorer than married people (Baertl-Helguero *et al.* 2014). This dummy variable thus captures the multi-dimensional social and economic marginality experienced by women heading households alone.

In sum, then, the statistical analysis strongly supports the contention that economic concerns have a major effect on subjective dimensions of wellbeing beyond economic confidence itself. Within the subjective, it is people's economic confidence that has the strongest association with how happy they say themselves to be. In turn, proxies for objective wealth and income are significant predictors of IWB – and indeed happiness – with wealth having by far the greater effect once other control variables are introduced. The strongest effect of economic status is on economic confidence, which in turn we have seen to be the domain which correlates most strongly with happiness. However, the effect of economic status stretches beyond economic confidence into almost all other domains of IWB. This seems to suggest that pursuing a multi-domain approach to subjective dimensions of wellbeing can capture better the effects of various 'objective' factors on how people are thinking and feeling about different aspects of their lives than depending on a single happiness item.

Re-thinking economics and subjectivities: Qualitative perspectives

Our statistical results demonstrate the great importance of economics to subjective dimensions of wellbeing, but they cannot tell us *how* this importance is configured. The whole logic of the tests we have undertaken assumes an external, causative relationship between an 'independent' and 'dependent' variable (see also Ramirez forthcoming). This is the kind of relationship that often appears as the 'social determinants of' health or wellbeing.

Our qualitative data, however, suggest a rather different kind of relationship, one that is more internal and constitutive, with economic identities implicated in the production of the self. This resonates with the theorising of WeD mentioned above, that wellbeing is comprised of intertwined material, relational and subjective dimensions.

There is not space within this chapter to develop the argument in detail, but we present three snapshots that may take it some way forward. The first is the way that notions of love and material provision are intertwined within (male) gendered identities around 'taking care'. The second is the centrality of reciprocity and the sense of a *moral* economy. The third is the suggestion that people use economics as an expressive idiom in talking about the self.

Gendered identities in 'taking care': Love and provision

The notion of 'taking care' is a very powerful one in Chiawa. It arises most immediately in the context of parental and marital relationships, but extends into broader, mainly but not exclusively kin-related, responsibilities. Being the provider, the one who 'takes care' is particularly central to adult male gender identities. Consider how this man describes how his moral and social identity is built through his giving of care to his family:

> I am taking care of my wife; I am taking care of my son; and also I am taking care of my mother; my own brothers and sisters who are in the village. I buy my mum some clothes, some blankets, I also send some money there and even there in the village most people really seek to say that 'this mother's son is taking good care of her. He must be a loving and caring son.' So I do take care of my mother and my brothers and sisters and also of my wife and my own son. At least other people are able to tell themselves that this person is a 'father' to his family.
>
> (MM 145)

Iris, whose husband's poor mental health meant he had been unable to provide for her or their children, similarly chose to emphasise a man's duties as the way things ought to be:

> What I can say for somebody to be living a good life is when one is in a marriage; first of all, your husband must stand up and say 'I have a wife whom I need to take care of.' Second also, one must be ready to bear responsibilities on his children. Also one must be ready to send his children to school so that if things fail you can say that things failed because of this reason, it's not that you neglected them. I am also saying things might be different on how people view it from the community and I don't know how they view it but the way I see things someone must really love and appreciate what he has in his life.
>
> (MW 90)

While this could be read as quite a conventional patriarchal script, in the context of the interview as a whole, it becomes clear that this would over-simplify. Her husband's mental illness had meant that Iris had to take on all the responsibility for running the household, and within her means, she was ably providing for herself and her children. Her statement here thus stands as part resistance and critique, part grief and longing for the more supportive relationship she would have liked to have had.

Beyond Iris's personal circumstances, however, her statement also signifies how marriage – especially when 'in the home you don't fight' – is central to understandings of wellbeing in Chiawa. Here again the relationship is seen in active voice, it is not something inert or static but realised through the mutual giving and receiving of care. This association of marriage with wellbeing has material dimensions. As mentioned above, as a group, single women are doing worse than married people on virtually every economic indicator. In life history interviews, single women also talked a great deal about the social marginality that they felt, experiencing suspicion and hostility from married women and sexual predation from married men. Interestingly, the issue of 'taking care' was a strong theme in single women's explanations of both why they might, and why they would not, seek to marry again. While some hoped for a new husband who would look after themselves and their children, a larger number stated that they would not re-marry, in the belief that another man would never take care of their children as his own.

Reciprocities and moral economy

The emphasis on taking care is part of a broader vision of a moral economy. People did not envisage themselves, for the most part, as self-interested, individual rational economic actors. Rather, the purpose of wealth was not to accumulate as an individual, but to provide for and share with others. While caring for one's immediate family might be common across most, if not all, human societies, the web of care that people envisaged in Chiawa stretched far more widely. As one man powerfully summed up:

> Well, if one is to live a good life in our community... I think first of all one must have enough food for his family... for himself and his family. And must also have something to share with the community, because like you don't just say, 'No, this is for my family alone', but you've also got some other relatives, some friends who can come and ask for things.
>
> (MM 54)

The modal form of exchange, therefore, is not the market transaction, but the gift. This is not to romanticise economic relationships, or to suggest that Chiawa operates as a 'traditional', pre-capitalist economy. Rather, the point is that the primary emphasis remains on the relationship between people, instead of, as in neo-classical understandings of the economic subject, between people and things. As economic anthropology has argued, however, there is within gift-giving a 'euphemized' (Bourdieu 1977) transactional element which is hidden by the passing of time between gift and return. In Chiawa, this intervening period may be extraordinarily extended – one man told us how as a child he lived for ten years with an uncle to fulfil a deal made with his father years before his birth.

A critical aspect of this moral economy is the sense of generalised reciprocity – that what goes around, comes around. Within this, the material and the relational are again closely intertwined. The following statement expresses this well:

> By helping both the sides I was not looking at my direct personal benefit because they being relatives, I felt maybe at one point that you never know who is going to help whom; because maybe if I helped my relatives maybe at some point they also help me or my children, or maybe their children who help my children. My wife's relatives also look at me as being a good person. Also, you never know who is going to be helped between my children and them.
> (MM 132)

This statement mixes together moral action and self-interest in a way that emphasises the voluntary nature of participation and thus re-inscribes the speaker's agency in his conformity. Other statements, however, bring out some of the tensions between the moral injunction to 'take care' and the material capacity to do so. The statement below was given in the context of describing how it is determined who will take on responsibility for children after their parents have died. In theory at least, moral considerations should trump material ones. When the elders sit to decide who should take the place of the mother or father, they consider the personal qualities of the individual, not his or her material circumstances. The critical thing is to be (seen to be) someone with a heart for others. In straitened times, this can set up a real tension between moral and relational considerations on the one hand and financial capacity on the other. The sense of tension between what is felt inside and what it is felt possible to express socially is palpable:

It is quite tricky in the sense that support becomes difficult even if you have one child you are taking care of especially looking at the economic situation especially here in Chiawa. And then eventually you are not prepared, you are given these children so somehow it becomes difficult although we say it is easy. It is quite difficult to say it is difficult because you feel people might say that you don't want to look after the children so even though the difficulty is there you say it's ok because you want to let people see that you want to keep the children but inwardly you feel that you can't look after the children.

(MM 124)

Economics as an expressive idiom

We mentioned above the way that people would often respond in terms of their economic circumstances to questions we had intended would capture their social relationships or self-worth. This tendency to speak of the self in economic terms was evident in qualitative interviews also. One explanation might be that people were producing themselves as 'poor', in response to their perception of our identities as rich potential sponsors or donors. There is no doubt that many people did indeed see us in this way. However, the predominance of economic references spread far beyond such contexts. Consider the following two descriptions by older, now single, women of their marriages. In the first case, Gertrude is reminiscing about her early days of marriage and the happiness she experienced.

> G: At that time [my husband] would go away [to work] for maybe a month without returning home.
> Shreya: And you would be alone all through this time?
> G: Yes.
> S: How did that make you feel?
> G: I was happy because I knew that he was out there looking for money that was going to help us.

(SW 38)

The second woman, Hattie, is describing how she divorced her husband after being unhappily married for many years:

> Shreya: Okay... you had divorced him. Was it easy to take that decision?
> H: It wasn't hard for me to take the dowry back because I had played through thick and thin through good 16 years. I didn't even have a chitenge[10]; I would do piecework for me to get one. I just started

living on piecework as (if) I had no husband until it just came to my mind after 16 years 'this is too much and I cannot withstand it any longer'. So I decided to do that and drop him.

(SW 39)

In each of these interviews, the experience has been described in emotional terms and in each the context (early married life, the breakdown of a marriage) would seem to lend itself to a psychological or emotional reflection. When the interviewer seeks to explore this further, however, the respondents take an unexpected turn: they foreground the economic aspect of their subjectivity, rather than the affective.

There are a number of possible ways to interpret this. As mentioned above, in line with Maslow (1954), it could be that these women were simply so poor that the material and economic inscribed the horizon of their worlds. Alternatively, it could be that people in such contexts are simply unused to speaking directly of their feelings, and/or that norms of propriety, self-deprecation, or a wish to retain privacy made them unwilling to speak in a more intimate way. To resolve these questions would require more detailed research. It is worth noting, however, that both these potential explanations locate the constraint within the Chiawa context.

There are two alternatives which problematise instead our initial point of entry.

First, within social psychology there is a syndrome called the 'fundamental attribution error' (Ross 1977). This refers to the tendency to over-attribute others' behaviour to their personal intentions or character, rather than recognise the situational factors that might be responsible. This is in contrast to the tendency to emphasise external factors when explaining one's own behaviour. For example, when other people arrive late for a meeting, people attribute it to their lack of concern for others, but when they are late themselves, they blame the traffic. Miller (1984) found that this tendency was not evident in her studies in India, suggesting that the error may be characteristic of cultural settings that emphasise individualism rather than others. This opens the possibility that the psychological subject of SWB might be an artefact of a Western 'culture-based syndrome'[11]: whereby exaggerated emphasis is placed on the individual and his or her character and mentality, resulting in the importance of material and situational dimensions of life being systematically under-valued.

Second, Scheper-Hughes (1992: 185–186) emphasises that for people 'who live by and through their bodies in manual and wage labour...socioeconomic and political contradictions often take shape in the "natural" contradictions of sick and afflicted bodies'. Following Boltanski (1984), she contrasts this with the fact that 'In the middle classes personal and social distress is expressed psychologically rather than physically, and the language of the body is silenced and denied.' It is this middle-class idiom that has been normalised within biomedicine, psychiatry and anthropology, labelling as 'somatization' the manifestation of social ills in bodily dysfunction, which is seen as an indirect, more primitive means of expression. While this paper has concentrated on the way people in Chiawa talk of their economic circumstances rather than their bodies, the materiality that is common across the two cases again gives pause for thought about the biases 'we' bring to the field, assuming that a psychological form of expression constitutes the norm.

Conclusion

For these communities in Chiawa where material hardship is common, economics provides a primary reference point when people talk about wellbeing. This is evident in the ways that people respond when asked what wellbeing means to them. Beyond this, however, economic capacity (or the lack of it), economic provision (or the lack of it) and economic endeavours are mentioned frequently even when the topic of conversation apparently relates to some quite different sphere of life. This seems, then, to confirm the findings of the literature on economics and SWB, that for poorer people their economic status is a strong predictor of how they evaluate their lives. Our statistical analysis reinforced this. Across the sample as a whole, we found that amongst the IWB domains, economic confidence had the strongest association with happiness. The analysis also showed that objective economic capacity had a significant effect on both IWB and happiness, even when other demographic variables were taken into account.

The main purpose of this chapter, however, is to re-focus from this familiar argument over numbers, to consider the kind of *subjects* that are being presented. Our suggestion is that in Chiawa at least, people often express their subjectivities in economic terms. This is in marked contrast to the rather disembodied, psychological subject generally assumed in psychological and subjective wellbeing discourses.

Mixed methods were used to explore economic subjectivities. Quantitative and qualitative data and analysis were found to strongly reinforce one another, both pointing to the importance of economic capacity to subjective dimensions of wellbeing. This overall congruence notwithstanding, the ways that qualitative and quantitative methods represented the relationship between economics and subjective dimensions of wellbeing were quite distinct. While the statistical analysis has the strength of being able to quantify results across the whole sample, it also has the weakness of having to construct relationships in external terms. As argued in Chapter 1, its tendency is to objectify. The qualitative analysis is weaker in being grounded in the experience of particular individuals rather than the group as a whole, but is stronger in being more sensitive to the ways that people seek to express themselves and how they understand their lives. This again emphasises the economic, but suggests that it cannot be separated out as *an external influence on* wellbeing, but rather is integral to people's understanding of relationality and personhood, a key element in the constitution of wellbeing itself.

In terms of policy and practice, the clear implication is that a commitment to basic economic and social rights should remain at the heart of development intervention. But it does not imply surrender to analytical approaches which would privilege a narrow understanding of the economic as simply concerned with the market or the 'rational' allocation of scarce resources amongst individualised actors. Rather, it suggests that we should follow economic anthropology and the nascent anthropological literature on happiness and wellbeing within Africa to bring economics, the body, the mind and materiality more clearly into the social world. We close with two examples of this. In the first place, Jackson (2011: 59) describes how not having enough to eat is linked for the Kuranko in Sierra Leone to moral and ethical breakdown:

> Without rice, people say, they starve. But hunger is also a metaphor. First, it is a metaphor for what is most difficult in life, and for the tenacity and strength of suffering. Hence the ironic response to the question 'Are you well?' ... 'I am as well as hunger', meaning I am *very* hale and hearty. Second, the hungry time signifies any situation in which generosity goes by the board. It suggests an ethically compromised situation, characterized by self-interestedness and regressive behavior, when adults behave like children.

In the second place, James Ferguson (2006: 72) describes on a broader canvas the intertwining of moral and material, economic and social:

> the production of wealth throughout wide areas of southern and central Africa is understood to be inseparable from the production

of social relations. Production of wealth can be understood as prosocial, morally valuable 'work,' 'producing oneself by producing people, relations, and things' (Comaroff and Comaroff 1991: 143). Alternatively it can be understood as anti-social, morally illegitimate appropriation that is exploitative and destructive of community.

Acknowledgements

This chapter would not have been possible without the work of many others. Foremost are Shreya Jha, who led the fieldwork on which it reports, and Stanley O. Gaines Jr., who provided the statistical analysis that validated the IWB model. Thanks are also due to Andrea Baertl-Helguero who undertook the initial analysis of the field data. In Chiawa, special thanks are due to Joseph Kajiwa, who was the lead local researcher in both rounds. He was supported by Goodson Phiri in both rounds, and Kelvin Matesamwa in 2010 and Stephen Kalio in 2012. Our thanks also to other members of the field team, Susanna Siddiqui (2010) and Jonnathan Mtonga (2012). We are also grateful to Uma Kambhampati (University of Reading) for very helpful comments on an earlier draft.

Notes

1. This work is supported by the Economic and Social Research Council/Department for International Development Joint Scheme for Research on International Development (Poverty Alleviation) grant number RES-167-25-0507 ES/H033769/1.
2. This is the title of a chapter in Graham (2011), for example.
3. Further details on the FA procedures followed are available from Viviana Ramirez on request.
4. The domain scores were calculated through a regression method that weighted each item according to the strength with which it loaded onto the factor in the FA.
5. See Ramirez (forthcoming) for a similar analysis with data from two communities in Mexico.
6. This means that there is less than a one per cent chance that this association has occurred by chance.
7. For details on this categorisation, see Baertl-Helguero, White and Jha (2014: 37).
8. For more details on the types of assets, see Baertl-Helguero, White and Jha (2014: 35).
9. This variable also reflects very few unmarried men who had been divorced or widowed since the first round of our survey in 2010.
10. A wrap that women wear over their skirt or trousers.

11. This term is used within medical anthropology to describe disorders which are recognised in particular local contexts but cannot easily be translated into Western bio-medical categories.

References

Ahmed, S. (2010) *The Promise of Happiness*. Durham and London: Duke University Press.
Baertl-Helguero, A., White, S. C. and Jha, S. (2014) *Wellbeing Pathways Report. Zambia Round Two*. Available at: www.wellbeingpathways.org
Boltanski, L. (1984) *As Classes Sociais e o Corpo*. Rio de Janeiro: Graal.
Bourdieu (1977) *Outline of a Theory of Practice*. Cambridge: Cambridge University Press.
Central Statistical Office (2010) *2010 Census of Population and Housing*. Lusaka. Available at: http://www.zamstats.gov.zm/ [accessed 12 July 2015].
Comaroff, J. and Comaroff, J. (1991) *Of Revelation and Revolution, Volume 1: Christianity, Colonialism, and Consciousness in South Africa*. Chicago: University of Chicago Press.
Craib, I. (1994) *The Importance of Disappointment*. London: Routledge.
Devine, J. (2002) Ethnography of a Policy Process: A Case Study of Land Redistribution in Bangladesh. *Public Administration and Development* 22(5): 403–414.
Devine, J. and White, S. C. (2013) Religion, Politics and the Everyday Moral Order in Bangladesh. *Journal of Contemporary Asia* 43(1): 127–147.
Diener, E. and Suh, E. M. (eds.) (2000) *Culture and Subjective Well-Being*. Cambridge, MA and London: The MIT Press.
Diener, E., Ng, W., Harter, J. and Arora, R. (2010) Wealth and Happiness across the World: Material Prosperity Predicts Life Evaluation, Whereas Psychosocial Prosperity Predicts Positive Feeling. *Journal of Personality and Social Psychology* 99(1): 52–61.
Easterlin, R. A. (1974) Does Economic Growth Improve the Human Lot? pp. 88–125 in P. A. David and M. W. Reder (eds.) *Nations and Households in Economic Growth: Essays in Honor of Moses Abramovitz*. New York: Academic Press, Inc.
Ferguson, J. (2006) *Global Shadows. Africa in the Neoliberal World Order*. Durham and London: Duke University Press.
Gough, I. R. and McGregor, J. A. (eds.) (2007) *Wellbeing in Developing Countries: New Approaches and Research Strategies*. Cambridge: Cambridge University Press.
Graham, C. (2011) *The Pursuit of Happiness: An Economy of Wellbeing*. Washington: Brookings Institution Press.
Grossberg, L. (1996) Identity and Cultural Studies – Is That All There Is? pp. 53–60 in S. Hall and P. du Gay (eds.) *Questions of Cultural Identity*. London: Sage.
Hall, S. and du Gay, P. (1996) *Questions of Cultural Identity*. London: Routledge.
Jackson, M. (2011) *Life within Limits. Wellbeing in a World of Want*. Durham, USA: Duke University Press.
Kahneman, D. (2012) *Thinking Fast and Slow*. London: Penguin.

Kahneman, D. and Deaton, A. (2010) High Income Improves Evaluation of Life but Not Emotional Well-Being. *Proceedings of the National Academy of Sciences of the United States of America* 107(38): 16489–16493.

Mama, A. (1995) *Beyond the Masks: Race, Gender and Subjectivity*. London: Routledge.

Maslow, A. H. (1954) *Toward a Psychology of Being*. 2nd ed. New York: Van Nostrand Reinhold.

Mazrui, A. A. (2001) Pretender to Universalism: Western Culture in a Globalising Age. *Journal of Muslim Minority Affairs* 21(1): 11–24.

McBride, M. (2001) Relative-Income Effects on Subjective Well-Being in the Cross-Section. *Journal of Economic Behavior & Organization* 45: 251–278.

Miller, J. G. (1984) Culture and the Development of Everyday Social Explanation. *Journal of Personality and Social Psychology* 46(5): 961–978.

Moore, H. (2007) *The Subject of Anthropology: Gender, Symbolism and Psychoanalysis*. Cambridge: Polity Press.

PADHI (2009) *A Tool, a Guide and a Framework: Introduction to a Psychosocial Approach to Development*. Colombo, Sri Lanka: University of Colombo. Social Policy Analysis and Research Centre.

Putnam, R. and Leonardi, R. (1994) *Making Democracy Work: Civic Traditions in Modern Italy*. Princeton: Princeton Paperbacks.

Ramirez, V. (forthcoming) *The Roles of Human Relationships in Wellbeing: The Case of the Oportunidades Social Programme in Mexico*. Unpublished PhD thesis, University of Bath.

Ross, L. (1977) The Intuitive Psychologist and His Shortcomings: Distortions in the Attribution Process. pp. 173–220 in L. Berkowitz (ed.) *Advances in Experimental Social Psychology 10*. New York: Academic Press.

Rowlands, J. (1997) *Questioning Empowerment: Working with Women in Honduras*. Oxford: Oxfam.

Ryan, R. and Deci, E. (2000) Self-Determination Theory and the Facilitation of Intrinsic Motivation, Social Development, and Well-Being. *American Psychologist* 55: 68–78.

Scheper-Hughes (1992) *Death without Weeping: The Violence of Everyday Life in Brazil*. Berkeley and Los Angeles: University of California Press.

Stevenson, B. and Wolfers, J. (2008) Subjective Well-Being and Economic Development: Reassessing the Easterlin Paradox. *Brookings Papers on Economic Activity*. Spring: 102. Available at: http://www.brookings.edu/~/media/projects/bpea/spring-2008/2008a_bpea_stevenson.pdf [Accessed 12 July 2015].

White, S. C. (2010) Analysing Wellbeing: A Framework for Development Policy and Practice. *Development in Practice* 20(2): 158–172.

White, S. C., Gaines Jr. S. and Jha, S. (2014) Inner Wellbeing: Concept and Validation of a New Approach to Subjective Perceptions of Wellbeing – India. *Social Indicators Research* 119(2): 723–746.

White, S. C. and Jha, S. (2014) The Ethical Imperative of Qualitative Methods in Understanding Subjective Dimensions of Wellbeing in Zambia and India. *Journal of Ethics and Social Welfare* 8(3): 262–276.

Wilk, R. and Cliggett, L. (2007) *Economies and Cultures. Foundations of Economic Anthropology*. Boulder, CO: Westview Press.

6
'The Weight Falls on My Shoulders': Close Relationships and Women's Wellbeing in India[1]

Shreya Jha and Sarah C. White

Introduction

'The weight falls on my shoulders' is the way a young married woman, Mangali,[2] chose to sum up her relationship with her husband on the first occasion Shreya met her, in rural Chhattisgarh (India) in 2011. The statement was striking, because in a few words it challenged a host of norms and assumptions about gender, marriage, etiquette and wellbeing. In a cultural context that values male dominance and women's deference, it was a direct claim of female centrality. Against expectations in the empowerment literature that women's agency is something to celebrate, Mangali posed her responsibility as burdensome and counter to her own desires. Where social norms counsel discretion and acceptance of one's lot, Mangali voiced a barely veiled criticism of her husband and an open statement of her own discontent with relationships at home, and that to a virtual stranger.

This chapter draws on mixed method research in Chhattisgarh, 2010–2013, to explore the associations between close relationships and wellbeing, and how methods of research are implicated in the results they produce. The chapter begins with a brief introduction to the literature on women's wellbeing and close relationships, particularly in the context of South Asia. It then introduces the methodology of the present research and describes the challenges we encountered in devising a robust scale to measure subjective dimensions of wellbeing in the context of close relationships. We present some of the results we generated and our response to and interpretation of these. While we reflect on quantitative data, we do so within an interpretivist paradigm, rather than seeking to use quantitative analysis to drive the argument.

The second part of the chapter returns to the case of Mangali and that of another unusually 'empowered' woman in the same community. Concentrating on these two case studies enables us to go into some of the complexity of specific examples which may be lost in the overall numbers. This is particularly evident in the second case study which includes the dimension of time, since it was built up through numerous research encounters over a 30-month period. Nonetheless, concentrating mainly on two individuals clearly limits the kind of generalisation that the chapter can aim to make. The intention is not to claim that these women are typical of the community to which they belong; they are interesting precisely because of how atypical they are. The evidence presented here does however suggest two points of broader applicability. Methodologically, it draws attention to the difference between high quantitative scores given in response to direct survey questions about close relationships, with much more equivocal qualitative accounts. This suggests the difficulty of getting accurate quantitative data on the quality of relationships and the importance of qualitative methods to balance and aid interpretation of quantitative scores. Substantively, the chapter questions the way that relationships are often presented as having an 'effect on' wellbeing, with both relationships and wellbeing imagined in rather static and reified terms. These women's narratives support instead a view of wellbeing as a process of active construction, in which women's everyday management and negotiation of relationships play a significant part.

Women's wellbeing and close relationships

The importance of relationships is widely recognised across the wellbeing literature. Ryan and Deci (2001) posit 'relatedness' as one of the three basic psychological needs in their self-determination theory (SDT). They add that it is when a relationship satisfies these three needs of autonomy, competence and relatedness that it can be thought of as contributing to people's wellbeing. Ryff (1989) and Ryff and Singer (2008) include 'positive relations with others' as one of the six domains in their model of psychological wellbeing (PWB).[3] Seligman (2011) includes positive relationships as one of the five elements in his 'wellbeing theory' and sees relationships as critical to evolutionary survival and human flourishing.[4]

Amongst relationships considered to be important to wellbeing, there is a particular focus on marriage, which (reflecting its origins in the Global North) centres mainly on the couple as dyad, rather than a broader-based alliance between kin. The association between marriage and wellbeing is generally claimed to be significant and positive (Glenn 1975, Myers 1999). However, Gove et al. (1983) caution that the connections between marriage and PWB are poorly specified, with quality of relationship being potentially more important, especially for women, than marital status per se. The economists Stutzer and Frey (2006) also question the assumed direction of influence as they analyse 17 years of the German Socio-Economic Panel survey.[5] They argue that happier people are more likely to get married, rather than that marriage makes people happier.[6]

Studies of wellbeing in the South Asian context confirm the broader picture of the importance of relationships to wellbeing. Biswas-Diener and Diener (2001, 2006), for example, found in two studies of people at the margins in Kolkata, India[7] that people recorded very high satisfaction scores for their social and family lives. In the first study, satisfaction scores on a scale of 1 to 3 were 2.50 for family and 2.40 for friends (Biswas-Diener and Diener 2001: 343). In the second study, on a scale of 1 to 7, the respondents in Kolkata scored their social satisfaction at 5.08 and family at 5.93 (Biswas-Diener and Diener 2006: 195). The authors suggest that this indicates a trade-off between material and social needs: 'to the extent the poor can utilise their strong social relationships, the negative effects of poverty are counterbalanced' (Biswas-Diener and Diener 2001: 347). While we welcome the recognition of a more social dimension within a literature that tends to be over-individualised, our discussion in this chapter suggests that this conclusion may be premature. As described below, qualitative evidence suggests a rather more ambivalent picture rather than a felicitous trade-off between material and social spheres.

White (1992) suggests that good relationships with key family members (particularly husbands and fathers-in-law) are important in enabling women in rural Bangladesh to expand the horizons of their economic activities. This contrasts with the received wisdom in much empowerment literature that increased voice in the family is an *outcome* of women's earnings. Camfield et al. (2009), again in Bangladesh, use mixed methods research to discuss the significance of relationships to wellbeing. Confirming the general consensus on the importance of relationships, they add that qualitative analysis can provide additional insights especially regarding *the form* that such influence takes. Their qualitative data indicated that close relationships intertwine affective and economic dimensions in the household, as love is shown through provision and mutual care (see also White and Ramirez, this volume).

While emotional ties are a source of happiness, there is also a strong social and status dimension. Thus a household head who rated his happiness highly linked this to the fact that there was consensus in their household and everyone obeyed him (Camfield *et al.* 2009: 82). Sons and daughters-in-law similarly linked their happiness at least in part to looking after their parents (in-law) well; this is important both in itself and because being able to manage these relationships successfully enhances reputation in the community (Camfield *et al.* 2009: 82–84). Such expressions of family life indicate that close relationships are not simply 'personal' or 'natural', but strongly governed by social norms and expectations. One dimension of this that bears significantly on narratives of wellbeing is a strong emphasis on presenting the family in the best possible light; this is discussed next.

Ahmed (2010: 45) points to the ideological weight carried by the family as 'a happy object, one that binds and is binding'. As Uberoi (1994: 2) describes, this is strongly marked in India, making discussion of any shortcomings highly sensitive:

> It is as though critical interrogation of the family might constitute an intrusion into that very private domain where the nation's most cherished cultural values are nurtured and reproduced, as though the very fabric of society would be undone if the family were in any way questioned or reshaped.

Palriwala (1999: 49) describes family and community in India as encapsulating 'the most sacred and natural of relationships – between children and parents, wife and husband, sister and brother, devotee and god'. She goes on, however, to note a fundamental ambivalence, as the family is both 'the community of cooperation and the community of sanction' (Palriwala 1999: 54). Rowlands (1997: 125) echoes this as she discusses how intimate relationships may be simultaneously supportive and disempowering in the context of Honduras. Her study of women's empowerment confirms the findings of others that it is in the sphere of intimate relationships that women find it most difficult to express agency, communicate their need for change and bring about desired change (Murphy-Graham 2010, Rowlands 1997).

In South Asia at least, the *ideology* of the 'happy family' joins together with the *material* centrality of the family in securing welfare and the *social* importance of family and marriage particularly, as a key site for the reproduction and reconfiguration of gender and other forms of social difference such as caste and class (Abeyasekera 2013). Not surprisingly, this results in tensions between public presentations and lived experiences of conjugal relationships. Women behave in ways that can be eased into locally prevalent discourses of ideal wives/mothers/women as a means of avoiding censure while still managing to achieve their aims. Thapan (2003: 81) found that women and girls in Delhi slums strongly identified their own wellbeing with that of their families. Nonetheless, she suggests:

> While providing security, fulfilment, and identity to women, marriage is also a context within which many of them find their opportunities and options limited. I found that women engage in a twin-track process of compliance and resistance, submission and rebellion, silence and speech, to question their oppression in the family, community, and society. Resistance can be overt and vocal, or muted, expressed in everyday life, in 'gestures, habits, desires – that are grounded in the body... as the sources of resistance and protest'.
>
> (Kielmann 1998: 129 in Thapan 2003: 77)

Sanctions against exposing any imperfection in the family unit mean that women's manoeuvring in close relationships is frequently obscured. Agarwal (1996: 430) emphasises that 'appearance of compliance need not mean that women lack a perception of their best interests; rather it can reflect a survival strategy stemming from the constraints on their ability to act overtly in pursuit of those interests'. Jeffery and Jeffery (1996), narrating women's lives in rural North India, describe how even when women openly defy gender norms within conjugal relationships they generally seek to legitimise this in some way, commonly for instance by invoking 'for the sake of the children', thus justifying those actions by apparently conforming to idealised norms of motherhood.

This brief review of a broad literature demonstrates a wide consensus that family relationships, and particularly marriage, are important to wellbeing. While we have concentrated here on social and psychological dimensions, marriage and family are also critical to the achievement of material wellbeing. Paradoxically, however, the very centrality of family and marriage relationships to wellbeing may make them difficult to investigate, as they present such a concentrated site of social, psychological and economic investment. The following sections describe how we encountered some dimensions of this and the implications for different methods of wellbeing research.

Methodology

The study presented here was part of the 'wellbeing pathways' research described in White and Ramirez (this volume) and followed the same methodology.[8] It investigated both how people were doing in 'objective' terms (livelihoods, health and education, plus access to government services) and 'subjectively' how they were thinking and feeling about their lives. In exploring subjective dimensions of wellbeing, we developed the concept 'inner wellbeing' (IWB) to describe what people feel and think themselves able to do and be. IWB comprises seven interconnected domains, of which close relationship is one.[9]

This chapter draws on an integrated, mixed method approach over two main research periods, February to May 2011 and 2013, plus an initial short visit in November 2010. Shreya Jha led the field research team of four local peer researchers, whom we employed with the assistance of a local non-governmental organisation (NGO), Chaupal. They provided critical support in introducing us to the research area, helped with interpretation of the local dialect and undertook many of the surveys themselves. Sarah White as project director visited for shorter times.

In-depth qualitative grounding and piloting were used to generate questions which would enable us to track both 'objective' and 'subjective' dimensions of wellbeing. For the IWB section, we began with six items (November 2010) which we reduced to four items for the first main round of fieldwork (2011). At that time we had eight domains and were concerned at the burden on respondents of retaining a larger number of items in each. After analysis of our first round of data, we finally settled on seven domains with five items in each (2013). A fuller account of the development of the survey and the statistical validation of the IWB model are given elsewhere (White and Jha 2014, White et al. 2012a, 2012b, White et al. 2014). Survey data were generated through individual interviews – 339 in 2011 and 368 in 2013. One hundred and eighty-seven people (55 per cent) of those surveyed in 2011 were surveyed again in 2013.

Both the organisation of the survey and our personal approach were designed to reflect a conversational style which would create space for people to speak in detail and for the interview to assume a natural flow (see Bryman 2001: 93–97). We also recorded observations on informal conversations to help contextualise the narratives. To deepen our understanding of local constructions of wellbeing, we did in-depth qualitative interviews with people who seemed both 'typical' and 'atypical' of the area to comprehend the diversity of people's lives. Qualitative data include 151 survey notes and full transcriptions of 30 interviews. The in-depth interviews were open-ended conversations which were partially structured around themes that had arisen in earlier conversations with the same people, but also broadened to include people's life stories so as to accommodate topics that might not otherwise have arisen. In most cases, the in-depth interview was with someone with whom a relationship had already been established through the survey interview.

The study context[10]

The research took place in four villages in Sarguja district, Chattisgarh state, where the population was predominantly Adivasi or 'tribal'.[11] While the villages differ in terms of ease of access, environmental location (close to a river, hill or forest), degree of poverty and dominant community, overall the villages are extremely poor, and until a recent food-security programme, people frequently had to go hungry. Literacy levels are very low, with more than half of the respondents never having gone to school. The mainstay of the economy is (mostly rain-fed) agriculture, and most people do some farming, supplemented by casual labour and gathering non-timber forest products. Despite being formally outside the caste system, caste-type practices are followed. Marriage is patri-local, with women moving to live with their husband's family, often in a joint family context, at least at first.[12] Our 2013 survey found 19 per cent of respondents lived in joint households (including more than one married couple), with a further 14 per cent in extended households (including one married couple plus at least one other adult, but not a second married couple), 52 per cent were in nuclear households (one couple and unmarried children) and 11 per cent in sub-nuclear households (a couple or single person without children) (Fernandez *et al.* 2014: 18).

Both of the case-study women are from the locally dominant Kanwar Adivasi community. Conventionally, gender relations are thought to be more egalitarian in Adivasi than in other parts of Indian society. Xaxa (2004) is one of several writers who question this. While Xaxa points out that several factors do indeed differentiate Adivasi from 'mainstream women', he cautions against reading any single difference as sufficient to make generalisations either regarding Adivasi women's equal position vis-à-vis Adivasi men or to their being in a relatively better position than non-Adivasi women. Far from being the 'untouched tribes' of anthropological legend, Xaxa points out that broad changes in political economy and society have affected Adivasi communities in both negative and positive ways, resulting in very heterogenous experiences and situations.

Constructing the close relationships domain

Seeking to measure psychosocial wellbeing amongst people who were completely unused to this type of survey proved extremely challenging. Our aim was to devise questions that resonated with how people talk and think locally, rather than simply to apply a framework that had been developed in a very different context. Even when you try to make the content of such questions culturally appropriate, however, their form still requires people to abstract from and generalise about their lives, to choose from a graduated set of responses the one which seems to fit their experience best. None of this is easy. Even given this general difficulty, however, it was the domain of close relationships that proved by far the hardest to capture. In part, this reflected the ways that this area of life is governed by particularly strong norms about what should be said, as introduced above. But it was also because people were simply not used to discussing their marriage and family relationships in such direct terms. We thus struggled to devise appropriate questions. To give an example, during piloting in Sarguja, we were trying to ask a woman about her experience of love and support in her family – a standard 'quality of relationships' dimension in Western surveys. She responded in three ways. First, she said she always worried about her husband going to another village, that he would drink there and maybe fall down, and what would happen to him. If her husband were at home then she would have cooked for him and fed him and known he was safe at home, but if he was out then she worried about him and could not sleep. Second, she said she was married in front of several people. Finally – and in some exasperation with us – she said surely he loved her since they had been living together so long and had had five children together! We eventually settled on four questions, which are given in Table 6.1.

Analysis of the 2011 data showed that three of the four items (numbers one, two and four) correlated significantly with each other. This

Table 6.1 Close relationship items in round one fieldwork (2011)

1. Do you feel that there is unity in your family?
2. If problems arise in your family, how often are you able to discuss and sort them out?
3. How often is it that your family requires you to do things that you don't want to do?
4. How much do people in your house care for you?

was confirmed through exploratory factor analysis (EFA) which tests the way that responses across the range of items group together, suggesting that they reflect a number of distinct underlying factors or domains. We were therefore able to be confident that these three items together constituted the close relationships domain. The exception was the third item, which sought to raise possible tensions between personal priorities and family demands. This item did not only fail to fit within the close relationships domain, but nor did it fit within the IWB scale as a whole, as it correlated significantly only with three of the other 31 items and did not load onto any factor in the EFA. Nevertheless, validating a domain with three out of four items was, in statistical terms, a success, as it is common to have to drop items which do not fit (see White and Ramirez, this volume).

A rather different issue was the high level of scores for this domain, and following on from this, our questioning about what lay behind the consistent pattern of response in these three items. Did it reflect exceptionally positive experiences of relationships, or simply the strength of a 'happy family' ideology? Taking a simple average of the item scores within each domain, the mean for the close relationships domain was extremely high, at 4.62 out of 5 compared with an average of 2.47 across the other domains.[13] This was at odds with our own experience in other qualitative research in India and Bangladesh and observations and interview-based evidence within this same study. We therefore believed that the major reason for this was the strong positivity bias suggested above – whatever their actual experience, people thought that family unity was what should be projected. In the second round of the survey, we re-used the questions that had 'worked' (i.e. correlated with one another) in 2011, though with some re-wording. We also sought to develop some new questions which we hoped would not trigger the same associations. The 2013 close relationship questions are presented in Table 6.2.

Table 6.2 Close relationship items in round two fieldwork (2013)

1. How well do you get along amongst yourselves?
2. If there is a problem in your family, how easily can you sort it out?
3. When your mind/heart is troubled/heavy, do you feel there is someone you can go to?
4. How much do people in your house care for you?
5. How uneasy are you made by the amount of violence in your home?

Analysis of the data from round two (2013) showed that the original three items continued to correlate consistently with one another. Now appearing as items one, two and four, they clearly associate with ideologies of the happy family, consisting of how people get along, care for each other and resolve any problems that arise. The items were again scored very highly, with a mean of 4.53 between them, compared with a mean of 3.16 of the 30 items across the other domains. By contrast, the two new items were scored very low, at 2.83 and 2.75, respectively.

The statistics showed that again we had one item that did not correlate significantly with any of the others in the domain.[14] This was item three, 'When your mind is troubled, do you feel there is someone you can go to?' This is the one item that does not refer specifically to family or household relationships. Qualitative comments confirmed that people did not tend to associate talking of troubles with the close family. Instead, people tended to talk of family relationships in terms of (reciprocal) roles and responsibilities and hence the pragmatic need to co-operate. This emphasis on structural relationships may be intensified in smallholder farming communities like these, where the family household constitutes the primary unit of production and consumption. A common response to the second question, for example, was 'If we fight then how do we work together and run the household?' Interdependence is similarly stressed in another response from a man to the same question: 'When we fight, she stops cooking, then I cook, if we don't eat, how do we work?' In such contexts, as the case studies suggest below, agency may be expressed through silence, rather than speech (see also White, Fernandez and Jha, forthcoming).

The patterns of response to the item on violence showed significant correlations with the second question, about being able to resolve conflicts in the family. Where question two was scored high overall, however, the one on violence was scored low. This merits some attention. We had tried earlier to have a question on violence, but found that it was met simply with denial – there was no problem in their family – and hence very high scores. This denial of domestic violence even in communities where it is known to be prevalent is a common difficulty with surveys. This question took a different tack, assuming the presence of violence and asking how people felt about it. It was striking that this met with very few denials, and where people did say that there was no violence in their house, they substantiated the claim in ways that made it seem genuine. While there were some cases of women being violent (usually, though not only, to other women), the vast majority of instances of violence mentioned involved men.

What was particularly interesting was that men answered this question significantly more negatively than women. This ran counter to the general pattern that men's IWB answers tended to be significantly more positive than women's. For the violence question, the mean score for men was 2.43, while that for all women was 3.04, breaking down into 2.97 for married women and 3.55 for single women. Statistical analysis confirms that responses to this question were significantly and positively correlated with both gender and marital status.[15] While it is commonly known, of course, that men feel remorse for their violence in the home which they yet continue to perpetrate, the suggestion from this data that violence has a more negative effect on men's sense of wellbeing than it does on women's indicates interesting potential for a new approach to mobilisation amongst men against gender-based violence. Amongst women, even when they expressed strong concern about the level of violence in the household, this tended to be balanced by anxieties about what would happen to the children if the relationship ended: 'If I leave them then a step-mother may not look after them as well'; 'If I remarry then a step-father will not look after them as well.'

In summary, then, we were unable to establish a close relationship domain within the IWB model that avoided the positivity bias of the 'happy family'. The items which consistently correlated with one another and emerged as a factor in factor analysis were those that attracted the higher scores. In one way, this did not matter. Although the scores were an average of around 25 per cent higher than in other domains, there was still sufficient variance in scores between people for the domain to 'work' as a measure of IWB. It does, however, constitute a warning against taking such scores at face value in comparing the level of wellbeing in one domain against another. We return to this point in the conclusion.

Case studies

In this section, we return to Mangali and introduce our second major character, Gulabi, to enable us to explore at closer quarters the associations between close relationships and wellbeing. We consider two issues, first, the implication of methods in rendering differing accounts of wellbeing and second, the substantive processes that produce wellbeing through family relationships.

Mangali

Mangali is approximately 35 years old, a married woman living in a nuclear household with her husband and five daughters. Their home is within a large house built around a central courtyard. Other parts of the house are occupied by her parents-in-law and her brothers-in-law and their families, with each sub-unit cooking and budgeting separately. Mangali does household work and farming and their five daughters all go to school.

This section draws on a single interview which Shreya had with Mangali. Shreya was accompanied by Pritam, one of our local peer researchers who had already completed a survey with Mangali. As described further below, Pritam happened to be from Mangali's natal village, making the association between them that of elder sister to younger brother. This helped in establishing an easy research relationship with her.

The interview began unusually. The intention had been to speak with Mangali's husband, but instead he sent Mangali out to see what Shreya wanted. Perhaps frustrated with this immediate context, Mangali said that she was forced to take the lead in anything that needed to be done: 'Typically in a married couple it is the man's job to talk first and take the lead when deciding anything and going out to do any work, but in our case it is always I who has to do all of this.' The contrast with the tight-lipped standard answers that we usually encountered when asking about close relationships was so striking that Shreya decided to continue the interview with her.

Although Shreya did not know it at the time, in the survey that Mangali had completed a few days earlier she had already shown her difference from her peers in her willingness to signal some degree of disharmony in family relationships. She gave scores of 4 out of 5 for two of the close relationship items (family unity and family care), 3 out of 5 for one (resolving problems in the family) and 2 for the other (being required to do things she didn't want to do). Even if we exclude this lowest scoring item on the basis of its lack of correlation with the other items (see above), this makes an average of 3.67 for the close relationships domain as a whole. This is markedly lower than the close relations average of 4.62 for the whole sample.[16] It is also much of a piece with Mangali's other domain scores, which ranged from 2.25 (social connections) to 3.75 (economic confidence), with a mean of 2.97. In brief, Mangali's close relationship domain score bucked the usual trend. It was not much higher than the mean of her other domains, forming part of a cluster of three positive domain scores (two at 3.67 and one at 3.75).

As her narrative unfolded, Mangali developed further the fact of having to take the lead in her marriage, and the burden she felt this to be.

> M: ....not from today but from the time he married me...see there is nobody to support me. If there is an argument or anywhere (that) we have to go, whether in the village, to the shop, or in the neighbourhood...but he will not take the lead. He will keep the money but he will not be the one to say anything when he is in the shop. I'll tell you one thing; in a husband–wife relationship it is supposed to be the husband to take the weight but here all the weight falls on my shoulders. He will earn money but if he doesn't talk to anybody then I have to be the one who has to do the work.

As noted in Introduction, such direct criticism or admission of discomfort in family relationships was extremely rare, even in the joint family.[17] Much more common were general statements from which a particular experience could be inferred: 'Where do husbands and wives not argue a little bit?' Mangali also challenged convention as she made it clear that it was her idea that she and her husband should separate from his parents and form a nuclear unit of their own. Breaking up the joint family is something that daughters-in-law in India are often blamed for, but rarely claim as their own initiative. Mangali does, however, conform to gendered narrative rules in justifying her behaviour as motivated by her children's interests, rather than her own:

> M: ...it wasn't the parents-in-law who made me like this or my husband but the children that made me think. I decided that I would educate them, bring them up well and somehow ensure that I can give them a good future.

While she criticises him, the love of her husband has clearly been an important resource:

> S: And did you say that it has been like this from the time you got married?
>
> M: Yes, from the very beginning. But at that time I didn't want to take the lead because my parents-in-law were also there and they didn't like me...but my husband loves me. So then I thought, 'Doesn't matter if they [parents-in-law] don't like me, the two of us will live in peace and make our lives comfortable.'

Mangali in fact suffered serious abuse, including physical violence, from her mother-in-law during her early marriage. Material and emotional supports from her natal family have been important in enabling her to set up and sustain an independent household with her husband. That both she and her husband know she could, if necessary, leave and return to her natal family, also gives her an important source of power. This reflects what Sen (1987) calls the 'breakdown position' in his analysis of intra-household relationships in India as 'co-operative conflicts' – a woman who has a viable alternative if the relationship breaks down is in a much stronger position than one who does not. While overall she and her husband get on well, Mangali admits there are times when they argue. Reflecting the pattern mentioned above, however, she refers to the necessity of guarding her tongue in view of their need to work in co-operation:

> M: No, we care for each other but, of course, there are times when we fight. Sometimes I may say something harsh but then we would not be able to work together.

Mangali also says she does not discuss these matters with others in the village, even women her own age, although all women refer obliquely to similar issues.

> M: I never tell anybody about what is in my heart and sometimes it can eat me up inside. (Whenever) everything comes out then...

What emerges from the combination of qualitative and quantitative data is therefore a complex picture. In terms of the 'real' quality of her relationship with her husband, the overall impression is generally positive: Mangali feels loved and valued, and has a great deal of room for manoeuvre, even if she feels ambivalent about this. The unusual terms of their marital relationship, however, in which she takes the conventionally male role of the one who leads and negotiates on their joint behalf, seem to give her a certain freedom when it comes to the ideologies that govern the family, a readiness to 'tell it like it is', both in direct conversation and through the numerical scores. The fact that her close relationship domain score was rather lower than the average should not therefore be read as an indication of a poorer quality of relationship, but of her greater freedom with respect to the ideology. This should not be taken too far, however. Mangali's stated caution about telling others in her neighbourhood about 'what is in her heart' demonstrates that she was fully aware of the need to maintain the façade of female submission and the happy family, and the social peril that could be occasioned by sharing her disappointments with others.

The fact that Mangali was ready to share so openly with the research team seems to reflect a combination of factors. The first is that Pritam, who had interviewed her for the survey and accompanied Shreya on the occasion reported here, was from Mangali's natal village. In North Indian culture there is a strong contrast between a woman's marital village as one of constraint and conditionality, and her natal village as one of freedom and acceptance. The motif of 'older sister–younger brother' which Mangali drew on in characterising her relationship with Pritam is one of particular ease, closeness and safety in intimacy. The second factor is Mangali's perception of Shreya as both an outsider and a similarly empowered woman, able to move about and talk to people as she wished. The third is the character and skill of Shreya and Pritam, eager to hear Mangali's story and ready to listen with empathy and understanding.

Gulabi

In 2011, Gulabi was 39 years old, a married woman in one of the leading families of her village. Unusually, she had grown up in the main district town. This made for difficulties when she first moved to the village, because she was not accustomed to the same kind of housework, and faced a lot of teasing for being over-educated and under-skilled in domestic tasks. She lives in a joint household with her husband, parents-in-law and three sons. She completed middle school (class eight) before her marriage 20 years ago and in 2012 completed her school-leaving exam (class 12) through open school.[18] Both she and her husband, Devsaya, have worked with a local community-based organisation (CBO) for many years. At the time of our first interview, Gulabi had recently been elected as *sarpanch*, the leader of the most immediate rung of local government, the *panchayat*.[19] Gulabi is thus very unusual, occupying a key public role that would not traditionally have been open to her, either as an Adivasi, or as a woman. Their association with the CBO has also made both Gulabi and Devsaya familiar with ideas of development and women's empowerment and they use this language when talking about their work.

We met Gulabi numerous times. Here we describe three surveys, one in-depth interview and one of many informal conversations with her. We first met in November 2010, when she and her husband had been asked to introduce us to their village as a potential research site. On this occasion, Gulabi was quite reserved, deferring to Devsaya in discussions with us, with him answering questions posed to her and taking us around the village. Our first interview with her took place the next day. On her own with us she came across much more strongly and we began to get a sense of the person she was.

In terms of the quantitative data, Gulabi conformed perfectly to the 'happy family' ideology. In all three surveys, from pre-piloting through the two rounds of fieldwork, she answered all of the core family relationship items with a resounding five. In the main fieldwork surveys, the only item which she gave a lower score (1) was in 2013, 'When your mind is troubled, do you feel there is someone you can go to?' Like Mangali, she emphasised the need to keep any troubles to herself and the danger of scandal if she were to talk 'outside'. As discussed above, this item cannot be considered to belong within the close relationships domain for these communities.

Table 6.3 and Figure 6.1 present Gulabi's domain scores in 2011 and 2013.[20] These clearly illustrate how Gulabi's life has expanded with the

Table 6.3 Gulabi's domain scores, 2011 and 2013

Domain	2011	2013
Economic confidence	3.75	3.4
Agency and participation	4.5	4.4
Social connections	4.5	4.6
Close relationships	5	5
Physical and mental health	2	2.75
Competence and self-worth	3	4.2
Values and meaning	3.5	3.25

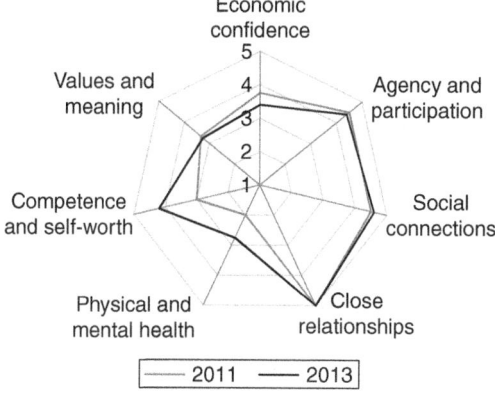

Figure 6.1 Gulabi's domain scores, pivot graph, 2011 and 2013

sarpanch role. In sharp contrast to most other women, her scores for the more social and political domains – agency and participation and social connections – are very high. Interestingly, the largest change between the two surveys is in her sense of self-worth, which is markedly higher in 2013. But overall there is considerable consistency between the two sets of scores. In both, physical and mental health comes out as by far the lowest – in fact, the only negative score (3 being the mid-point). This was confirmed by Gulabi's frequent comments about the amount of work that she had to do as she sought to balance her household responsibilities with the demands of her political role as *sarpanch*. In both surveys, she is only moderately positive about her economic position. She explained this by reference to the demands of her role in the CBO and as *sarpanch*, restricting the amount of attention she could give to farming. She was interestingly ambivalent in her scores in the values and meaning domain, which aims to gauge how people reflect on their life in more cosmic terms. While we did not discuss this with her, this might be read as an indication of a conviction that it is her own effort, rather than a divine gift or good fortune, that is responsible for what she has achieved in life, and the sense of continuing struggle that remains.[21]

Gulabi's comments explaining her scores were also interesting. Confirming the argument made more broadly in this volume, these reveal links between material, relational and subjective dimensions of wellbeing. In piloting, she responded to the statement 'There is little harmony in our home' by saying that there is harmony now because they are economically better off, which makes life less stressful. In response to the statement 'I feel alone even when there are people around', she referred to hard times in her early married life when they were struggling financially and nobody, not even her natal family, offered help and support even when she had asked for it.[22]

On the face of it, then, Gulabi's quantitative data indicate an empowered woman who is strongly supported within her close family, enabling her to take on an unusually prominent public role. The picture that emerges from the qualitative evidence, however, is rather more complex.

Conditional harmony

The first aspect of this complexity, which first emerged during piloting, was the extent to which the 'good relationships' were dependent on Gulabi's own self-regulation. In explaining harmony in the home, she says she constantly checks herself from doing anything that she feels would displease Devsaya. If she did by chance offend him, then he would tell her and she would be careful to avoid such behaviour in the future. In the 2011 survey she explained that she would never hold on to grudges: where could she possibly go if she were to hold on to her anger? She added that the idea of not having 'her own' place made her feel helpless. This is perhaps a reference to the strained relations with her natal family, who had failed to help her when she was in need. She also said that she would lose her honour and self-respect if she were to run away or talk outside about difficult situations in the home.

A qualitative interview in May 2011 provided the context for Gulabi to describe to Shreya in more detail how self-restraint, of both herself and her husband, played a critical role in producing good relationships in the home. It began by discussing Gulabi's early married life.

> S: You talked about how you were unable to do all the work in the beginning and he had also thought that you are of a good household and you should stay in and manage the household but when your sisters-in-law and others would taunt you about being the educated daughter-in-law who couldn't do anything then what would he say?
> G: He wouldn't pay attention to all those things. (*S: And did you ever tell him about these things?*) No, I wouldn't ever say anything. (*S: You would keep it to yourself...*) I am not able to and he would not have been able to tolerate it... neither have I ever complained to him, nor to my parents 'so-and-so says this or that'. I have never done any of that.
> S: When you say that he would not have been able to tolerate it what do you think would have happened?
> G: Then there would have been a fight, he would have said something to me... I don't say anything to him and nor does he say these things to me. I don't complain to him.
> S: So you feel it might cause him to fight with them and then you could face the repercussions?
> G: Yes, you never know, they could turn around and point a finger at me. I tolerate as much as I can.
> S: And when it is no longer tolerable?
> G: Then at that time then I may say something, sometimes others may say something.
> S: Have there been occasions when you have been forced to say something? (*G: Yes occasionally...*) But you have noticed that he gets annoyed when you complain about such things...
> G: Yes, he gets irritated so I don't say anything but he also never complains about anything to me.

The picture that emerges from this exchange is rather different to the simple presentation of positive relationships that is conveyed by the quantitative scores. It draws attention to the limits, the hidden terms which must be observed, the conditionality of the 'happy family' which rests on the compliance of some to the satisfaction of others. While a happy family is surely to be wished for, it also rests on the threat of sanction, with repercussions for both individual and family honour if it is contravened. Even for a remarkably empowered woman like Gulabi, what is required from her is restraint. There are two particular factors in her personal history that reinforce this. The first is that Gulabi experienced violence in her natal family, and has quite consciously sought to avoid any behaviour that might trigger violence in her marriage. She is grateful to Devsaya that he has never been violent to her, and also that he supports her as a woman in a public role, paying no heed to what others might say. In addition, she is conscious that as daughter-in-law to the village headman she belongs to a family that commands prestige locally. Lack of restraint on her part would therefore occasion considerable shame. The broader point is that the high survey scores are not just the result of a 'natural' state of good family relationships; instead these relationships are achieved through constant negotiation and engagement in which some people carry a greater burden than others.

Work

As noted above, workload was a major issue for Gulabi, and it was in relation to this that some tensions in the house first emerged. In her 2011 survey, she gave as evidence how people in the house cared for her, the fact that there was no pressure on her to do household work and that she did only what she was able to do. In relation to the health domain, however, she contradicted this, as she responded to a question about tension that she constantly had headaches because of the amount of work she had to do. Once she finished her work for the *panchayat* and CBO, she had to attend to the household work. This reflects both her sense that it would be unfair to leave it to her elderly mother-in-law and her wish to avoid giving any cause for censure.

The issue of workload framed the final interview between Shreya and Gulabi, which took place in 2013. Gulabi insisted that Shreya hold the interview at that time because she was not sure when she would next get time to sit. Immediately after the survey finished, her mother-in-law asked Gulabi something, to which she replied that she had completed the task. Once her mother-in-law was out of hearing, she turned to Shreya, almost rolling her eyes, and said, 'They don't like it.' She continued that her parents-in-law resented the fact that she worked outside the home with the CBO and *panchayat*, expressing their displeasure indirectly over the fact that she was not always around to complete all the household work. She added that she woke up at 3.30 am during the farming seasons and worked incessantly till about 10 pm, appealing to Shreya plaintively, 'What more can I do?'

Her husband then arrived, and Gulabi resumed the thread of her conversation. She started by describing tension in the household in a somewhat indirect manner. She said that they were able to manage the household expenses because they both worked, otherwise it would be difficult. She also added that Devsaya however did no household work. She spoke once more of her parents-in-law's annoyance at her working, but that she did not bother much about it because she knew that Devsaya supported her. Her work had also been vital to their ability to manage financially, especially in the earlier days of their marriage, when they were really struggling. However, she added that Devsaya told her she must sort out these matters herself and not involve him in them. Confirming the point made above concerning her own self-regulation, Gulabi then went on to say that when they had a difference of opinion, she would keep quiet and wait until he was ready to listen to her, and it was only then that she would voice her own feelings.

Although on the one hand Gulabi was talking to Shreya, she was also directing her remarks to Devsaya, almost as if she was making Shreya a witness to a conversation between the two of them. Devsaya remained silent throughout but acknowledged that the remarks were also directed at him by nodding or smiling at times. Gulabi appeared watchful. It seemed that (at least) two things were going on. First, Gulabi appeared to be seeking a public validation of her role in contributing to the household, especially as she repeatedly emphasised that she took on most of the household tasks in addition to her work outside the home. Secondly, it appeared as if Gulabi might have been using Shreya's presence to make it safer to voice what are somewhat 'unacceptable' opinions. Shreya's particular positionality is relevant here. She was an outsider, an independent and educated woman, who would have been strongly identified with the notions of women's empowerment that both Gulabi and Devsaya were familiar with due to their work in the CBO. All of this, along with Devsaya's own personality, would have made it very unlikely that he would have reprimanded Gulabi in Shreya's presence.

The depth of Shreya's interaction with Gulabi, using a variety of research instruments across two and a half years, gives us unusual scope to explore the genesis of accounts of wellbeing. There is a marked contrast between the maximum scores that Gulabi consistently gave to all the core family relationship items and her much more ambivalent qualitative narratives. The difference with Mangali, whose quantitative scores were much closer to her verbal accounts, suggests that Gulabi's sense of status required her to conform to the ideologically approved appearance of the 'happy family' when approached through the brute form of direct questions. Where there was more scope for nuance and ambiguity, and perhaps where the personal relationship with Shreya was more to the fore, a more ambivalent, polyvocal account could be presented.

A further issue is the identity of the researchers. The importance of the connection between Mangali and Pritam, as coming from the same village, is noted above as introducing an ease and confidence into the research relationship. Shreya's identity is also an important part of the story, as her views and perspectives affect how she received and interpreted responses and this in turn shaped the further questions she asked. Having trained and worked as a counsellor has a significant impact on how Shreya conducts herself in an interview setting. This is especially relevant to the domain of women's close relationships which Shreya's counselling experience has shown to be fraught with tension. Thus she works to keep a neutral tone so as not to suggest she is endorsing any 'right' view of marriage or the family, and the tenor of her questions may be to uncover complexity. This opens the possibility of co-construction, that what Gulabi and Mangali revealed to Shreya was as much a response to what she asked, as her questions were a response to what she 'sensed' they may have been saying.

Time is also an important character in these accounts. The relationship between Shreya and Gulabi developed over time through repeated meetings, both fleeting and longer conversations. Over the course of these meetings the tone of the conversation changed, so that with each successive interview there was a greater degree of revelation. This was especially marked in the last informal conversation. Through this process it became possible to discern something of the everyday practice that goes into the construction of wellbeing: the reproductive labour of servicing the household; the social labour of sensing and accommodating oneself to the bounds of what is normative; and the personal labour of consuming one's disappointments and harms in silence and moving on.

Conclusion

This chapter has brought together quantitative and qualitative data to investigate in the context of rural Chhattisgarh the widely remarked associations between close relationships and wellbeing. It began by noting the particularly privileged place of the family in South Asian society, which gives people – and especially women – a strong incentive to preserve the ideology of the 'happy family' and to represent their behaviour and experience in terms that conform to this ideal.

It then discussed the challenges involved in developing a quantitative scale that could track how people are thinking and feeling about their close relationships. A quantitative measure demands that people answer along a particular continuum, whereas their views about that particular issue may be qualified by other factors. It also requires a summative score which cannot reflect the diversity within each person's life or how different situations in a person's life may make them act or feel differently (Bryman 2001). Despite our reservations, we did manage to produce items which statistical analysis of correlations and factor analysis suggested belonged together as a close relationships domain. We were concerned, however, that the much higher scores in this domain compared with others suggested either a very high intrinsic quality of relationships or a high level of satisfaction with them. Both of these interpretations were at odds with other qualitative evidence.

Interestingly, very high satisfaction scores are also common in relationship studies in the West (Stanley Gaines, personal communication). Researchers have thought that this was due to the fact that those with more positive relationships would be more likely to volunteer for a relationship survey. Our suggestion is rather different, that the high scores reflect the strength of the 'happy family' ideology and its centrality to understandings of wellbeing. Paradoxically, then, it may be that the very centrality of family relationships to social reproduction and to wellbeing makes it hard to produce an accurate metric for them. Personal factors also play a role in shaping what scores are given. In our case studies, Mangali's lower scores for the close relationship domain did not seem to reflect less happy relationships but a greater freedom with respect to the ideology, and Gulabi's consistently high scores seem to reflect her strong awareness of social prestige and weaker breakdown position. Overall, the analysis here constitutes a warning against taking such scores at face value in comparing levels of wellbeing, between domains, between people, or between contexts.

The second part of the paper presented case studies of two unusually empowered women. These provide an opportunity to listen to the way they described their lives in their own terms rather than being constrained by how the survey 'allows' people to answer, muffling the specific tones of their own voice. While one woman spoke in an unusually open way from the outset, with the other, it took the passage of time and many meetings for her to gradually reveal a quite complex, polyvocal narrative.

The studies drew attention to a number of issues which bear on women's wellbeing in close relationships in this context and point to directions for future research. The first is violence. The quantitative survey produced the interesting finding that men's violence in the home has a more negative effect on men's sense of wellbeing than it does on women's. This indicates possible scope for a new approach to mobilisation against gender violence amongst men. Both women, however, had experienced violence in the family earlier in their lives and it had had long-lasting consequences. For Mangali, it was one of the reasons for moving to live separately with her husband away from his parents. For Gulabi, it instilled a sense of caution and wariness, to behave in such a way that violence would not become an issue in her marital home.

The second theme that arose in characterising women's wellbeing in close relationships was work. Thapan (2003: 81) emphasises the importance of work to the sense of wellbeing amongst women in Delhi slums:

> Any sense of well-being they had came, to a large extent, from their engagement with, and commitment to, their work.

While Thapan here is referring implicitly to paid employment, the links between work and wellbeing in our research were more varied. It was striking, for example, how often men and women referred to work and the need for co-operation in and between various forms of labour, in describing the dynamics of their close relationships. This again suggests the intertwining of material, relational and subjective dimensions of wellbeing that is a recurring theme throughout this volume. Within the case studies, Mangali stressed the 'work' of having to take the lead in representing the family and negotiating on their joint behalf, contrasting their practice with what she felt was the appropriate gender division of labour. Gulabi stressed frequently the amount of work she had to do and this was also quite visible in our many encounters with her. Work in the house was required of her not only to ensure the material reproduction of the home and family, but also as a form of labour in upholding the quality of relationships. Work outside the house she also justified in terms of her family responsibilities, but there was a much greater sense that this was something (also) for her personal fulfilment, rather than something simply done under compulsion.

The third theme concerns speech and silence. Constructions of relationship wellbeing in the West place considerable emphasis on the relationship as a place of spoken intimacy. In this research, both qualitative and quantitative data and analysis suggest that in this community, there is much greater emphasis on the shared intimacy of understanding that does not need to be put into words, of the materiality of living side by side and providing care to one another, and indeed the hazard of speaking what is in one's heart. Doing, not talking, seems to provide the dominant idiom of family relations in this context. This clearly requires further research, but it again indicates the importance of grounding measures of wellbeing within a particular context, rather than assuming a 'universal' model will be appropriate for all.

This chapter clearly illustrates the implication of research methods in the accounts of wellbeing they produce. The particular relationship that is established between researcher and respondent is also of great importance. Although the chapter presents only parts of both women's narratives, in both cases, there are continuities between what they say in response to survey questions and in qualitative interviews. In addition to using the quantitative data in a conventional way at the aggregate level to test a hypothesis, this suggests there is merit in subjecting the numbers to a more qualitative approach, reading an individual's scores against their larger narrative which unfolds over time.

Finally, this chapter confirms the general observation that close relationships are of great importance to wellbeing. It draws attention in addition, however, to the conditional character of harmony in the home, and the material and emotional labour that women put into sustaining this. This reinforces arguments made elsewhere in this book about the importance of viewing both wellbeing and relationship as process rather than state, and indeed of the fact that such processes are not neutral, but deeply implicated in power.

Acknowledgements

This chapter would not have been possible without the work of many others. These are Stanley O. Gaines Jr., who provided the statistical analysis that validated the IWB model and undertook the descriptive analysis of the 2011 quantitative data; and Antonia Fernandez, who undertook the descriptive analysis of the 2013 quantitative data. In Chhattisgarh, special thanks are due to Chaupal and Gangaram Paikra for supporting the research, and to our local team of peer researchers: Pritam Das, Usha Kujur, Kanti Minjh, and Dinesh Tirkey; plus Susanna Siddiqui and Abhay Xaxa (2011 only) and Kanhaiya Yadav and Laxman Singh (2013 only).

Notes

1. This work is supported by the Economic and Social Research Council/Department for International Development Joint Scheme for Research on International Development (Poverty Alleviation) grant number RES-167-25-0507 ES/H033769/1.
2. Pseudonyms have been used following convention.
3. The other domains are self-acceptance, autonomy, environmental mastery, purpose in life and personal growth.
4. Seligman's other elements are positive emotion, engagement, meaning and accomplishment.
5. The findings are based on a single self-report item on satisfaction with life.
6. The logic, they argue, is that more introverted and dissatisfied people will find it harder to find a partner, while happier people are more attractive and fun to be with (Stutzer and Frey 2006: 329). An alternative explanation could be that people with lower expectations are more likely to settle into marriage, and also to report themselves as satisfied with their lives!
7. Kolkata was formerly known as Calcutta. This is the term that appears in these articles.
8. See http://www.wellbeingpathways.org.uk for more information.
9. The other domains are economic confidence, agency and participation, social connections, physical and mental health, competence and self-worth, and values and meaning.
10. For a detailed description of the Indian field sites, see White *et al.* (2012a).
11. The term 'Adivasi', literally meaning original inhabitants, refers as a whole to communities that have traditionally lived in and depended on the forests for their livelihoods. While it is sometimes used interchangeably with the officially designated term 'Scheduled Tribes', which marks Adivasi communities for special benefits from the government, the two terms are not necessarily coterminous (Bijoy 2003).
12. As elsewhere in North India, a man may move to live with his parents-in-law if they have land but no sons, so he can provide labour on their land.
13. The domain score for close relationships is based on the three items that emerged through factor analysis, as discussed above. The mean scores across the other domains similarly exclude a few rogue items shown by correlations and factor analysis.
14. Factor analysis suggests that it belongs to the social connections domain.
15. Our sample was composed of married men and women and single women, so this finding is not able to capture any differences between men by marital

status. Nevertheless, gender is significant at p < 0.01 (coefficient 0.1661) and marital status is significant at p < 0.05 (coefficient 0.1208).
16. Analysis of the 2011 data, the year of Mangali's interview, showed that gender/marital status did not predict the close relationships domain score, though it did predict significantly IWB considered as a single factor and some of the other domains (White *et al.* 2012a: 53–54). The fact that the 4.62 average close relationship domain score includes both men and women does not therefore form part of the explanation of why Mangali's score should be so different from the norm.
17. The narrative of mothers-in-law and daughters-in-law not getting along is part-and-parcel of joint family life in India. It is understood that daughters-in-law bear their mothers-in-law's abuse as long as they are in a subservient position in the household. This changes with the passage of time, most usually when the mother-in-law is widowed (see Kandiyoti 1998, Palriwala 1999).
18. The open school system allows candidates to appear at school examinations through a self-study programme rather than mandatory school attendance and is especially favoured by people who have been unable to complete their school at the appropriate age.
19. The *panchayat* is the lowest rung of the local self-government institutions; members are elected directly by the *gram sabha* which comprises all the adult (18+ years of age) members of the village community. *Panchayat* members are involved in overseeing the delivery of almost all government welfare schemes, especially the flagship rural employment guarantee (MNREGS) and subsidised food distribution (PDS) (but not restricted to these). They are also in charge of making the lists of people targeted by these schemes, which makes them quite powerful locally.
20. As described above for the close relationship domain, the 2013 survey built on learning from 2011, so some of the items making up the domains were different in the two years. In 2013, we also had five items per domain, rather than four. As with Mangali's domain scores, these reflect the items that were validated through factor analysis.
21. In 2013, the items for this domain were: how well are your gods and goddesses looking after you? How lucky have you been in your life? How much peace do you experience in your mind/heart? To what extent would you say that you fear harm from witchcraft or evil powers? To what extent do you feel that life has been good to you?
22. This suggests the importance of economics to subjectivities, as argued with respect to Zambia in Chapter 5.

References

Abeyasekera, A. (2013) *The Choosing Person: Marriage, Middle-Class Identities and Modernity in Contemporary Sri Lanka*. Unpublished PhD thesis, University of Bath.

Agarwal, B. (1996) *A Field of One's Own: Gender and Land Rights in South Asia*. New Delhi: Cambridge University Press.

Ahmed, S. (2010) *The Promise of Happiness*. Durham and London: Duke University Press.

Bijoy, C. R. (2003) The Adivasis of India. A History of Discrimination, Conflict and Resistance. *People's Union for Civil Liberties Bulletin*. February. Available at: http://www.pucl.org/Topics/Dalit-tribal/2003/adivasi.html [Accessed 12 July 2015].

Biswas-Diener, R. and Diener, E. (2001) Making the Best of a Bad Situation: Satisfaction in the Slums of Calcutta. *Social Indicators Research* 55: 329–352.

Biswas-Diener, R. and Diener, E. (2006) The Subjective Well-Being of the Homeless, and Lessons for Happiness. *Social Indicators Research* 55: 185–205.

Bryman, A. (2001) *Quantity and Quality in Social Research*. Abingdon: Routledge.

Camfield, L., Choudhury, K. and Devine, J. (2009) Well-Being, Happiness and Why Relationships Matter: Evidence from Bangladesh. *Journal of Happiness Studies* 10: 71–91.

Fernandez, A., White, S.C. and Jha, S. (2014) *Wellbeing Pathways Report. India Round Two*. Available at: http://www.wellbeingpathways.org/images/stories/pdfs/working_papers/India_T2_report_FINAL_whole.pdf [Accessed 12 July 2015].

Glenn, N. (1975) The Contribution of Marriage to the Psychological Well-Being of Males and Females. *Journal of Marriage and Family* 37(3): 594–600.

Gove, W., Hughes, M. and Briggs, C. (1983) Does Marriage Have Positive Effects on the Psychological Well-Being of the Individual? *Journal of Health and Social Behavior* 24(2): 122–131.

Jeffery, P. and Jeffery, R. (1996) *Don't Marry Me to a Plowman! Women's Everyday Lives in Rural North India*. Boulder, CO and Oxford: Westview Press.

Kandiyoti, D. (1998) Gender Power and Contestation: Rethinking Bargaining with Patriarchy. pp. 135–151 in C. Jackson and R. Pearson (eds.) *Feminist Visions of Development: Gender Analysis and Policy*. London: Routledge.

Murphy-Graham, E. (2010) And When She Comes Home? Education and Women's Empowerment in Intimate Relationships. *International Journal of Educational Development* 30(3): 320–331.

Myers, D. G. (1999) Close Relationship and Quality of Life. pp. 374–391 in D. Kahneman, E. Diener and N. Schwarz (eds.) *Well-Being: The Foundations of Hedonic Psychology*. New York: Russell Sage Foundation.

Palriwala, R. (1999) Beyond Myths: The Social and Political Dynamics of Gender. pp. 49–79 in N. Kabeer and R. Subramanian (eds.) *Institutions, Relations and Outcomes: A Framework and Case-Studies for Gender-Aware Planning*. New Delhi: Kali for Women.

Rowlands, J. (1997) *Questioning Empowerment: Working with Women in Honduras*. Oxford: Oxfam.

Ryan, R. M. and Deci, E. L. (2001) On Happiness and Human Potentials: A Review of Research on Hedonic and Eudaimonic Well-Being. *American Psychological Review* (52): 141–166.

Ryff, C. D. (1989) Happiness Is Everything, or Is It? Explorations on the Meaning of Psychological Well-Being. *Journal of Personality and Social Psychology* 57(6): 1069–1081.

Ryff, C. D. and Singer, B. H. (2008) Know Thyself and Become What You Are: A Eudaimonic Approach to Psychological Well-Being. *Journal of Happiness Studies* 9(1): 13–39.

Seligman, M. (2011) *Flourish: A Visionary New Understanding of Happiness and Wellbeing*. London/New York: Free Press.

Sen, A. (1987) Gender and Co-operative Conflicts. *Wider Working Paper 18*. Helsinki: World Institute for Development Economics Research.

Stutzer, A. and Frey, B. (2006) Does Marriage Make People Happy, or Do Happy People Get Married? *The Journal of Socio-Economics* 35(2006): 326–347.

Thapan, M. (2003) Marriage, Well-Being, and Agency among Women. *Gender and Development* 11(2): 77–84.

Uberoi, P. (1994) Introduction. pp. 1–44 in P. Uberoi (ed.) *Family, Kinship and Marriage in India*. New Delhi: Oxford University Press.

White, S.C. (1992) *Arguing with the Crocodile: Gender and Class in Bangladesh*. London and New Jersey/Dhaka: Zed Books/University Press.

White, S. C., Gaines Jr. S., Jha, S. and Marshall, N. (2012a) Wellbeing Pathways Report: India Round 1. *Wellbeing and Poverty Pathways*. University of Bath. Available at: http://www.wellbeingpathways.org/images/stories/pdfs/working_papers/indiatime1report.pdf

White, S. C., Gaines Jr. S., Jha, S., Marshall, N. and Graveling. E. (2012b) Wellbeing Pathways Report: Zambia Round 1. *Wellbeing and Poverty Pathways*. University of Bath. Available at: http://www.wellbeingpathways.org/images/stories/pdfs/working_papers/zambiatime1report.pdf

White, S. C, Gaines, S. O. and Jha, S. (2014) Inner Wellbeing: Concept and Validation of a New Approach to Subjective Perceptions of Wellbeing: India. *Social Indicators Research* 119(2): 723–746. DOI: 10.1007/s11205-013-0504-7.

White, S. C. and Jha, S. (2014) The Ethical Imperative of Qualitative Methods in Developing Measures of Subjective Dimensions of Wellbeing in Zambia and India. *Ethics and Social Welfare* 8(3): 262–276. DOI: 10.1080/17496535.2014.932416.

White, S. C., Fernandez, A. and Jha, S. (forthcoming) Beyond the Grumpy Rich Man and the Happy Peasant: Using Mixed Methods to Explore Policy Impact on Subjective Dimensions of Wellbeing. *Oxford Development Studies*.

Xaxa, V. (2004) Women and Gender in the Study of Tribes in India. *Indian Journal of Gender Studies* 11(3): 345–367.

Part II
Qualitative Research

7
The Dynamics of Relational Wellbeing in the Context of Mobility in Peru

Rebecca Huovinen and Chloe Blackmore

Introduction

Relationships are recognised as an important dimension of wellbeing across each of the four concepts outlined by White (Chapter 1, this volume): subjective wellbeing, psychological wellbeing, capabilities and relational wellbeing. This chapter explores the relational wellbeing of residents of Esperanza, a shantytown on the outskirts of Lima, Peru in the context of mobility and relationships across distance. Much of the wider migration-development debate has focused on flows of remittances and, to a lesser extent, on diaspora resources (Castles and Delgado Wise 2007, De Haas and Rodríguez 2010). Yet many have acknowledged the need to move beyond this socio-economic focus (Castles and Delgado Wise 2007, DeWind and Holdaway eds. 2008, International Organization for Migration [IOM] 2010) and support for a wellbeing perspective is beginning to gain momentum (IOM 2013, Wright 2010, 2011, 2012, Wright and Black 2011). While the focus in the migration-development debate and the wider migration literature is on *international* migration (IOM 2005, King and Skeldon 2010, Laczko 2008), the majority of poor people in developing countries move within rather than between countries (de Haan and Yaqub 2009, King and Skeldon 2010, Migration, Globalisation and Poverty [MGP] 2009, Sorensen *et al.* 2003).

In Peru, mobility has become a necessary and integral aspect of livelihoods (Leinaweaver 2008, Paerregaard 1997, Sorensen 2002). Moving is part of the search to get ahead (*salir adelante*) (Huovinen 2013, Takenaka and Pren 2010). People talk about leaving the community, going to another place, coming and going between places, between here and there, going to live in other places, going away and being away. These expressions convey a sense of routineness, naturalness and normality of movement in people's lives. These movements are often multiple and complex, beginning from a young age, and give the impression that individuals and their families are involved in an ongoing journey entailing multiple movements over the course of their lives.

Mobility inevitably entails a rupture in relationships with close family, separating parents, children, siblings and others with implications for wellbeing. Drawing on in-depth 'mobility stories', this chapter explores the relational dynamics of mobility in Peru. It illustrates how key relationships with family matter to people especially in the context of insecure community relations, how people rework their relationships with family when they become separated through mobility and the sense of responsibility and commitment to care in these relationships, which is strongly gendered. The relational is closely intertwined with the emotional and material and is experienced differently by men and women and at different stages in the lifecycle.

In contrast to the wider migration literature which has tended to place emphasis on the positive, harmonious, resilient and cohesive nature of migrant network ties (see Åkesson et al. 2012, Tapias and Escandell 2011), the chapter paints a picture of struggle and fragility, and a sense that people could not always accomplish what they desired in (re)establishing family relationships and maintaining connections across distance. An in-depth look at the relational offers a more nuanced understanding of relationships than the instrumental concepts of social capital or social resources often used by development researchers. Here, the relational emphasises power hierarchies and axes of difference (White 2010). It brings sensitivity to relations being a source of harm, conflict and constraint as well as of care and support, and shows the contradictory demands often placed on women in relation to their natal kin and their own partner and children.

Esperanza

This chapter draws on in-depth fieldwork carried out by the first author of this paper, Rebecca Huovinen, in 2007. With the assistance of a local field researcher, Lida Carhuallanqui, a series of 52 narrative interviews were carried out based on the 'mobility stories' of residents of Esperanza, a shantytown on the outskirts of Lima, Peru. The settlement of Esperanza was established with support from the municipality of

Lima in 1985 and was initially occupied by 10,000 families from other lower class settlements in eastern Lima. In exchange for a moderate sum and membership of an accredited Lima-based migrants' association, families were given the right to a piece of land on which to build a house (Meneses 1998). The settlement grew rapidly in the 1990s and into the new millennium, with newcomers constantly arriving. In 2005, the population was estimated to be at least 112,410 (Alvarez and Arroyo 2005). A sample survey[1] collected in 2004 found that the majority (72 per cent, $n = 133$) of Esperanza residents were born in a department outside of Lima. Esperanza thus represents a place of high mobility.

Peru is administratively divided into 25 departments which are subdivided into 195 provinces and 1,833 districts. It is made up of three broad geographical landscapes which divide the country into the *costa* (coast), *sierra* (highlands) and the *selva* (rainforest). The coast refers to the narrow coastal plain and the western slopes of the Andes up to a height of 1,950 m; the *sierra* to the Andes Mountains above 1,950 m; and the *selva* to the eastern slopes of the Andes and the Amazon headwaters (Lloyd 1980).

Poverty is widespread in Esperanza, with many living close to the official extreme poverty line (Copestake *et al.* 2008). While homes in the most developed central or lower areas have gradually replaced their bamboo/straw matting with bricks and cement, adding upper floors as they become more established, homes in the higher, expanding zones are constructed from rustic materials including wood panelling and bamboo/straw matting. The central areas have secured access to electricity, water, sewerage/sanitation and many have a phone connection, whereas the higher areas lack access to these services. There is a public hospital, health posts, private health facilities and a proliferation of educational facilities, both public and private institutions for primary, secondary and higher education (Alvarez and Arroyo 2005). The settlement is well connected to central Lima and surrounding areas – minibuses and mototaxis operate within the settlement taking people to the central highway, and from the highway, there are frequent minibuses/buses into central Lima taking around two hours. Issues of alcoholism, violence, gangs, crime, drug consumption and drug trafficking are all prevalent within the community (Alvarez and Arroyo 2005).

Mobility stories

The interviews took the form of mobility stories or 'personal stories' (Ryan 2004) about the different places people had lived over the course of their lives. A key factor shaping the development of this method was the first author's previous research with the Wellbeing in Developing Countries (WeD) research group in Peru. This research used semi-structured interviews to explore goals, aspirations and expectations of movement and the extent to which these had been achieved. It was striking how much people talked about the dynamics of interpersonal relationships, particularly family relations (see Lockley et al. 2008). There was a strong 'relational layer' in the narratives (Mason 2004). However, this rather prescribed and structured approach at times deflected from and restricted the extent to which respondents' own stories could be told. The research reported here thus took a less structured approach to elicit free-flowing narratives in order to excavate the layers of mobility in people's lives. Mobility stories sought to gain a 'movie' of mobility experiences as on-going moments, a dynamic lived experience through time, rather than focusing on a 'snapshot' (or specific mobility event) (McGregor 2007: 25–26). They also sought to bring 'others' (even distant ones) more vividly into the movie. Narratives are 'shaped by the environments in which they are formed' (Burrell 2006: 16); therefore stories are not just about 'the personal', decontextualising individual lives, but also about the personal in the broader socio-cultural context (Mitchell 2006). In interpreting people's stories, therefore, I was concerned to locate experiences of movement within the wider socio-cultural environment to explore how this context impacts on their understandings (Grbich 2007).

The interviews were mostly unstructured with a checklist of broad thematic areas and probe questions if needed. Some interviews became more structured when individuals were less comfortable speaking at length about their lives and needed more direction and prompting than others. This was more common amongst male interviewees than female. Following the collection of basic demographic details, interviews began by inviting people to talk about the different places they had lived over the course of their lives. As others have found (e.g. Mason 2000), this proved to be a good and familiar medium for people to organise and talk about their life stories. It also provided an appropriate medium for people to talk about more 'private' issues including personal relations and domestic life (Kothari and Hulme 2004). Interviews also covered experiences of living apart from family, who interviewees turned to when they needed help and the ways in which people maintained relations with family, especially close family, from whom they were spatially separated. Family was defined broadly to include inter- and intra-generational relatives, across locations (Ryan et al. 2009). This included at times extending to more distant relatives who were felt to be particularly close and to those who were felt to be 'like family', even though not conventionally defined as kin (Mason and Tipper 2008).

The people interviewed mostly came from one neighbourhood in the higher areas of Esperanza with more recent arrivals. Some residents of the central, more established area were also interviewed. The interviewees differed in terms of gender, age, lifecycle stage and time of residence in the community. The majority were Catholic, had a low level of education and were doing low-paid, insecure and temporary jobs as and when they could find them. Women tended to be based at home looking after children and pursuing economic activities around childcare and domestic activities. A large proportion of the working population left the settlement daily or weekly for central Lima to work mainly in factories, retailing and domestic service (Alvarez *et al.* 2008). The majority of interviewees (69 per cent) originated from the *sierra* region of Peru or had parents who came from there (15 per cent). Most had lived in Esperanza for six years or more at the time of research.

Relational anchoring

The intrinsic importance of relationships with family emerged through the mobility stories of Esperanza. Samuel is 47 years old and single. He grew up in Cerro de Pasco (highlands, Department of Pasco, c. 300 km from Lima), the youngest of seven siblings, where he stayed until he was 20 years old. He then made a series of movements before settling in Esperanza at 36 years of age where he now works as a teacher. Samuel's mother and two of his six siblings still live in the village; his father has died. Samuel's other siblings are spatially dispersed, one lives in an urban area of Cerro de Pasco, one sister is in Huancayo and two sisters are also living in Esperanza. He explains the importance of his family, despite being geographically distant from them.

> There's nobody like family, family protects you, takes care of you, worries about you, at least you have someone no? Someone you can trust... if there's a family behind you, you have someone to share with, someone to be happy with and you don't feel alone, no?... family is fundamental, it is where one can fulfil oneself.

The term 'relational anchoring' is useful here. It was introduced by Auyero and Swistun (2008) in their research in an Argentinean shantytown to explain how residents have become attached to and taken roots in the neighbourhood through work, family and friendship networks. Activities of building families, enjoying friends and working are identified as 'anchoring routines' and these routines work to root residents in the community. However, anchoring points change over time (e.g. through the life course and inter-generationally) and across space (e.g. as people themselves move and as relatives become spatially dispersed through mobility). In the context of mobility, relational anchoring can also describe the ways in which relations with close family living outside of the community are re-worked. Relational anchoring is conveyed in the Esperanza narratives by a sense of togetherness and closeness and is based on relations of affection, love and warmth (*cariño*). This sense of anchoring is not solely restricted to kin relations but also develops through 'having lived together' or 'been raised together'. It expresses a sense of belonging and attachment, and reveals how these key relations are central to one's sense of self.

Family relations are important to wellbeing in a number of ways. As Samuel identifies above, family relations are often viewed as the only trustworthy ones. This is particularly important as community relations in Esperanza are felt to be insecure, characterised by a widespread lack of trust and suspicion. Family relations are also a key, and often only, source of economic support. Yet the meaning of family extends beyond mechanisms for transfers, reciprocal exchanges and flows of resources or remittances. It is the intrinsic emotional value and meaning derived from family relations which gives a sense of anchoring to people's lives. Family are an important source of wellbeing in their own right (Lloyd-Sherlock and Locke 2008). Interestingly, the Andean conceptualisation of poverty is intimately linked with a lack of kin relations. Translated literally, *waqcha* refers to a person who has very little or nothing (materially), but is also a person who has nobody, no family or relatives, or very few relatives (Altamirano 1988, Degregori *et al.* 1986, Programa de las Naciones Unidas para el Desarrollo [PNUD] 2002, Skar 1994). By contrast, *apu* refers to a person who not only has material wealth, but also a large network of kin that can be relied upon (Isbell 1977).

The importance of relational anchoring is signified by the emotional disruption associated with movement and separation from family. This is expressed in the interviews in terms of 'having *pena*', a socially-culturally elaborated profound sense of sorrow and extreme sadness, which may persist long into the future (see also Tousignant and Maldonado 1989, Van Vleet 2008). Bertha is 65 years old and a widow, she was born in Junin (highlands, c. 300 km from Lima) and she made several moves within the highlands with her husband for his work and returned to Junin following his death. Bertha moved to Lima at the age of 48 to live with her sister and her daughter; ten years later she moved to Esperanza where she now lives with her son. Another son also lives in Lima. Bertha's village of origin in Junin remains a key anchoring point in her life. She is particularly close to her maternal uncle (*tio*) who lives there whom she calls 'dad' or her '*tio papa*'. Bertha shows how *pena* can motivate connection.

> Sometimes in his dreams he thinks about me, me as well, sometimes. I call him by surprise. He says to me, 'daughter, how are you?' 'I'm well dad', I say... 'I dreamt about you, you were sad', he tells me. 'No dad, I'm well', I tell him... he misses me a lot, a lot.

Pena and worry are intimately linked and motivate connection through phone calls and visits. When communicating with her *tio papa* Bertha feels *tranquila* (content/tranquil), an emotion which contrasts with *pena*. *Tranquila* reflects a sense of emotional wellbeing, characterised by calmness, peace of mind, a feeling of contentment and of being without problems. News from her sister who lives in another district of Lima about her *tio papa* also eases her *pena*.

> I feel *tranquila*, sometimes my sister arrives with the news that she went to Junin and he's [her *tio papa*] *tranquilo*... and it alleviates me a lot, it relieves me.

Pena also evokes collective response. Bertha shows how expressing *pena* mobilises her family to draw around her, to help her to overcome her *pena*.

> My son [says] let's go, let's go, you're sad, let's go, go to Junin, take this money and go to Junin... they [her children] look after me. 'Mum, you have *pena*, you have *pena* about your house, your uncle, the cemetery. Go!'

Tousignant and Maldonado (1989) also found in Ecuador that those suffering from *pena* attract attention from others; *pena* encourages people to improve relationships with the social network and family. Bertha's son who she lives with acts to try to overcome her *pena* by giving her money to travel back to her village. When returning to Lima she feels happier and more content in herself. During visits, Bertha gives fruit, sweets or bread to her *tio papa*'s family. She explains, 'I never arrive empty handed,

I always arrive with my hands full', and 'that makes them feel more and love me more'. There were numerous references in the narratives of giving gifts/money as expressions of love, care and affection, and the emphasis is often on the symbolic act of giving rather than the material value.

Childhood, abandonment and ambiguous relations

In Esperanza, many of the narratives revealed ambiguities and contradictions in finding and maintaining a sense of relational anchoring. They paint a picture of considerable struggle which is experienced differently at different stages in the lifecycle and by men and women.

A common pattern in the interviews was of child or youth mobility where children and young people are separated from their parents and go to live and work with *tias* and *tios*, often when parents have many young children who they cannot support. It reflects widespread and deeply rooted cultural practices in the Andes of adoption, fostering, 'child circulation' and using children, especially daughters, as domestic labour (Anderson *et al.* 2006, Carrasco 2010, Deere 1990, Leinaweaver 2008, Weismantel 2001). This is especially common in the context of poverty and insecurity. Anderson *et al.* (2006) have introduced the notion of the '*sistema de tias*' (system of aunts) to show how networks of *tias* have become institutionalised in child domestic labour. The *tia* is not always a 'true' *tia*, a parent's sibling, but often a more distant relative, for example a parent's cousin, or a fellow *paisana* (from the same village) known in the rural community. In some cases, the precise relation of the '*tia*' was not clear.

The expectation is that children and young people go to live with an aunt, working in the home, looking after children, or working in the family business and in exchange receive food, shelter, the opportunity to study and sometimes payment. It is important to recognise the heterogeneity of experiences of these living situations. Some (mainly males) reflected more positive experiences in the homes they lived in: they went to 'good' aunts or uncles indicating that they experienced the 'warmth and affection of a family' or were 'like friends', shared activities together (e.g. eating together, watching TV), were treated well and were able to study. Although some males did express sorrow, suffering and isolation, their narratives were notably more positive and shaped by a masculine discourse of becoming economically independent. This could be partly because men are less conditioned to express emotion in this way (see Lloyd-Sherlock and Locke 2008). Nevertheless, they tended to emphasise the freedom and independence gained through working from an early age and 'making one's own life', not needing to be dependent on others. These male interviewees appeared to be currently managing financially with steady work or running their own businesses. For example Nicolas started working from the age of eight and spent his adolescence living apart from his parents and siblings. He explains how he used to be enslaved by work, working day and night without rest, but that now he's enjoying life, he's made progress, has his own home and business, is living well and that he feels content (*tranquilo*) with his position in life.

While this movement of children can work well for some, many (mainly women) reported that they were given little or no time to study due to long working hours, received no or very little payment and frequently experienced abuse (physical, sexual and emotional), humiliation and maltreatment. The ambiguity of these living situations emerged strongly in the narratives. It was often unclear whether the living situation was one of 'staying with relatives', or a position of domestic service, as it often had elements of both. In these situations, interviewees spoke of creating 'family-like' relations, for example, being 'like a daughter' or calling those they lived with '*tia*' or 'like a mother', trying to form a close, personal relationship (see also Gill 1994, Young 1987). This seemed particularly significant in contexts of abandonment and rupture in close family relations and reveals the need to establish relations and to build a moral proximity of responsibilities and obligations, relations that one can rely on and that act 'like family'.

Lucia is 35 years old and lives with her children in Esperanza; she runs a small shop from her home and this is her only source of income. Her husband left the country several years ago to work in Ecuador. At first he made return visits and contributed to the household income but he is no longer in contact with her and their children. Lucia was born in Lima. When she was five years old her mother died and a few years later her father took her and her sister back to live in his village of origin in Cusco (c. 1,100 km from Lima). Lucia's father was violent and physically abusive towards her. From the age of nine, Lucia embarked on a cycle of mobility, moving to the city of Cusco and then back to Lima, rotating around various aunts (*tias*) and uncles (*tios*), some of whom were distant relatives and others who were *paisanos* (from the same village in Cusco). She recalls these moves as an escape from her father and talks about her childhood and youth as a time of immense sadness. This pain has continued in her life.

> ...it stays with you, from childhood it stays with you, for me as well, I always remember...I don't want to keep on remembering though,

it's something awful that you feel in your heart [crying], I don't want to remember.

Lucia's mobility story is framed by her search for affection (*cariño*) in the different homes she moved to. In each home she lived in, Lucia tried to gain the love and affection of those she was living with, by working hard, being helpful and obliging. Lucia explains:

> I wanted them to love me, seeing as I didn't have *cariño*, well I did from my mum when she was alive, my father was distant, I wanted to feel *cariño* and my father said they're going to love you, so I was helpful.

Tamagno (2002) has identified the discourse of 'winning somebody's affection' as a cultural strategy of adjustment and adaptation in the context of movement, to enable people to establish and maintain social relations. Tamagno argues that winning the affection and love of others 'has been fundamental to surviving in the midst of difficult family situations and frequent moves' (Tamagno 2002: 108) and that the feelings generated by being accepted, winning *cariño*, or being rejected are fundamental to the children's wellbeing.

Working hard to make others love her involved Lucia in forms of exploitation, submission and unequal relations which convey the 'ambiguous affections' in these family environments (Goldstein 2003), relations that were at times both affectionate and exploitative. Some however, never felt 'like family', especially when a child was living with more distant relatives or non-relatives and with a greater social/class distance.

While longing for love can mean children put up with abuse for many years, there often comes a point when they have had enough. Lucia, who moved to Lima to her *tia* Maria at 11 years old, identifies a key turning point in her life when she 'woke up' to the way she was being exploited by her *tia* and became more assertive. At 15 years old she decided to leave her *tia* Maria.

> I left from there because...I realised...I started to complain a little because they exploited me a lot, too much. So as I already started to wake up...I wanted to escape.

Other women similarly described a degree of agency as they related the ways they contested, confronted and 'escaped' from exploitative and abusive living situations, moving onto other homes, from *tia* to *tia*. Agency is widely recognised as an important dimension of wellbeing (Devine *et al.* 2008, Ryan and Deci 2001, Sen 2009). However, often the women moved on to a similar situation, experiencing similar levels of maltreatment and abuse, being trapped in cycles of mobility and vulnerability. Lucia moved on to another *tio*, her father's half-brother, in Lima where she did not adapt or find *cariño*. She then went in search of her old neighbour Juana in La Victoria, Lima. It was here that she finally found and experienced the *cariño* and nurturing, the sense of anchoring, that she had been searching for.

> At this time I didn't say mum, *tia* I said to her, *tia* Juana, *tia* Juana, *tia* until there, since I was 16 years old, when I lived with her, then I knew that, it's like, how can I tell you, it's to live like [crying] like you have to live without maltreatment, without... [crying]... even the shampoo, my *tia* never let me wash my hair with shampoo always with Ace [detergent for washing clothes]... whereas with her I began to know... how a mum is, or how a family actually is, how they love you, not washing with Ace, she gave me shampoo... well I was 16 years old and they, they treated me how it should be and I liked that. From there, how I was living with my mum, I started to live.

The impact on Lucia's wellbeing of finding *mama* Juana and receiving the *cariño* and quality of treatment that she needed is evident. Her closeness to *mama* Juana was also related to her shared knowledge, experiences and memories of her biological mother when she was alive. They used to live next to each other before her mother's death. This maternal connection seems significant to Lucia and is a theme which emerged strongly in other narratives, illuminating the importance of emotional attachment and nurturing in the mother–child relation (Boyden and Mann 2005). In the absence of a mother, a maternal connection in other relationships is particularly significant, for example a maternal grandparent, maternal aunt or uncle, or as in Lucia's case, shared experiences and memories of a mother. Juana had been a close friend of Lucia's mother – they were 'like a family'.

However, despite finding a sense of anchoring with Juana and what appears to be a less exploitative work situation, this relation was not without ambiguity. Lucia highlights the limits or boundaries to her relation with *mama* Juana. Although she is 'like a daughter', she is not 'as a daughter'. Lucia does not share the material benefits and commitments that *mama* Juana shares with her 'true' daughters, for example, in terms of supporting her education or buying her new clothes. This was particularly evident when Lucia's future husband went to visit *mama* Juana to seek her permission for their marriage. Lucia and her husband tried actively to cement the relationship with Juana, to ask her to be the godmother (*madrina*) for their marriage, which entails an obligation to sponsor the wedding and to help the couple set up a household and keep it together (Isbell 1977). However, Juana declined and persuaded Lucia to ask her *tia* Maria, her mother's cousin who raised her for five years instead. As a single mother with four daughters, Juana probably could not afford to take on this financial commitment to the couple. This episode reveals the difficulty in breaking away from adverse and problematic relations when there are no other key relations to call upon, requiring Lucia's continued dependence on her aunt, from whom she had previously tried to escape. It also shows the moral content embedded in blood ties which is difficult to create and enforce in non-kin relations.

While a mother's absence in particular was deeply felt, much was left unsaid in the narratives in relation to a father's abandonment. This suggests a tacit acceptance of a father's absence in contrast to an expectation of 'always present' mothers, nurturing, caring and physically present. These gendered differences in how separation from mothers and fathers is experienced compare with other studies which find that children talk about the lack of care received from their mothers while rarely blaming their fathers (Parreñas 2005, Zontini 2010). In narratives where a father's absence was spoken about, although some lamented the lack of a father's affection, in general a father's absence was couched in terms of a lack of provisioning, in particular not providing an education for their child and the chance to become professionals, to 'become someone', which is consistent with the wider socio-cultural idiom of making progress through education. Felix (40 years old) was 'abandoned' first by his father who left his mother when she was pregnant with him and subsequently by his step-father. He comments that he was like 'a second household head', taking care of his siblings as detailed below. Felix feels that if his father had been present during his childhood he would have become a professional and taken a different pathway in life. The absence of his father is directly linked to his own struggle to fulfil notions of the responsible economic provider.

Lucia still talks of a 'lack' in her life, and her narrative, like others, shows a deep, enduring *pena* dominated by continued suffering, loneliness and isolation. This deep sense of emotional pain and upset is closely related to fragility and rupture in close kin relations. These narratives of childhood show how memories, past experiences and relationships, especially with close family members, influence current emotions and perceptions of current wellbeing (Lloyd-Sherlock and Locke 2008). Lucia's continual suffering cannot be divorced from the material conditions in which she lives. Lucia feels that she has had to continually struggle and fight in her life to make ends meet. This raises the issue of how people feel about their present affecting how they read their pasts and future (White 2008). Lucia's feelings of 'falling down', sorrow and suffering are intertwined with her lack of material resources, struggles to get by materially, as well as about her damaged relationships, maltreatment during childhood and abandonment by her husband. Almost all those who express an enduring sorrow and isolation were amongst the poorest, living in the higher zones of the community and were still struggling to establish themselves, access basic services and find stable work.

Middle years and conflicting anchoring points

For people in their middle years, conflict between different emotional anchoring points emerged as a strong theme. Maintaining anchoring to one's natal family (parents and siblings) and deepening anchoring to one's family of reproduction (partner/spouse and children) create competing and conflicting demands on people's limited and stretched resources. This results in a sense of tension within and between households, as sentimental and economic attachments to parents and siblings compete with developing economic, social and affective relationships with one's spouse and children (Van Vleet 2008). A strong morality of care, based on the cultural value of reciprocity, emerged in the narratives. A sense of shared responsibility amongst siblings towards parents, and within the family more generally, is expressed through making collective contributions to family members in need (*hacemos la bolsa*) and a rotation of care (caring *por turno*). Single siblings are viewed as the most available ones to provide hands-on care and support, and many (men and women) recalled sending money and goods, sometimes everything that they earned, back to their parents and siblings in places of origin when they were single.

Sofia is 25 years old. She moved to Esperanza from Apurimac (in the rainforest, c. 1,100 km from Lima) at the age of 15 years and has lived there for ten years. One sibling has now moved to live with her; her parents and other siblings have remained in Apurimac. Sofia emphasises how her need to focus her resources on the needs of her own household means that she struggles to afford the travel costs to visit her parents and to help with the coffee harvest. She also feels pressure to return with gifts for her relatives.

> When you go, I always want to go to my mum but at least taking something, no?... always your brothers and sisters are waiting, 'my sister she'll be bringing me [something]', when you arrive they start to look, imagine if you arrive with nothing.

Victor (42 years old) was born in Cusco. He moved 1,100 km to Lima with his older brother when he was eight years old and a couple of years later he moved to Puerto Maldonado (in the rainforest, c. 1,500 km from Lima) for work. Victor returned to Lima when he was 15 years old and has since made multiple moves around different districts of Lima. He explains that before he married he used to return to Cusco to visit his mother every year and that he always took many gifts for her (groceries, fruit). However, now because of his work, lack of time and his commitments to his daughters who live in Lima with his first partner, and his current partner and her children with whom he lives in Esperanza, he has not returned to visit his mother for several years. Two of Victor's older siblings still live in Cusco and 'watch over' his mother. His father has passed away. His other siblings live in different districts in Lima and a brother in Chincha (on the coast). Victor explains how amongst his siblings living in Lima,

> ...always we have a meeting between all the siblings here in Lima each three months, we all give a sum, what we can, we take it in turns, rotate,... we never forget her.... we don't say 'you brother this much', no, what we can. For example, in these three months I'm able to give more and the other trimester I can give less, it's like this.

This sense of shared responsibility of care for mothers (and fathers) simultaneously reinforces the ties to one another as siblings. For example, Samuel explains that the one time in the year when all his family get together is for his mother's birthday. His mother is elderly (87 years old) and he is concerned about how her death will impact on the relationship amongst his siblings.

> What unites us the most, what unites us greatly is our mum, no?... and when she dies, we're going to disintegrate maybe, or we're going to become distanced.

The need to focus on one's family of reproduction (partner/spouse and children) is to a certain extent expected and accepted, but this appears to be more the case for sons than for daughters. There seems to be a tacit acceptance of sons giving less support 'because he has his wife and children' or 'because they are married' yet there is still an expectation of the availability of a daughter who has a husband and children. As Pedro (60 years old) comments, 'There are sons who don't care a lot, daughters, yes, they're always with their mum.' Sons are viewed (and experienced by some) as being more likely to evade their responsibilities when they have their own family. In general, however, the sons/brothers that were interviewed did present themselves as continuing to support their parents/siblings, even when this brought tension and conflict within their own households. This points to the strong 'moral sway' of blood ties (Fonseca 1991).

Nicolas (38 years old) was born in Lima; his parents originated from the southern *sierra*. He is one of ten siblings, two of whom have migrated abroad. He started working from the age of eight years old and spent his childhood and adolescence moving around various relatives in other districts of Lima and in the highlands south of Lima. A masculine discourse of the loyal son/provider shapes Nicolas' narrative. Nicolas conveys how his continued financial support to his parents has created conflict with his wife as they were 'lacking' in their own household. He recalls when his father became ill and he covered the cost of his medicines.

> My partner didn't think the same, no, 'why must you give to him [his father]'? .... They're my parents, they have given to me, and now they need me.

Following his father's death, Nicolas' mother, who lives in another district of Lima, became ill:

> What happened? I decided to draw out everything that I have, all for my mum ... to cover her energy, her electricity, her water ... I have to give my mother what I have.

This caused further conflict with his wife because they needed the money in their own home.

Nicolas emphasises that he was the one who went out to work, to make a living, implying that it was his money and his decision about how it was spent.

In common with other narratives, Nicolas reveals strong notions of male dominance and authority (*machismo*) within the household. This leaves women with less control over resources and less say over where the money goes. As a result, their gendered roles as wives and mothers are fraught with contradiction. While there are clear notions that daughters should be dependable, reliable and 'available', women's subordinate position in their marital households means they face great difficulty in living up to these expectations and maintaining relations with their natal kin. Although many men did not appear to deny a woman's support to her family, they expressed the view that the husband/male partner has the power to decide and determine the type and level of support given, and that women must seek a man's permission and authorisation. As a result, women sometimes have to resort to subterfuge to continue to support their relatives, hiding what they are doing from their husbands/male partners. Justina (22 years old) explains, 'A daughter always, even hiding it from her husband, so that she gives (money, goods) to her mum.' When husbands/male partners do support a woman's relatives (e.g. through buying medicines, clothes, or having them to stay in the household), women consider themselves to be fortunate, the exception rather than the norm.

For some, in the context of an acute lack of material resources, the demands from competing anchors to one's immediate family and to kin become too great, leading to a withdrawal from relations, a 'forced isolation'. *Pena* is accentuated when people cannot maintain relations and fulfil their responsibilities as they desire. Irene (65 years old) is originally from the rainforest; she moved to Lima to join her children after separating from her husband. She then moved to Esperanza 11 years later with her son and looks after two of her grandchildren while her son works long hours as a driver. Irene identifies her step-mother as a key figure in her life, and details the love, care and nurturing she received from her. However, Irene feels guilt and sorrow that she does not have the resources to keep in touch with and help her step-mother. She cannot reciprocate the care that she received from her as a child. Irene cries in the interview as she comments,

> ...she brought me up, she provided for me, but I can't go to bring her here like she had me, I long to have her here, but one needs more resources... how much I want to make it up to her, to give her some support.

Felix (40 years old) was born in Cañete (coast, c. 160 km south of Lima); his parents both originated from the highlands (Huaraz and Ayacucho).

He moved to Lima in his adolescence and has lived in Esperanza for ten years. Felix depends on temporary jobs in construction, as a porter in markets and as a bus-ticket collector to provide for the household. His wife stays at home looking after their son and suffers from ill health. Felix reveals how his struggle to meet the daily subsistence needs of his own household has forced him to withdraw support and connection from his mother who lives in Cañete. Felix feels emotional pain that he has not visited his mother for several years. He expresses how when he returns to visit his mother in Cañete he cannot go with 'empty hands'.

> When I go, I can't go with empty hands.... Because your mum is going to ask you for a T-shirt, shoes, no? Mums ask you for things...you have to take her clothes, fruit, oil, whatever little thing...When you go to visit you must take something even if it's just fruit, you must take something.

Felix is struggling to fulfil notions of the loyal son/provider as well as the independent husband/father provider. Perhaps part of his distance from his family is an unspoken sense of failure and shame that he has not made progress and cannot return with his 'hands full'. However, his narrative also reveals underlying tensions in his family relations.

Felix is the second oldest sibling in his family. He did not finish primary school and left in order to work to support his siblings, including agricultural labour and working in a fruit market in Lima. This reflects a socio-cultural pattern of children's early participation in family economic strategies. From an early age children are expected to be hardworking, contributing to the household income, and have various household and work-related tasks (Anderson 2007). Felix emphasises the sacrifice he made to help his siblings, to take them forward (*sacarles adelante*), sacrificing his own education. There is a strong hierarchy of responsibility of care flowing from older to younger siblings which is exemplified by an older child becoming 'like a father or mother' to their younger siblings, and then in the next generation, to nieces and nephews. This was frequently mentioned in the narratives. Felix comments how his wife complains,

> 'What have you done in your youth? What have you done? Where is your money?' My money is in my siblings, that's where my money is.

Two of his step-siblings have become professionals; one a teacher, the other a nurse. Felix has a strained relationship with his one blood sibling (older) who he describes as irresponsible, not working, but just staying dependent on Felix's help (the goods and money he sent). He seems tired of being the one to hold the family together. It may also be that by detailing his sacrifices and these tensions Felix legitimises his withdrawal from these relations. As Felix's case has started to show, the unfolding of relationships reveals the underlying relational conflict and tensions which underpinned his initial move to Lima.

Conclusion

This chapter gives a detailed, more holistic insight into relational wellbeing in the context of mobility. The use of unstructured and free-flowing narratives in researching wellbeing allowed interviewees to 'wander off' in their own minds, creating depth in the data which might not have been able to emerge with a more structured line of questioning. A criticism often made of wellbeing approaches is that an individual focus fails to take into account structural influences on experiences; it understates the significance of structures (Wright 2012). However, narratives have revealed elements of structure as it is lived, drawn out by the person in the broader socio-cultural context.

In particular, the notion of relational has drawn out the intertwinement and interplay of the material, relational and subjective dimensions of wellbeing. While there is something intrinsic about the importance of family and family-like relations, these relations are closely entangled with material and emotional realities. For many it is the economic opportunities and the hope of a better life which lead to mobility in the first place, and gifts are a key part of expressing love and affection and maintaining anchoring routines in the face of separation. Yet material and practical constraints shape what people can accomplish. This was particularly the case in narratives of the middle years where anchoring to kin (parents and siblings) and to one's immediate family (partner and children) created competing and conflicting demands on their limited and stretched resources. For others, material hardship leads to a forced isolation from family when they feel unable to meet demands from kin and may become dependent on exploitative relationships. These dynamics unsurprisingly exert a strong influence upon people's emotions and their sense of self, with pain experienced during childhood and youth sometimes enduring through adulthood. Yet emotions also motivate anchoring routines which in turn strengthen relational wellbeing.

The picture is a complex one which contrasts with the positive, cohesive, resilient and harmonious nature of ties amongst spatially dispersed families depicted in much of the literature. The narratives revealed struggles, tensions and constraints in the reworking of these relationships. The chapter has shown that there is a 'dark side' of family (and family-like) relations which can entail violence, exploitation, harm and abuse (White 2010). Female narratives were more commonly characterised by an enduring *pena* and they experienced more vulnerabilities and ambiguities compared with male narratives. This reflects women's positioning in a culture of *machismo*, their indigenous origin, their lower socio-economic class and continuing poverty. It also points to the importance of considering time in studies of wellbeing as people's sense of wellbeing can be highly conditioned by experiences in the past and/or expectations of the future.

Finally, also in need of greater recognition within the wellbeing literature are the marked differences in people's expectations and experiences of relationships according to their stage of the lifecycle and their gender. This chapter has explored some of the ambiguities experienced during childhood, as well as tensions for men and women during their middle years. For example, a tacit acceptance that sons may become more focused on their wife and children, relinquishing support to parents and siblings, is contrasted with an embedded notion of 'always available' daughters, dependable and reliable. However, there is an inherent contradiction here that, due to a woman's positioning in the household where a culture of *machismo* prevails, she faces a greater struggle to live up to these expectations and maintain kin relations. A further contradiction is the embedded notion of 'always present' mothers, caring, nurturing and physically present in a socio-cultural context of common, habitual practices of early parent–child separation and 'childgiving'. Gender and lifecycle need to be taken much more seriously as structuring factors in the experience of wellbeing.

Note

1. This was part of the Wellbeing in Developing Countries (WeD) research. The support of the Economic and Social Research Council is gratefully acknowledged.

References

Altamirano, T. (1988) *Cultura Andina y Pobreza Urbana: Aymaras en Lima Metropolitana*. Lima: Pontificia Universidad Catolica del Peru (PUCP) Fondo Editorial.

Alvarez, J. and Arroyo, M. (2005) *Perfil de la comunidad autogestionaria de Nuevo Lugar*. Internal document. Bath: WeD ESRC Research Group.

Alvarez, J., Arroyo, M., Carhuallanqui, L., Copestake, J., Jaurapoma, M., Lavers, T., Obispo, M., Paucar, E., Reina, P. and Yamamoto, J. (2008) Resources, Conflict, and Social Identity in Context. pp. 31–60 in J. Copestake (ed.) *Wellbeing and Development in Peru: Local and Universal Views Confronted*. New York: Palgrave Macmillan.

Anderson, J. (2007) Urban Poverty Reborn: A Gender and Generational Analysis. *Journal of Developing Societies* 23(1–2): 221–241.

Anderson, J. Pacheco, R. and Velarde, C. (2006) *El trabajo infantíl domestico en el Perú. Informe Perú – Proyecto Tejiendo Redes*. Lima: Organizacion Internacional del Trabajo (OIT)/Programa Internacional para Erradicacion del Trabajo Infantil (IPEC).

Auyero, J. and Swistun, D. (2008) The Social Production of Toxic Uncertainty. *American Sociological Review* 73(3): 357–379.

Åkesson, L., Carling, J. and Drotbohm, H. (2012) Mobility, Moralities and Motherhood: Navigating the Contingencies of Cape Verdean Lives. *Ethnic and Migration Studies* 38(2): 237–260.

Boyden, J. and Mann, G. (2005) Children's Risk, Resilience, and Coping in Extreme Situations. pp. 3–25 in M. Ungar (ed.) *Handbook for Working with Children and Youth: Pathways to Resilience across Cultures and Contexts*. London: Sage Publications.

Burrell, K. (2006) *Moving Lives: Narratives of Nation and Migration among Europeans in Post-War Britain*. Aldershot: Ashgate.

Carrasco, L. N. (2010) Transnational Family Life among Peruvian Migrants in Chile: Multiple Commitments and the Role of Social Remittances. *Journal of Comparative Family Studies* 41(2): 187–204.

Castles, S. and Delgado Wise, R. (2007) Introduction. pp. 1–13 in S. Castles and R. Delgado Wise (eds.) *Migration and Development: Perspectives from the South*. Geneva: International Organization for Migration (IOM).

Copestake, J., Guillen-Royo, M., Chou, W.-J., Hinks, T. and Velazco, J. (2008) Economic Welfare, Poverty, and Subjective Wellbeing. pp. 103–120 in J. Copestake (ed.) *Wellbeing and Development in Peru: Local and Universal Views Confronted*. Basingstoke: Palgrave Macmillan.

Deere, C. D. (1990) *Household and Class Relations: Peasants and Landlords in Northern Peru*. Berkeley, CA: University of California Press.

Degregori, C. I., Blondet, C. and Lynch, N. (1986) *Conquistadores de un Nuevo Mundo: de Invasores a Ciudadanos en San Martin de Porres*. Lima: Instituto de Estudios Peruanos (IEP).

de Haan, A. and Yaqub, S. (2009) *Migration and Poverty: Linkages, Knowledge Gaps and Policy Implications*. PP SPD40, Geneva: United Nations Research Institute for Social Development (UNRISD) Programme Papers on Social Policy and Development.

de Haas, H. and Rodríguez, F. (2010) Mobility and Human Development: Introduction. *Journal of Human Development and Capabilities: A Multi-Disciplinary Journal for People-Centred Development* 11(2): 177–184.

Devine, J., Camfield, L. and Gough, I. (2008) Autonomy or Dependence – Or Both? Perspectives from Bangladesh. *Journal of Happiness Studies* 9(1): 105–138.

DeWind, J. and Holdaway, J. (eds.) (2008) *Migration and Development within and across Borders: Research and Policy Perspectives on Internal and International Migration*. Geneva: IOM (International Organization for Migration) and New York: SSRC (Social Science Research Council).

Fonseca, C. (1991) Spouses, Siblings and Sex-Linked Bonding: A Look at Kinship Organisation in a Brazilian Slum. pp. 133–160 in E. Jelin (ed.) *Family, Household and Gender Relations in Latin America*. London: Kegan Paul.
Gill, L. (1994) *Precarious Dependencies: Gender, Class, and Domestic Service in Bolivia*. New York: Columbia University Press.
Goldstein, D. M. (2003) *Laughter out of Place: Race, Class, Violence, and Sexuality in a Rio Shantytown*. London: University of California Press.
Grbich, C. (2007) *Qualitative Data Analysis: An Introduction*. London: Sage.
Huovinen, R. (2013) *Mobile Lives in Peru: The Dynamics of Relational Anchoring*. PhD thesis, University of Bath.
International Organization for Migration (IOM) (2005) *Migration, Development and Poverty Reduction in Asia*. Geneva: IOM.
International Organization for Migration (IOM) (2010) *Mainstreaming Migration into Development Planning: A Handbook for Policy-Makers and Practitioners*. Geneva: IOM.
International Organization for Migration (IOM) (2013) *World Migration Report 2013: Migrant Well-Being and Development*. Geneva: IOM.
Isbell, B. J. (1977) Those Who Love Me: An Analysis of Andean Kinship and Reciprocity within a Ritual Context. pp. 81–105 in R. Bolton and E. Mayer (eds.) *Andean Kinship and Marriage*. Washington, DC: American Anthropological Association.
King, R. and Skeldon, R. (2010) Mind the Gap! Integrating Approaches to Internal and International Migration. *Journal of Ethnic and Migration Studies* 36(10): 1619–1646.
Kothari, U. and Hulme, D. (2004) *Narratives, Stories and Tales: Understanding Poverty Dynamics through Life Histories*. GPRG-WPS-011, University of Manchester: Global Poverty Research Group.
Laczko, F. (2008) Migration and Development: The Forgotten Migrants. pp. 7–11 in J. DeWind and J. Holdaway (eds.) *Migration and Development within and across Borders: Research and Policy Perspectives on Internal and International Migration*. Geneva: IOM (International Organization for Migration) and New York: SSRC (Social Science Research Council).
Leinaweaver, J. B. (2008) *The Circulation of Children: Kinship, Adoption, and Morality in Andean Peru*. London: Duke University Press.
Lloyd, P. (1980) *The 'Young Towns' of Lima: Aspects of Urbanisation in Peru*. Cambridge: Cambridge University Press.
Lloyd-Sherlock, P. and Locke, C. (2008) Vulnerable Relations: Lifecourse, Wellbeing and Social Exclusion in a Neighbourhood of Buenos Aires, Argentina. *Ageing and Society* 28(6): 779–803.
Lockley, R., Altamirano, T. and Copestake, J. (2008) Wellbeing and Migration. pp. 121–151 in J. Copestake (ed.) *Wellbeing and Development in Peru: Local and Universal Views Confronted*. Basingstoke: Palgrave Macmillan.
Mason, J. (2000) *Deciding Where to Live: Relational Reasoning and Narratives of the Self*, Working Paper 19. Leeds: Centre for Research on Family, Kinship and Childhood, University of Leeds.
Mason, J. (2004) Personal Narratives, Relational Selves: Residential Histories in the Living and Telling. *Sociological Review* 52(2): 162–179.
Mason, J. and Tipper, B. (2008) Being Related: How Children Define and Create Kinship. *Childhood* 15(4): 441–460.

McGregor, J. A. (2007) Researching Wellbeing: From Concepts to Methodology. pp. 316–350 in I. Gough and J. A. McGregor (eds.) *Wellbeing in Developing Countries: From Theory to Research.* Cambridge: Cambridge University Press.

Meneses, M. (1998) *La Utopia Urbana: El Movimiento de Pobladores en el Perú.* Lima: Brandon Enterprises Editores.

Migration, Globalisation and Poverty (MGP) Development Research Centre (2009) *Making Migration Work for Development.* Sussex: University of Sussex.

Mitchell, W. P. (2006) *Voices from the Global Margin: Confronting Poverty and Inventing New Lives in the Andes.* Austin: University of Texas Press.

Paerregaard, K. (1997) *Linking Separate Worlds: Urban Migrants and Rural Lives in Peru.* Oxford: Berg.

Parreñas, R. S. (2005) *Children of Global Migration: Transnational Families and Gendered Woes.* California: Stanford University Press.

Programa de las Naciones Unidas para el Desarrollo (PNUD) (2002) *Informe Sobre Desarrollo Humano Peru 2002: Aprovechando las potencialidades.* Lima, Peru: PNUD.

Ryan, L. (2004) Family Matters: (E)migration, Familial Networks and Irish Women in Britain. *The Sociological Review* 52(3): 351–370.

Ryan, L., Sales, R., Tilki, M. and Siara, B. (2009) Family Strategies and Transnational Migration: Recent Polish Migrants in London. *Journal of Ethnic and Migration Studies* 35(1): 61–77.

Ryan, R. M. and Deci, E. (2001) On Happiness and Human Potentials: A Review of Research on Hedonic and Eudaimonic Well Being. *Annual Review of Psychology* 52: 141–166.

Sen, A. (2009) *The Idea of Justice.* London: Allen Lane.

Skar, S. L. (1994) *Lives Together – Worlds Apart: Quechua Colonization in Jungle and City.* Oslo, Norway: Scandinavian University Press.

Sorensen, N. N. (2002) Representing the Local: Mobile Livelihood Practices in the Peruvian Central Sierra. In N. N. Sorensen and K. F. Olwig (eds.) *Work and Migration: Life and Livelihoods in a Globalising World.* London: Routledge.

Sorensen, N. N., Van Hear, N. and Engberg-Pedersen, P. (2003) The Migration-Development Nexus: Evidence and Policy Options. In N. Van Hear and N. N. Sorensen (eds.) *The Migration-Development Nexus.* Geneva: United Nations and International Organization for Migration.

Takenaka, A. and Pren, K. A. (2010) Leaving to Get Ahead: Assessing the Relationship between Mobility and Inequality in Peruvian Migration. *Latin American Perspectives* 37(5): 29–49.

Tamagno, C. (2002) 'You Must Win Their Affection...' Migrants' Social and Cultural Practices between Peru and Italy. pp. 106–125 in N. N. Sorensen and K. F. Olwig (eds.) *Work and Migration: Life and Livelihoods in a Globalising World.* London: Routledge.

Tapias, M. and Escandell, X. (2011) Not in the Eyes of the Beholder: Envy among Bolivian Migrants in Spain. *International Migration* 49(6): 74–94.

Tousignant, M. and Maldonado, M. (1989) Sadness, Depression and Social Reciprocity in Highland Equador. *Social Science and Medicine* 28(9): 899–904.

Van Vleet, K. E. (2008) *Performing Kinship: Narrative, Gender, and the Intimacies of Power in the Andes.* Austin: University of Texas Press.

Weismantel, M. (2001) *Cholas and Pishtacos: Stories of Race and Sex in the Andes.* Chicago, IL: University of Chicago Press.

White, S. C. (2008) *But What Is Wellbeing? A Framework for Analysis in Social and Development Policy and Practice.* WeD Working Paper 43/Paper for Regeneration and Wellbeing: Research into practice, University of Bradford, 24–25 April 2008, University of Bath: Wellbeing in Developing Countries (WeD), ESRC Research Group.

White, S. C. (2010) Analysing Wellbeing: A Framework for Development Policy and Practice. *Development in Practice* 20(2): 158–172.

Wright, K. (2010) It's a Limited Kind of Happiness, Barriers to Achieving Human Wellbeing through International Migration: The Case of Peruvian Migrants in London and Madrid. *Bulletin of Latin American Research* 29(3): 367–383.

Wright, K. (2011) Constructing Migrant Wellbeing: An Exploration of Life Satisfaction amongst Peruvian Migrants in London. *Journal of Ethnic and Migration Studies* 37(9): 1459–1475.

Wright, K. (2012) *International Migration, Development and Human Wellbeing.* Basingstoke: Palgrave Macmillan.

Wright, K. and Black, R. (2011) Poverty, Migration and Human Well-Being: Towards a Post-Crisis Research and Policy Agenda. *Journal of International Development* 23: 548–554.

Young, G. (1987) The Myth of Being 'Like a Daughter'. *Latin American Perspectives* 14(3): 365–380.

Zontini, E. (2010) Enabling and Constraining Aspects of Social Capital in Migrant Families: Ethnicity, Gender and Generation. *Ethnic and Racial Studies* 33(5): 816–831.

8
Tensions in Conceptualising Psychosocial Wellbeing in Angola: The Marginalisation of Religion and Spirituality

Carola Eyber

Introduction

Within the humanitarian aid sphere, the provision of mental health and psychosocial support to displaced populations has been a growing field over the last two decades, albeit a contested one. Bio-medical discourses dominate the field through conceptualising the distress and suffering in the form of mental disorders such as traumatic stress, anxiety and depression (Bolton *et al.* 2004), and proposed interventions draw on theories of cognitive, behavioural and psychotherapy in efforts to alleviate this suffering (Jordans *et al.* 2009). Juxtaposed against this bio-medical trauma model are the efforts of more holistically oriented practitioners who seek to improve psychosocial wellbeing rather than treat mental disorders. Many of these practitioners are of the opinion that local context and cultural perspectives need to be taken into account when trying to understand the impact that displacement and conflict have on wellbeing (Miller and Rasco 2006, Wessells and Monteiro 2006). In contrast to the individualist orientation of bio-medical approaches, attention has focused on the coping strategies that communities make use of in dealing with the problems and distress caused by war (Honwana 1997, Wessells and Monteiro 2000). Such work has typically argued that concepts of mental health and distress vary between cultures and that local concepts have to be given precedence over bio-medical and Western models if understanding and insight are to be gained into the meaning attached to certain illnesses or symptoms

(Dawes and Honwana 1996). Authors such as Wessells and Monteiro (2000) have further maintained that local healing practices themselves should be recognised as effective treatment strategies that constitute the primary resource for the majority of communities affected by war. Honwana's (1997, 1999) work, for instance, focuses on indigenous concepts of mental health in Mozambique and Angola which she argues are intricately related to cultural and spiritual paradigms and local cosmology. Some problems which may be interpreted as mental illness by psychiatrists are seen as spiritual difficulties caused by the angry, vengeful spirits of those who have been killed unjustly or who have not received proper burials, and recourse is to be found in the performance of community rituals that cleanse and purify those affected by the spirits.

The work of Honwana (1997) and Wessells and Monteiro (2000) highlights some of the spiritual dimensions of illness and distress related to war, referring for example to the inter-relationship between witchcraft, political conflict and mental illness. However, the approach taken to these issues subsumes a large variety of perspectives and healing systems under the 'umbrella' of culture and traditional practices. The effect of this is to neglect an important and influential resource which is often made use of by war-displaced people themselves, namely religion. The tendency to collapse religious and spiritual issues into the broad category of cultural practices and beliefs is widespread amongst academics (for example Peddle *et al.* 1999, Summerfield 1999) as well as amongst psychosocial practitioners and humanitarian aid organisations. Little attention has been paid to the way in which religious matters affect the meanings attached and the expressions given to suffering, or the way in which everyday practices and notions of wellbeing are intertwined with religious and spiritual aspects of life. This paper analyses some of the possible reasons that religion[1] and spirituality are being ignored in the dominant conceptualisation of psychosocial wellbeing or subsumed under the notion of cultural practices. It also argues that ignoring religion and spirituality undermines the commitment to take local understandings of wellbeing as an essential starting point for understanding the suffering of displaced populations. As such, this chapter examines how the 'who and how' dimension of the knowledge-construction triangle (see White, Chapter 1 of this volume) influences the particular account of wellbeing we produce and critically questions the potential political implications of this. The chapter first provides a brief overview of the interaction of development and humanitarian aid with religion, then presents findings from ethnographic research conducted in Huila, Angola, during the armed conflict, and analyses how this relates to conceptualisations of wellbeing. Finally, the instrumental view of religion will be discussed in relation to the findings and existing theories in the field.

Development, humanitarian aid and religion

In order to gain insight into this neglect of religion in people's responses to suffering and conceptions of wellbeing, one has to contextualise the provision of psychosocial support within the broader humanitarian aid and development field. The field of humanitarian assistance has a longstanding practice of ignoring religion and the role it plays in people's lives due to the assumption that as societies develop and modernise, they would 'naturally' undergo a process of secularisation (Deneulin and Rakodi 2011). Secularism is based on two ideas: firstly that religion is backward and traditional and would therefore be replaced by a more reasonable worldview as societies become modernised, and secondly that it is primarily a private matter of individual preference rather than an aspect that affects public and political life. Ager and Ager (2011) go so far as to claim that secularism is the 'religion of development', meaning that neo-liberal notions of progress, development and positive social change are associated with an unquestioned commitment to a 'rational' and secular worldview. Neo-liberal notions of the importance of economic and material dimensions of life have reinforced the marginalisation of religion. Finally, uncertainty as to how to deal with the 'irrational' aspects of religion has resulted in development workers sidestepping many aspects of religious expressions and manifestations in the lives of the people they seek to assist.

However, in recent years a change has been noted, with development and humanitarian organisations increasingly recognising that they cannot ignore an aspect of many people's lives that they themselves identify as a central principle of action and core to their understandings of wellbeing (Deneulin and Rakodi 2011, Schafer 2010). The assumptions of secularisation theories have not been born out in that religion and spirituality continue to shape the everyday lives of many people in low- and middle-income countries, as well as in high-income countries (Devine and White 2013). In particular, development agencies have started to recognise the role that religious organisations play in providing economic, social and developmental assistance to people on the ground (see Bompani 2010 for an example of the role of independent Christianity in South Africa; the International Federation of the Red

Cross' [IFRC] World Disaster Report 2014, and the United Nations High Commissioner for Refugees [UNHCR] 2014 amongst others).

The reluctance of specifically mental health and psychosocial practitioners to engage with issues of religious and spiritual beliefs may also be attributable to other factors. The medical and clinical training that many practitioners undergo assumes a rationalist, evidence-based approach to mental health and psychosocial wellbeing which excludes perspectives on spirituality and religion. Also, many psychologists and psychiatrists 'do not consider it appropriate to encourage discussion of religious or spiritual issues with their patients' (Dein *et al.* 2010: 63) because they feel that such discussion can be easily construed as abuse of power as therapists are seen to promote their own vested (religious) interests. While there are clearly ethical concerns about abuse of power in a therapeutic relationship, the exclusion of religious matters from this relationship constructs religious interests as personal and a matter of conviction as opposed to an issue that is seen by many as universal and collective.

The psychosocial field itself has had to struggle for recognition in the field of humanitarian assistance where material and physical needs of affected populations are deemed to be a priority and 'psychobabble'[2] is construed as being of much lesser importance. As Van den Berg *et al.* (2011: 66) explain:

> In the MHPSS [Mental Health and Psychosocial Support] field, we have faced challenges in finding a term, phrase or definition to describe the spectrum of what we do and believe in, particularly in gaining legitimacy with the 'non believers' among our humanitarian colleagues. We have worked a long time to demystify and label processes that are very personal and intimate in their nature, and that relate to feelings, beliefs, thinking and capacities, during times of great human suffering or in the face of inhumane experiences.

Incorporating religious and spiritual elements into psychosocial work could be perceived as 'reversing' the processes of demystifying the work and could possibly run the risk of losing some of this hard-gained legitimacy in the humanitarian field.

A final factor could be difficulties of translating recognition of the religious and spiritual lives of people into practical programming activities aimed at improving wellbeing. What would a psychosocial programme look like that incorporates religious issues into its activities? As Van den Berg *et al.* (2011: 67) state: 'This is potentially dangerous territory. Are we in a position to recommend religious or spiritual dimensions to healing and recovery, in the same way we advocate exercise, getting enough rest and avoiding excessive alcohol?' Clearly, these authors are of the opinion that the answer to this question is negative.

However, to ignore the religious facets of people's personal, social, cultural and political lives excludes a significant element in how people construct their own wellbeing. Religion and spirituality is evident in every aspect of daily life in many countries and constitutes as much part of everyday discussions as does talk about poverty, conflict, family problems, health and illness and other daily topics of conversation. If we are to take an emic perspective on how people conceptualise wellbeing we cannot afford to 'pick and choose' aspects of local understandings that we approve of, feel confident to handle, or can understand. Recognising such systematic forms of bias suggests the need to question critically how wellbeing knowledge is constructed and by whom, and to investigate the possible political implications that these dominant constructs may have.

Investigating wellbeing knowledge

I will use data collected in Angola[3] during a period of armed conflict to illustrate why excluding religious and spiritual perspectives on wellbeing constitutes a fundamental challenge for how we construct wellbeing knowledge. The ethnographic data presented here were collected during eight months of fieldwork in 2000 in the province of Huila in southern Angola.[4] They formed part of my doctoral research which made use of methods such as participant observation, semi-structured interviews and focus-group discussions in order to gain insight into local understandings of distress as well as strategies and resources for healing. In regard to investigating religious and spiritual practices and belief systems, participant observation proved to be a valuable methodology which allowed me to visit churches, healers and religious gatherings and participate in the religious activities and events.[5] Participant observation also involves the constant and extensive use of unstructured interviewing in the form of conversations with participants about various topics of interest. These were solicited or unsolicited accounts which provided both direct and indirect information about the setting, people's perspectives, concerns and explanations of practices. Building relationships with key informants was another aspect of the prolonged engagement in the communities I stayed in, and while I took note of ethnographers'[6] warnings against the over-reliance on key informants without triangulating the information obtained, these informants provided me with valuable insight into the dynamics and relationships between different sectors of the religious communities in the area. Semi-structured interviews with religious leaders and healers in the communities and focus-group discussions with members of various religious groupings yielded insights into the beliefs, practices, motivation, faith and hope attached to their religious participation. Frequently I conducted an 'introductory' interview with a religious leader and returned for a follow-up interview days, weeks or sometimes months later. Subsequent interviews were often combined with participant observation of some form of religious practice. The focus-group discussions were conducted in a semi-formal manner, arranged beforehand with one or two participants, asking them to invite others who wished to participate. A short list of open-ended questions guided the group discussions, and often the discussion took directions I had not anticipated. These unanticipated conversational turns sometimes provided surprising and valuable insights into community events or issues that I was unaware of and thus contributed significantly to my understanding of the social reality as the participants themselves constructed it.[7]

My previous experience of having worked with Angolan refugees in South Africa influenced my assumption that there would be variations amongst local perceptions of distress, wellbeing and healing which would be affected by the specific context and culture of different groups and locations. However, my pre-drafted research questions focused almost entirely on the cultural aspects of the explanatory models and treatment resources available in these communities; religion and spirituality did not feature specifically as a topic. I had thus a priori imposed my own limits on 'who and how' would contribute to the constructions of wellbeing knowledge that I wanted to investigate (see White, Chapter 1 of this volume). By initially excluding the spiritual dimension from my research, I placed boundaries around the types of accounts of wellbeing that I could elicit. However, because of the nature of the methodology I used (ethnography), these boundaries were rapidly breached as it became apparent that issues of health, illness and suffering were not only intimately related to cultural and traditional practices but also to spiritual and religious matters. When talking about the suffering caused by war, the *deslocados* (internally displaced people) made frequent references to God, faith-healing, the importance of the churches, prayer and help from church groups. I will now provide a brief overview of one particular aspect of this religious landscape that influenced constructions of distress and wellbeing.

The independent churches in Huila

The landscape of religion and spirituality in the province of Huila was not homogenous, but consisted of three broad sectors: the African traditional religions, established Christian denominations and the independent churches.[8] The focus here is on the perspectives and practices of one particular religious sector, the independent churches, and on the approach of independent churches to illness and the treatment options and help provided by them.

The rise of new religious movements in many parts of the world, and in Africa specifically, has been well documented over the last two decades (Bompani 2010, Bowie 2000, Geschiere 1997). Independent churches, which are not usually affiliated to any of the main governing international church bodies, form part of this. Different categories of independent churches exist in Huila, which can be broadly divided into the charismatic, 'born-again' churches, and the prophetic, indigenous churches.

The most well-known charismatic churches at the time of the research were the *Igreja de Mana* (Church of Mana), the *Igreja Universal de Reino de Deus* (Universal Church of the Kingdom of God [UCKG]) and the Pentecostal Church of Angola, all of which established themselves in Lubango and Matala, two major towns in Huila province, over the last four or five years. They placed special emphasis on the intervention and power of the Holy Spirit and practices such as speaking in tongues and being 'born again', a spiritual experience during which a person sheds his or her past life and becomes a new person through faith in Jesus Christ. Many churches preached the 'gospel of prosperity': faith in Jesus Christ would bring blessings of health, wealth and success. Born-again Christians were called to be successful in all areas of their lives because it was God's plan that humankind should prosper in all things. A central principle of faith is that God had met all the needs of human beings in the suffering and death of Jesus Christ, implying that every Christian shared the victory over sin, illness and poverty (Gifford 2004).

In relation to this latter doctrine, in order to participate in God's prosperity, Christians had to make an investment by giving 'seed money', a concept based on the New Testament verse which states: 'A man reaps what he sows' (Gal. 6:7, New International Version). Members of the congregation 'planted seeds' by giving money to the church, considered to be an act of faith that would be richly rewarded by God. A series of special blessings were performed by the pastors in the churches of Mana and UCKG during services, for example for those who wanted a car or who needed extra help with their business. In the UCKG, specific days were set aside for certain spiritual activities, for example Monday was a day for faith-healing, Tuesday for spirit exorcism and Wednesday for receiving blessings for prosperity.[9]

Prophetic movements and African indigenous churches are churches that have 'indigenised' Christianity by absorbing the Christian spirit into traditional African religious and cultural forms, thus creating new, Christian, African religious communities (Gifford 2004, Mbiti 1989). They were often formed as religious and political protests against the missionary churches, based on the belief that adherence to Jesus Christ as Lord rather than adherence to Western culture is a measure of Christian identity (Githieya 1997). They are usually founded by a strong, inspired prophet, who receives a message from God instructing him or her to break away from another church because of its unchristian practices. The founders have special spiritual powers that, in order to be practised and expressed, require the formation of a separate church organised around the prophet's person. In Huila, some of the most well-known of these were the churches of Simão Togo and Simon Kimbanigsta, as well as the *Igreja Cheio da Palavra do Deus* (Church Full of the Word of God). In addition, countless numbers of small churches led by *santas* and *santos* existed in almost every neighbourhood in Lubango. The word *santa* means 'saint' but was used more in the sense of a holy person who possesses the power of faith-healing. In Huila, *santas* were predominantly female and often built small church structures on their properties from which they conducted daily church services and healing activities.

The independent churches expected their followers to abide by a number of rules and taboos. These usually involved a complete abstinence from sexual relations outside of marriage, alcohol, tobacco, secular forms of entertainment and any form of traditional healing or divining. Eating of pork, and sometimes all meat, was forbidden by some. If someone had sinned against these prohibitions, they could be put on probation, suspended from church or excommunicated, depending on the severity of the sin. In the prophetic, indigenous churches, Old Testament texts and practices are often more prominent than those from the New Testament. Bible verses may be interpreted literally and are taken as directives from God. A characteristic of the independent church sector is, however, the variation and innovation in beliefs and practices amongst the churches.

The churches attracted different groups within communities: the charismatic movements appealing to urban youth and the prophetic churches to a cross section of ages and backgrounds. As with the mainstream churches, the role that the churches played in the lives of their members cannot be understood solely in religious and spiritual terms but include social, economic and political elements. The social life of members of the charismatic churches, for example, often revolved around the church where there were continuous rounds of Bible studies, prayer meetings, choir practices, revivals and evangelistic activities, thus providing a 'new spiritual family' within the religious group (Bompani 2010).

Conceptualisations of wellbeing and illness

The independent churches used spiritual explanations for understanding issues of health and illness, and the majority saw bio-medical factors as either irrelevant or as secondary to these. According to the 'gospel of prosperity', Christians should enjoy physical and mental wellbeing, and its absence indicated a spiritual problem. Illness, just as poverty, was attributed to a lack of faith, to sinful behaviour or to the invasion of the body or soul by satanic spirits. In the first two cases, illness was the consequence of someone turning away from God and was thus the fault and responsibility of the ill person. In the case of demonic possession or witchcraft, the person could not be held responsible for his or her illness and was considered to be a blameless victim. Some of the charismatic churches believed that all illness was caused directly by the Devil, as explained by the pastor of one of the large, popular churches in Lubango:

> I can't give what I don't have. It's the same with God: He can't give what He doesn't have. The illnesses don't come from God – it is the Devil who destroys, kills, robs. An illness destroys humans. If you have a house and it's all good and then you start breaking a window, break the door. Would you do this? No, you would not. It's the same with God: He created everything and the best thing He created is the human. He won't destroy this.
>
> (Pastor R., Lubango)

The churches believed that the basic premise for being cured was faith in God and in the healing power of Jesus Christ. Healing could occur instantaneously or gradually but would only occur if sufficient faith in God was present:

> Yes, the cure comes to those people who believe in Jesus. When Jesus comes to a person, the person receives everything: salvation,

liberation, healing. The person is liberated from this moment onwards. But this doesn't mean that from this moment on the person will not feel sick... I can't say that you will be healed on this day if you don't have the faith that God will do this.

(Pastor R., Lubango)

A number of further actions needed to be undertaken depending on the cause of illness: if the ill person had sinned, she or he had to confess the sins and make amends to the person wronged; if she or he was possessed, the demons had to be exorcised; and all ill people participated in faith-healing conducted by the church leaders or *santas*. Some independent churches, such as the UCKG in Lubango, for example, forbade their members to consult a doctor or visit a clinic or hospital, as medicines were considered unbiblical on the basis that Jesus healed only with the power of the Holy Spirit. Church members were encouraged to rely entirely on God's healing power which could be accessed through prayer, reading the Bible and the power of the church leader, and not through doctors:

> Sometimes the problem is that the person hasn't prepared the soul. At times God wants you to go to church to pray. You spend your life just with drinking and with adultery – you will not stay well. You are sick because of the result of your sins because God punishes you for these things... Many people are sick because of their sins – or because their soul is dirty, a dirty body and a dirty soul.
>
> (*Santa* T., Lubango)

Faith-healing formed a central part of each service and would take place during the worship or afterwards when people lined up in front of the pastor to receive blessings, the laying on of hands or prayers for their recovery. Often healing was done through the sprinkling of ashes, water or perfume that had been blessed by the pastor or *santa*. Faith-healing was an important way in which the prophet or the leaders of the church demonstrated their power and explicit closeness to God (Ben-Tovim 1987). The healers did not take credit for the miracles performed, however, as their powers came directly from God and the Holy Spirit:

> Who cures is God Himself. God only cures when you follow Him. If you don't follow Him you will be sick. The soul is like the body: the body needs to have breakfast, and then lunch and then dinner.

There is a time when you need to pray because the soul works as the body.

(Santa M., Lubango)

Some healers relied only on spiritual healing while others used herbal treatments as well; the latter were most common amongst *santas* who could undergo training periods similar to those of traditional healers, referred to as *curandeiros* in Angola, in order to learn the healing properties of plants, roots and herbs. Successful faith-healers acquired reputations that spread from one area or town to another, attracting new converts to their churches. Many people who had tried several different healthcare options and had not been cured approached the independent churches in the hope of being healed. *Santas* charged for individual consultations along similar lines as *curandeiros*.

While the charismatic churches rejected many of the traditional cultural practices of the local populations, they nevertheless used a supernaturalistic vision of reality and a discourse that included God and the Devil, miracles and an instrumental understanding of religion (Bowie 2000). This accorded well with aspects of traditional religious thinking, as well as with an understanding of wellbeing as a spiritual, social and physical issue. Similarities existed between traditional religious practices and those of the prophetic, indigenous churches, for example in the healing practices of the *santas* which may closely resemble those of *curandeiros*:

Q: How do you heal someone who is sick?

The spirit tells me that a sick person is coming. And if the patient has luck the spirit will also tell me what sickness this is. At times the spirit doesn't say what the illness is, I sit down and start to pray and then I discover what are the problems of this patient.

Q: Is this the spirit of God?

I cannot say if this is an evil spirit or a spirit of God. But I think it is the spirit of God because he never tells me to do something else apart from prayer. It's only prayer.

(Santa M., Lubango)

Bompani (2010) and Sindima (1994) suggest that the ability to bridge traditional and Christian beliefs and practices explains some of the success and growth of independent churches in many parts of Africa, as they offer people a religious space where both can be accessed.

The distinction between 'religion' and 'culture' is often unclear and not possible to make as they are closely intertwined. While each religious movement has what is often defined as 'original doctrines', these are influenced by context and historical time and many arguments ensue over how the culture of ancient and current times affect these doctrines.

Spirit exorcism formed part of most of the independent churches' understanding of spiritual and holistic health, as a constant battle was being waged between witchcraft, evil ancestral spirits and demons on the one hand, and the churches on the other. The battleground of this contest was not only the body of the ill person but also in the communities where members of the churches confronted and challenged people suspected of practising witchcraft. Demon possession expressed itself through illness but also through signs such as repeated miscarriages, an unhappy marriage or an addiction to alcohol. The practice of spirit exorcism was an important resource to local populations who were confronted with issues of witchcraft and spiritual forces in their daily lives and who not only found the existence of witchcraft affirmed in the independent churches, but were also provided with the means to combat it (Geschiere 1997). This was in contrast to the mainstream churches which often did not acknowledge the existence of witchcraft and some had dropped talk of the Devil and witchcraft from their discourses.

The independent churches overtly emphasised the spiritual dimensions of war and suffering, with charismatic churches attributing the war and its consequences to the Devil:

> The Bible teaches us that our enemy is not the human being. Our enemy is the Devil... The role of the Devil is to injure the hearts of people.... These injuries of the heart cause the terrible things we see in life: there are many people who do barbaric things, have no hope in life, people who are traumatised and injured by the Devil.... The Devil puts one man against the other. The mission of the church is to convince the people of this reality and show people this.
>
> (Pastor C., Lubango)

This perspective placed the war and its consequences into a realm in which the churches and their leaders were the experts. The *santas* and prophets often had more complex explanations of the war, attributing it to the greed of humans, witchcraft,[10] the neglect of God and His ways, and sin.

In the accounts I have provided, the voices of authority on spiritual matters were the religious leaders, and they were often invested in maintaining a consistent discourse on spiritual matters that their members adhered and subscribed to. Questions need to be asked about the forms of power involved in producing these dominant accounts of how to achieve and preserve wellbeing and the mechanisms used by religious leaders and members to 'patrol' these accounts. A number of church members reported, for example, that they would watch each other to see if they adhered to the churches' teaching and saw it as their role to admonish and guide members back to the correct spiritual path should they encounter 'straying' behaviour. Authority and 'true' accounts were thus maintained through various means by these churches.

The independent churches as a resource for healing

Attendance at the services of the charismatic churches and those of the *santas* was increasing in Huila during the years of conflict, with many churches filled to beyond capacity.[11] Many of those who attended these churches were previously members of other mainstream churches.

Members expressed support and faith in the particular approach of their church and many claimed to adhere strictly and exclusively to their church's perspectives on health and healing. Because complete trust in God's healing power was a requirement for a successful faith-healing process, members of the independent churches usually considered a pluralistic approach to healthcare counter-productive.[12] In some instances this meant that churches forbade their members to seek out any form of bio-medical care. However, some degree of medical pluralism did take place amongst congregations of independent churches. This became apparent in conversations with a few church members who noted that they had consulted the clinic or 'another healer' for an illness, as well as from conversations with *curandeiros* who occasionally treated members of independent churches.

In Huila, some antagonism and conflict existed between representatives of the different spheres of religious activity in some communities. The established churches often denounced the independent churches as heretics who had left the fold of Christianity, while independent churches were frequently hostile towards *curandeiros* and *adivinhadores*.[13] A 'competition' for adherents could ensue between churches where insults were traded and practices derided. In one area of Lubango, a small-scale battle raged between a *santa* and a charismatic church, each one denouncing the other for Devil worship and practising witchcraft, drawing community members into the conflict:

> The Devil creates things that are intended to make people concentrate on other things and not on God... And so what does he do: he creates *curandeiros, santas*, the astrologers who read the stars. And when you go there you find a Bible there. But they do not speak in the name of God, they speak in the name of the Devil... they are deceivers, liars.
>
> (Pastor S., Lubango)

While this research was conducted during a time of great adversity, participants insisted that religion and the worship of God was part of the everyday life of the *deslocados* and not just something to revert to in times of crisis and illness. One person expressed this by saying: 'We were already Christians before we [were displaced] and we continue to be Christians here. The suffering will not make us leave God' (Catechist M., Matala). People drew comfort from being part of a community of believers and the churches provided a sense of belonging in a society where war had disrupted family unity and relations:

> The war destroys. Up to now we never lived where we were born. A person was born in that province but you can't go there anymore because of the war. People live far from one another, the mother here, the grandmother there and the son in another place. Things here are complicated and the only thing that saves us is to join a church. In church you find friends with good sense and you become family, relatives.
>
> (C., Lubango)

The churches thus offered support, a sense of identity and community to the *deslocados*, in essence providing a safe haven and an account of reality that members were asked to subscribe to with varying degrees of commitment.

Religious and spiritual matters can never be divorced from the contexts in which they occur and cannot be understood in isolation from social, political and economic forces within societies and communities. They need to be situated within a wider field of power relations in which various competing discourses and practices exist, each providing certain resources but also raising complex issues and potential conflicts. The political implications of the dominance of certain religious discourses over others require careful analysis and critical questions need to be raised about the potential negative effects these may have, as religion and spirituality do not only have positive effects on wellbeing. Feelings of guilt, depression, abandonment, anxiety and worthlessness have been noted in some studies that investigated the correlation between spirituality and mental health (Schafer 2010). The intense commitment demanded from some churches has been perceived as placing excessive strain on some members who subsequently leave the congregation (Tankink 2007 in Schafer 2010). Public exclusion of church members who have 'erred' in their ways can be humiliating and distressing,[14] illustrating that a one-sided positive view on religious participation and belief does not capture individual and communal experiences. In addition, the fact that some churches prohibited bio-medical health care was seen as a negative and dangerous practice that was criticised by some community members.

While there is no doubt that there are positive aspects of being a church member, critical questions also need to be asked about the political dimensions of these accounts. For example, to what extent can these constructions of reality be questioned by members? What happens when bio-medical care is prohibited but members require it in order to be treated? What influence over members' agency do the churches have in relation to accessing other resources for wellbeing? These questions are relevant not only for examining who defines wellbeing in what way but also for discussing the engagement of development and humanitarian work with this religious sector.

An instrumental view of religion?

Rakodi (2012) argues that while development work has started taking account of the role that religion plays in people's lives, most of the studies focus on how religion can be *used* to achieve developmental objectives. The emphasis is on how religious participation enhances social relationships, facilitates economic networking opportunities and provides meaning and purpose. This instrumental view of religion ('what can religion do for people's wellbeing?') is limited in that religious participation is judged purely on what it contributes on material and social levels (Ager and Ager 2011). As an alternative worldview it is relegated to a marginalised position in relation to the dominant secular one, and this continues to be the case despite the increasing recognition that religion enjoys within the development field at present.

The material presented in this chapter can also be construed as taking an instrumentalist view of religion, as I have pointed out some very practical reasons for why people participate in independent churches in Huila province. However, recognising that people have a very practical orientation towards religious participation does not detract from the fact that religion and spirituality play a constituting role in people's worldview, *raison d'être* and their identity. Rather, the separation of practical and spiritual realms which is evident in much of Western thought is not one which is necessarily present in conceptualisations that emphasise a continuity of practical, material, social, moral, spiritual and other realms of life.

It can also be argued that most mental health and psychosocial support work shares such a functional view of wellbeing in that practitioners are interested in what makes people feel and function better. In this, and in many other aspects, psychosocial work and the work of religious organisations overlap and have, perhaps, some commonalities that are frequently overlooked. However, the differences in conceptualisations of wellbeing remain dominant. Recently, in a seminar on the role of religion in psychosocial work, a student adamantly declared: 'Religion has no role to play here, I don't want to have anything to with it and it should not be allowed in psychosocial programmes.' Equally, an Angolan woman who had completed a psychosocial training programme aimed at improving her communication skills with her children approached me and asked: 'What can I do with this certificate? I thought this programme would help me get a job so that my daughter can be better off.' For her, improving a particular aspect of psychosocial wellbeing was just as alien – and potentially useless – as religion was for my student. Thus, referring back to the triangle of knowledge construction (White, Chapter 1 of this volume), it is perhaps less the 'who and how' that is important in understanding notions of wellbeing but the 'where and with whom' that should determine what is relevant and meaningful to people. Constructions of wellbeing are judged according to how they relate to context and the relevance of the meaning they create.

It must also be noted that power plays a role in whose voice becomes dominant in constructing religious accounts of wellbeing and available resources for achieving or maintaining these. Religious leaders are important actors in the very conflicted and diverse religious terrain where different accounts of how to attain wellbeing compete with one another and community members are presented with a 'choice' of different versions, each accompanied by a variety of potential attainments (health, spiritual wellbeing, life after death, comfort, support, wealth, etc.) and the required religious and other practices that make these possible. Being located in a wider environment which was characterised by poverty and conflict and thus not conducive to facilitating wellbeing is likely to play a role as well. For development workers, this presents challenges in considering how to engage with the spiritual dimensions of people's lives and how to find common ground between their own accounts of wellbeing and those of the churches. What happens when development organisations cannot or do not want to support specific constructions of how to achieve wellbeing? How should development agencies work with religious leaders who they think do not provide effective treatment and who are consequently perceived to present a 'risk' to wellbeing? Is it not easier and safer to continue to ignore local spiritual constructions of wellbeing rather than enter into a minefield of political tensions in the religious arena of a community? These questions cannot be answered easily but challenge development workers to examine their own understandings of wellbeing and recognise them as that: constructions and not reality. The continued salience of religion and spirituality exposes the partiality of a modernist worldview that believes it owns the true account of wellbeing.

Conclusion

The independent churches combine elements of religion, spirituality and healing in innovative ways to address the problems and health concerns of their congregations. They play an important role not only as alternatives to an often inadequate healthcare system and an absent mental healthcare service in Angola but also in the social and communal life in the communities of the displaced. In addition, they offer clear and outspoken explanations of the war and the suffering it causes. This discourse does not draw primarily on medical, psychological or political frameworks but on spiritual and religious paradigms which in turn incorporate medical and political elements. Their perspectives resonate with the spiritual concerns that people have in relation to illness and the war which are often ignored by the bio-medical sector and only partially addressed by the established Christian denominations. The growing membership of the independent churches and their reciprocal relationship with civil society indicate that they are, and are likely to remain, important actors in local strategies of improving wellbeing in these impoverished communities.

The accounts and versions of wellbeing that are constructed by these churches are at times very different from those offered by bio-medicine, psychology and development work. Arguably, they offer a closer 'fit' with local context than other ways of presenting wellbeing, as they speak directly to the issues facing their congregations and offer a language of spirituality and efficacy that people relate to. However, all versions of reality are intricately entwined with politics, and questions of power, dominance and exclusion/inclusion are as central to these constructions as they are to those originating in bio-medical and psychology disciplines. Accounts of wellbeing thus need to be critically examined – not for the 'truth' – but for how other voices, options and resources are silenced and excluded, while at the same time acknowledging what they enable and construct and the extent to which they allow alternative interpretations of wellbeing to flourish.

Notes

1. There is no agreement over definitions of religion and spirituality. However, for the purpose of this paper, religion is defined as 'a set of core beliefs and teachings that amongst other things specify (or suggest) how to live in accordance with the principles of the faith tradition and how society should be ordered' (Rakodi 2012: 640). Spirituality is defined as the personal quest for understanding answers to ultimate questions about life, about meaning and about a relationship to the sacred or transcendent (adapted from Koenig *et al.* 2012).
2. This term was used by a Médecins Sans Frontières (MSF) staff member when explaining to me why the psychologist whom headquarters had sent to them in the field was useless to their operations.
3. The author acknowledges the assistance of Child Fund Angola (Huila) in facilitating the research process, with special thanks to Samuel Pinocas and Nazaret Zangui.
4. The *deslocados* amongst whom the research was conducted had mostly been displaced by attacks by the National Union for the Total Independence of Angola (UNITA) as a result of the war of 1992–1994 and the renewed outbreak of violence in 1998/1999. For many of them this was not their first experience of displacement as they had been subjected to brutal attacks and forced to abandon their possessions and lands many times over in the four decades of almost continuous armed conflict in the country. Research was undertaken in two areas of Huila: amongst self-settled *deslocados* in the town of Lubango and in government-run centres in the rural areas near Matala.
5. The methods of participation and observation work in a dialectic relationship, influencing one another and each gaining greater significance and appropriateness depending on the specific situation. Both methods were frequently used simultaneously but there were also instances where I assumed the role of observer without participating in activities.
6. For instance, Schensul *et al.* (2015); Suwankhong and Liamputtong (2013).

7. When investigating social constructions of wellbeing it is important to reflect on how I, as researcher, construct my own version of the participants' version.
8. The term 'established Christian denominations' is used here to refer to official churches recognised by the World Council of Churches and the Roman Catholic Church, in order to differentiate them from smaller, independent religious movements that may have originated in more recent times. These definitions are, however, in themselves problematic as they define newer, smaller religious movements in relation to the European-founded mission churches (Sindima 1994).
9. A tragic stampede in December 2012 in Luanda has led to the UCKG being banned by the Angolan government in February 2013. A rally had been called under the slogan 'Day of the end – come and put an end to all problems in your life, disease, misery, debt etc.' and the huge numbers of people who attended together with a lack of security and limited capacity of the stadium led to 16 deaths. See: http://www.portalangop.co.ao/angola/en_us/noticias/politica/2013/1/5/Government-suspends-Universal-Church,05a2018b-ebaf-4385-83ca-f2bb935a8759.html
10. Jonas Savimbi, the leader of the UNITA rebel movement, was widely believed to be practising witchcraft, based on accounts of defected aides and rumours about the murder of his own mother in order to make use of her spirit (Brinkman 2000).
11. This is true of all churches, including Catholic and Protestant ones.
12. This may place a burden of responsibility on a person who is ill if they believe that a lack of faith is the reason for non-recovery. Members of the congregation may be criticised for not placing enough trust in God's healing powers as exercised by the church leaders.
13. *Curandeiros* and *adivinhadores* play an important role as 'spirit specialists' who have the abilities to heal and divine through the power, knowledge and skill conveyed to them by specific spirits. These spirit specialists deal with a number of difficulties and illnesses that may arise as a consequence of war when aggrieved spirits may seek vengeance for injustice, witchcraft or neglect (Honwana 1997).
14. A friend in South Africa told me that she was made to kneel in front of the congregation and confess her sin when she fell pregnant while unmarried. She was also told to sit in the last row at the back for two years. Her anger and humiliation over this treatment led her to leave the church.

References

Ager, A. and Ager, J. (2011). Faith and the Discourse of Secular Humanitarianism. *Journal of Refugee Studies* 24(3): 456–472.

Ben-Tovim, D. I. (1987) *Development Psychiatry: Mental Health and Primary Health Care in Botswana*. London: Tavistock Publications.

Bolton, P., Wilk, C. M. and Ndogoni, L. (2004) Assessment of Depression Prevalence in Rural Uganda Using Symptom and Function Criteria. *Social Psychiatry and Psychiatric Epidemiology* 39(6): 442–447.

Bompani, B. (2010) Religion and Development from Below: Independent Christianity in South Africa. *Journal of Religion in Africa* 40(3): 1–24.
Bowie, F. (2000) *The Anthropology of Religion: An Introduction*. Oxford: Blackwell.
Brinkman, I. (2000) Ways of Death: Accounts of Terror from Angolan Refugees in Namibia. *Africa* 70(1): 1–24.
Dawes, A. and Honwana, A. (1996) Children, Culture and Mental Health: Interventions in Conditions of War. In *Children, War and Prosecution – Rebuilding Hope*. Proceedings of the Congress Maputo (December 1996) Maputo: Rebuilding Hope.
Dein, S., Cook, C. C. H., Powell, A. and Eagger, S. (2010) Religion, Spirituality and Mental Health. *The Psychiatrist* 34(2): 63–64.
Deneulin, S. and Rakodi, C. (2011) Revisiting Religion: Development Studies Thirty Years On. *World Development* 39(1): 45–54.
Devine, J. and White, S. (2013) Religion, Politics and the Everyday Moral Order in Bangladesh. *Journal of Contemporary Asia* 43(1): 127–147.
Geschiere, P. (1997) *The Modernity of Witchcraft: Politics and the Occult in Postcolonial Africa*. Charlottesville, VA: University Press of Virginia.
Gifford, P. (2004) Persistence and Change in Contemporary African Religion. *Social Compass* 51(2): 169–176.
Githieya, F. K. (1997) *The Freedom of the Spirit: African Indigenous Churches in Kenya*. Atlanta, GA: Scholars Press.
Honwana, A. (1997) Healing for Peace: Traditional Healers and Post-War Reconstruction in Southern Mozambique. *Peace and Conflict: Journal of Peace Psychology* 3(3): 293–305.
Honwana, A. (1999) Non-Western Concepts of Mental Health. pp. 103–119 in M. Loughry and A. Ager (eds.) *The Refugee Experience*. Oxford: Refugee Studies Programme.
International Federation of the Red Cross (IFRC) (2014) *World Disaster Report. Focus on Culture and Risk*. Geneva: IFRC.
Jordans, M. J., Tol, W. A., Komproe, I. H. and De Jong, J. V. (2009) Systematic Review of Evidence and Treatment Approaches: Psychosocial and Mental Health Care for Children in War. *Child and Adolescent Mental Health* 14(1): 2–14.
Koenig, H., King, D. and Carson, V. B. (2012) *Handbook of Religion and Health*. Oxford: Oxford University Press.
Mbiti, J. S. (1989) *African Religions and Philosophy*. 2nd ed. Oxford: Heinemann.
Miller, K. E. and Rasco, L. M. (2006) An Ecological Framework for Addressing the Mental Health Needs of Refugee Communities. pp. 1–64 in K. E. Miller and L. M. Rasco (eds.) *The Mental Health of Refugees: Ecological Approaches to Healing and Adaptation*. Mahwah, NJ: Lawrence Erlbaum Ass.
Peddle, N., Monteiro, C., Guluma, V. and Macaulay, T. (1999) Trauma, Loss and Resilience in Africa: A Psychosocial Community-Based Approach to Culturally Sensitive Healing. pp. 121–151 in K. Nader, N. Dubrow and B. Stamm (eds.) *Honoring Differences: Cultural Issues in the Treatment of Trauma and Loss*. Philadelphia: Bruner/Mazel.
Rakodi, C. (2012) A Framework for Analysing the Links between Religion and Development. *Development in Practice* 22(5–6): 634–650.
Schafer, A. (2010) Spirituality and Mental Health in Humanitarian Contexts: An Exploration of World Vision's Haiti Earthquake Response. *Intervention* 8(2): 121–130.

Schensul, S. L., Schensul, J. J., Singer, M., Weeks, M. and Brault, M. (2015) Participatory Methods and Community-Based Collaborations. pp. 185–212 in H. R. Bernard and C. C. Gravlee (eds.) *Handbook of Methods in Cultural Anthropology*. 2nd ed. Lanham, MD: Rowman and Littlefield.

Sindima, H. (1994) *Drums of Redemption: An Introduction to African Christianity*. Westport, CT: Praeger.

Summerfield, D. (1999) Sociocultural Dimensions of War, Conflict and Displacement. pp. 73–92 in A. Ager (ed.) *Refugees: Perspectives on the Experience of Forced Migration*. London: Pinter.

Suwankhong, D. and Liamputtong, P. (2013) Ethnographic Performance and Its Flexibility in Researching a Traditional Healing System in Southern Thailand. *Qualitative Research Journal* 13(3): 244–252.

The Holy Bible, New International Version (1984). Grand Rapids: Zondervan House.

United Nations High Commissioner for Refugees (UNHCR) (2014) *Partnership Note on Faith-Based Organisations, Local Faith Communities and Faith Leaders*. Geneva: UNHCR.

Van den Berg, S., Reiffers, R. and Sniders, L. (2011) A 'Psycho-Spiritual Approach': Beyond the Mental Health and Psychosocial Support Humanitarian Mandate? *Intervention* 9(1): 61–73.

Wessells, M. and Monteiro, C. (2000) Healing Wounds of War in Angola: A Community-Based Approach. pp. 176–201 in D. Donald, A. Dawes and J. Louw (eds.) *Addressing Childhood Adversity*. Cape Town: David Philip.

Wessells, M. and Monteiro, C. (2006) Internally Displaced Angolans: A Child-Focused Community-Based Intervention. pp. 67–94 in K. E. Miller and L. M. Rasco (eds.) *The Mental Health of Refugees: Ecological Approaches to Healing and Adaptation*. Mahwah, NJ: Lawrence Erlbaum Ass.

9
Picture This: Visual Explorations of Wellbeing in a Landmine-Contaminated Landscape in Cambodia

Gabrielle Davies

Introduction

Millions of people around the world are affected by the presence of landmines, which represent lasting legacies of war and conflict that continue to impact on people long after the guns fall silent. Improving the wellbeing of affected people is a key tenet of the mine action sector, but it is not clear how wellbeing is defined or the ways in which the wellbeing of people is expected to be affected by the presence of mines. Although a number of studies have explored the meso- and macro-level impact of landmines, there is a scarcity of research at the micro level (Roberts and Littlejohn 2005). In addition, as Harpviken and Millard (2000: 27) assert, further community-level studies are necessary as 'improved assistance to mine-affected communities must start with a deeper understanding of the situation faced by people living in these communities.' This forms part of the driving force behind my research which aims to deepen the understanding of the ways that the continual presence of landmines impacts on the wellbeing of affected people.

Wellbeing is a notoriously difficult concept to define and has different meanings for different people. How then would the many and varied understandings of wellbeing affect responses to mine contamination, clearance and development? In order to answer this question I incorporated a variety of participants in my overall research design: from mine action and development actors at international and national level, to local villagers living in a mine-affected community. Using a bricolage approach, my fieldwork consisted of a variety of qualitative data-generation methods. This paper focuses on one aspect of my fieldwork: the use of participatory photography and photo-elicitation interviews within a mine-affected community in Cambodia. It documents some of the trials, tribulations and triumphs of utilising a participatory and visual approach in the assessment of wellbeing. Ultimately it concludes that participatory photography provides a three-dimensional approach to discussions about what people need for life to be good that encapsulates the material, relational and subjective dimensions of wellbeing, as well as people's past, present and future aspirations, all in the space of one image.

The context: Cambodia, landmines and the fieldwork setting

Cambodia is situated in South-East Asia and has borders with Thailand, Vietnam and Laos. With a total population of approximately 14 million, 85 per cent of people live in rural areas and are predominantly engaged in agricultural activities, many as subsistence farmers. Ranking 138th out of 187 countries on the United Nations (UN) Human Development Index, Cambodia is recognised as one of the poorest countries in the world, with an estimated 45 per cent of the population living in poverty, the majority of which is found in rural areas (United Nations Development Programme [UNDP] 2013).

Decades of war have had a lasting impact on Cambodia, which remains one of the most heavily mine-contaminated countries in the world. Despite over 15 years of clearance activities, landmines continue to pose a daily threat to thousands of people. During the 30 years of conflict in Cambodia, all sides laid mines both offensively and defensively and the country is littered with numerous unmapped minefields. Over 30 different types of anti-tank and anti-personnel mines have been found and the contamination situation can best be described as diverse and complex, with multi-layering of minefield on minefield in some places. The most contaminated areas are located along the north-western border with Thailand, with five provinces being most heavily affected: Battambang, Batan Meanchey, Oddar Menachey, Preah Vihear and Siem Reap.

My fieldwork was undertaken for the most part in Battambang province in 2012. The first phase of in-country fieldwork consisted of conducting interviews with various national and international mine action actors in order to gather as many different perspectives and understandings of the way that landmines affect the wellbeing of people and to gain valuable background information on the situation in Cambodia. Having made connections with the majority of mine action organisations working in Cambodia, I was then able to negotiate access to a mine-affected community via the Cambodian Mine Action Centre (CMAC) who assisted in identifying and then taking me to visit the community with which I spent the following three months.

The village is situated approximately 55 km away from Battambang towards Pailin and is in a fairly remote rural location. It consists of 159 households and 602 people. The main occupation of the villagers is subsistence farming, predominantly rice, but also corn and in some cases, sesame. There is no electricity, no running water, and no health service in the village and generally it is a very hand-to-mouth existence. People have settled in the village from all over the country and for the most part their homes consist of small bamboo or wooden houses such as the one in Figure 9.1. The area was previously dense forest and was a thoroughfare for both government and Khmer Rouge forces so was (and still is) heavily contaminated with both anti-tank and anti-personnel mines and other explosive remnants of war (ERW). CMAC has undertaken three clearance sweeps in the village: the first clearing 15 metres from

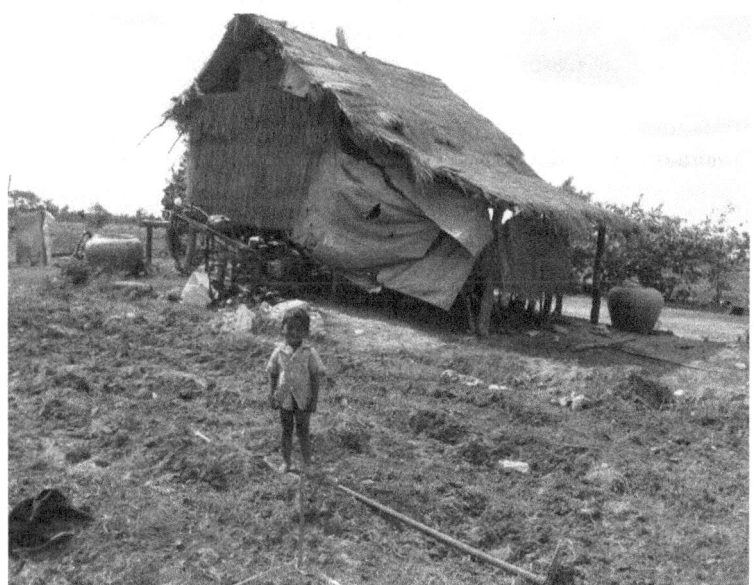

Figure 9.1   The home of one of the villagers

the main path through the village, the second clearing 50 metres from the path and the third clearing fields so that they could be cultivated. CMAC has also undertaken infrastructure and community development projects in the village and has built a road, ponds for water and engaged in agricultural training activities with the villagers. Landmines are still prevalent in the area and CMAC continues with clearance, having set up a base camp in the village two years ago.

In terms of mine contamination, some villagers had their land cleared several years ago, while others had their land cleared more recently, and some plots are yet to be fully cleared. The village therefore presented an interesting location in which to undertake my research as it enabled me to talk to people about how their lives were before clearance had taken place and how their lives have changed since clearance had been undertaken. I was also able to talk to a number of the de-miners and to observe the interaction between the villagers and the people responsible for making their land safe.

The village was established in 1997 and at that time consisted of only five families. The area had not previously been inhabited, and when the first settlers arrived it was densely forested and heavily contaminated with both anti-tank and anti-personnel mines as it had been a thoroughfare for both government and Khmer Rouge forces, and both sides had laid mines offensively and defensively. People had come to the area for one reason and one reason only: land. However, although land was available, it was densely forested and highly contaminated with landmines. Even though much of the forest has now been cleared, life remains extremely hard. The majority of people have no savings so face difficulties if an unexpected expense occurs, such as an illness in the family. Many people have left the village to work across the border in Thailand in order to earn money to send back to their families. All but one of the families I spoke to have microfinance loans, and in some cases, multiple loans which they have had for several years and have difficulty repaying. The guarantee for these loans is their land, meaning that should the microfinance organisations decide to foreclose, there are going to be many landless families in the area. The rains were also late coming so most of the rice that people had planted had died, and during my time in the village people were starting to go hungry as they had nothing left from their own produce and no money to buy any food. However, despite the evidence of material poverty, in terms of wellbeing, a very different picture can be painted. Sharing a small part of their lives for three months, the villagers showed me a perspective that was both positive and gently optimistic, and one that gave me an insight into the ways that landmines have impacted on their wellbeing and the enormous difference that clearance has made to their lives.

The approach: Bricolage and the inter-disciplinary nomad

Throughout my research I have adopted a bricolage approach. A bricoleur could best be likened to a maker of quilts or a film-maker (Denzin and Lincoln 2005): someone who draws the fabric of ideas from multiple places and sews or edits them together to make a finished product that is bigger than the sum of its parts. This is in keeping with who I am as a researcher and indeed, as a person. I have lived in numerous countries from Europe to Asia to Australasia and back again and have a somewhat esoteric employment history that encompasses both international development and international business. From these diverse experiences, I have learned to take inspiration where it falls and this is reflected in my research which draws from a number of different disciplines. As such, I class myself as an inter-disciplinary nomad and believe that by drawing together ideas and knowledge from a variety of different places I can collate them into a bricolage that reflects some of the multiple perspectives and ways of knowing inherent within any given scenario. In the research on which this chapter draws I am thus trying to capture the multiple viewpoints on mine contamination, de-mining and wellbeing and how these different understandings shape responses to landmine contamination, clearance and development (Davies 2015). This chapter focuses on one set of perspectives, those of the villagers and their understandings and experiences of living with landmines.

I follow the Wellbeing Pathways definition: 'Wellbeing is experienced when people have what they need for life to be good' (Wellbeing Pathways 2013: 3). While acknowledging the wide body of literature surrounding wellbeing, in my project I have drawn on the work of the Wellbeing in Developing Countries (WeD) Research Group, an Economic and Social Research Council (ESRC)-funded project at the University of Bath (Gough and McGregor eds. 2007). This presents a more holistic, inclusive and positive approach to research within an international development context, which can often stigmatise people through the use of negatively value-laden language such as poverty and social exclusion. Wellbeing is something that everyone aspires to, regardless of their sex, age, race, or material circumstances (White 2009). This approach to wellbeing also focuses more on people's strengths rather than needs and was therefore in keeping with my own conceptualisation of mine-affected people not as passive victims waiting for assistance, but instead as active agents in their own lives who continue to strive for a better quality of life despite their physical circumstances.

The WeD approach to wellbeing considers three inter-related dimensions: the material, the subjective and the relational. By exploring not only what people have (material wellbeing), but how they feel about what they have (subjective wellbeing), the emphasis is also firmly placed on wellbeing in relation to others (relational wellbeing) (White 2009). This reflects the relational approach to wellbeing identified in Chapter 1. We do not live in isolation, but share our lives and our experiences with others: from the closest family members, to friends and neighbours within the community, and on a wider scale, we are influenced by the values and cultures in which we are embedded and the rules and customs to which we are bound.

The centrality of land to the villagers' narratives made me realise that looking at human wellbeing in isolation was not enough; I needed to locate this within the context of the relationship to the environment. I have therefore linked the WeD concept of wellbeing to a broader socio-ecological approach of person-in-environment. That there is an important relationship between human wellbeing and the natural environment is now quite widely recognised, as in the Millennium Ecosystem Assessment (MEA). In my view, however, this relationship needs to be understood as much more than simply positioning the environment as a provider of services (MEA 2005). Instead, the relationship between people and the environment is dynamic and intertwined. Changes in the physical environment result in changes in the behaviour, attitudes and actions of people, and changes in the behaviour, attitudes and actions of people result in changes in the physical environment. The relationship is not linear, but iterative and systemic. Indeed, research with indigenous peoples demonstrates that there is also a spiritual and emotional connection between people and the environment, and that the wellbeing of people is inherently linked with the wellbeing of the environment (McGregor et al. 2003, Panelli and Tipa 2007). This, I would argue, can also be applied to rural agrarian populations more broadly. By considering the wellbeing of people and environment as intrinsically linked, a more rounded analysis of the different and varied characteristics of a mine-contaminated landscape can be presented that incorporates different ways of seeing and understanding the relationship between the natural and social world. Developing a term introduced by White and Jha (2014), I have labelled 'wellbeing ecology' this fusing together of wellbeing with a socio-ecological approach to environmental change.

The methodology

As a bricoleur, I find it difficult to work within the constraints of a fixed and rigid method of enquiry, and instead prefer to have the flexibility to adapt the project design to the situation and to use whatever methods are appropriate at any given time. To this end I used a variety of qualitative data-generation methods to try to capture the multiple stakeholder perspectives inherent within the project landscape. The use of purely qualitative methods was a deliberate choice, as it is my belief that there is an over-reliance on quantitative data, particularly within the mine action sector. In addition, as Camfield *et al.* (2009: 7) note, qualitative methods used to explore people's subjective experiences of wellbeing are essential and valuable in their own right and 'encompass areas of people's lives that are influential and important, but rarely measured (for example, spirituality and religious practice)'. With this in mind, and as a firm believer in research with and not on people, I felt that my time and resources would be better used concentrating on building relationships with the project participants and providing an active listening space for people to express themselves in the way that they wanted to. There is, of course, a place for quantitative statistics which can document the number of mines taken out of the ground, the amount of land cleared and the number of people who have benefited from clearance. However, numbers alone cannot truly capture the impact that clearance has had on people's lives. How do they feel about it? And what effect has clearance had on their wellbeing? It is often the small things that make a difference: having the ability to walk down a road without fear; being able to visit the temple to worship; letting your children play freely outside; and being able to offer water to your guests when they visit your home. These things cannot be adequately reflected through statistics alone, but must be complemented by narrative accounts and visual representations that paint a more holistic and in-depth picture of people's lived realities. With this in mind, I used a combination of semi-structured interviews, observation, participatory photography and photo-elicitation interviews in my fieldwork. It is to the use of participatory photography and photo-elicitation interviews with the villagers that I will now turn.

Participatory photography and photo-elicitation interviews

I decided to incorporate visual methods in my research because our experience of the world incorporates all of our senses and, as Lacey

(1998: 5) notes, 'Of all our senses, it is sight that gives us the most detailed information.' In addition, visual methods can reveal hidden or unanticipated things (Banks 2007). Although photographs are snapshots in time, and are open to interpretation, they can also show how we feel about certain objects, environments, activities and interactions that are sometimes difficult to articulate with words (Prosser and Schwartz 1998). This is particularly pertinent when researching wellbeing, as it is not a concrete or physical entity and is often difficult to capture with words alone. I therefore decided to use photography and photographs in my research as a means of trying to access a visual perspective of what wellbeing is for the participants.

Participatory photography is a research method that aims to 'see the world through someone else's eyes' (Thomas 2009: 1). It also represents a more participatory approach to research, as the participants are actively involved in the research process and the production of knowledge (Thomas 2009). In addition, as Noland (2006) argues, photographs can help us identify what people value, how they see others and how they view their world. By using as the basis for interviews photographs that have been taken by participants, there is a shift in the balance of power between the researcher and the participants, whereby the participants become the 'experts', leading the researcher through the images (Collier and Collier 1986). I was very aware that I was a Western outsider coming into the village and I wanted to try to reduce the perception of myself as 'expert', and instead make it clear that I was there to listen, watch and learn. By asking the participants to take photographs and to lead the discussions about them, the participants told their stories in a way of their own choosing, and we were able to jointly construct the meaning of the images (Harper 2002), thereby making it a more collaborative and participatory approach to research, which was in keeping with the ethos of my project. All of the photographs shown and described in this chapter have been taken by participants themselves.

The choice of participants was a key factor for the participatory photography. I had conducted over 30 individual and household interviews by that time and had found that the women tended to be more reserved and less articulate than the men when being interviewed, so wanted to see if taking a different approach would result in richer data, while ensuring that I maintained a gender balance and good mix of ages. In total, ten villagers took part in this aspect of the research: five women and five men, some of whom I had talked to before and some of whom I had not. The participants ranged from 24 to 68 years old and included a monk, a landmine survivor, relatively newly arrived residents and people who had lived in the village for over ten years. Despite the range in ages and the length of time they had lived in the village, there were a significant number of marked similarities between the photographs that were taken and the way that the participants spoke about why they had taken the pictures and what they represented in terms of their wellbeing.

I began this phase of the research by showing the villagers how to use the cameras while my interpreter provided a running commentary. We then stayed with them while they got used to the camera and took some initial practice shots. In some cases this took longer than others, as some of the villagers had never seen a digital camera before, let alone used one. One of my most abiding memories from my time in the village was watching the face of a woman in her late 60s as she learned how to use the camera and seeing her obvious delight at the images she was able to capture. We then asked each participant to keep the camera for several days and to take as many pictures as they wanted to of things, people and places that were important to them, their lives and wellbeing (translated into Khmer as 'having what you need for life to be good'). After I had printed out the images, in some cases up to two weeks after they had been taken, my interpreter and I then visited the participants in their homes to interview them about the images. Each photo-elicitation interview was digitally recorded with the permission of the participant. We began by asking the villager to talk us through each picture and to explain why he or she had taken it, what it meant to him or her and what it represented in terms of his or her wellbeing. I found that apart from one woman who provided very literal explanations of what the images represented, all of the other villagers articulated stories around each image, with some pictures, particularly of land, eliciting much longer and fuller narratives.

The trials and tribulations

Timing was a consideration for this part of the research. I had already been in the village for two months before I began the participatory photography, as I felt that it was important for the villagers to become used to my presence, cycling round the village on my clapped-out bicycle, stopping here and there to have a chat, before I asked people to take part. Living in a mine-contaminated village with no electricity (bar the occasional small tractor converted into a generator for the evening) in a fairly remote location also meant that I had to think about a number of practical challenges. After talking to several people who had been involved with photography projects in Cambodia, I opted to buy two battery-operated second-hand digital cameras. This meant that the participants could take as many photographs as they liked and were instantly able to see the images. It also meant that the photos could be transferred onto my computer without having to be scanned in. I tried photo-elicitation interviews using both the images on the computer and hard copies and found that participants were much more at ease with the printed pictures, as they were able to flick through all of the photographs and decide which ones to speak about and in which order. It also meant that I was able to give the participants the photos as a small thank you for taking part, which was greatly appreciated as very few people in the village had a camera and photos were in scarce supply.

Talking about wellbeing can be an emotional experience. Asking people to think about their lives invariably brings to the fore the challenges and difficulties that they are facing. Taking the photographs proved to be a positive experience for all of the participants, but talking about the images and delving deeper into their lives was more challenging for both the participants and myself. My aim was to provide a safe space where the participants could tell me about their lives, but it is very difficult to conduct a private interview in a communal setting. You are never alone in the village, and interviews tended to attract other people, be it family members or neighbours. Although this was the norm for the villagers who seemed to live their private lives in the public domain, for me it raised a number of ethical issues. How could I maintain confidentiality? Would the participants feel able to speak freely if they had an audience? What should I do if other people insisted on answering some of my questions instead of the person I was aiming to interview? The first-ever photo-elicitation interview I conducted provided multiple examples of the potential difficulties. The participant was Mrs NA, but several members of her family had taken pictures, and we all crowded into her small bamboo hut to look at them on my computer. Understandably there was much excitement to see the photos, and indeed the short videos they had made of the noodle-making process. However, this also resulted in everyone talking at the same time about what the images showed, making it difficult to probe any deeper meanings behind the pictures. I therefore realised that it was better to provide the people with copies of the images prior to arranging the photo-elicitation interview so that the villagers had a chance to go through the pictures and consider what they wanted to say about them. This was an invaluable lesson, and on subsequent occasions I made sure that I had allowed the villagers time and space to view and share their photographs before having to speak about them.

The timing and location of the photo-elicitation interviews was extremely important and I tried to ensure that we negotiated a time and setting, invariably in the homes of the participants, that would be relatively free of interruptions and where the participants felt comfortable discussing their lives with me. In some cases I decided to curtail the interview and return at a later time or date if it became clear that the interviewee was uncomfortable. Overall, however, the photo-elicitation interviews were successful, proving to be interesting, informative and in depth.

The triumphs

The most powerful part of the participatory photography was in helping me to see wellbeing more through the eyes of the participants. Any preconceived ideas I had about what wellbeing was for the villagers and how the presence of mines had affected this were firmly set aside as the villagers led me through the images, explaining what they represented and why they were important. It was sometimes surprising to hear the explanations behind the pictures. For example, the image of a bowl of Cambodian noodles in Figure 9.2 was taken by the monk who described how on a literal level it meant sustenance for him, but on a deeper level, it related to the relationship he had with his parents who had died, as they used to make and sell noodles in order to support the family. It also represented an aspiration for the future, as he intended to make and sell noodles if he ever left the pagoda, which would enable him to live and to honour the memory of his family. The noodles were therefore an image of his past, his present and his future and interwove the material, subjective and relational aspects of his wellbeing.

The photographs represented a different perspective from which to view wellbeing. By using participatory photography I was able explore the way that people framed their lives, using the images as the basis for free-ranging discussions that were led by the villagers. This presented a contrast to the individual and household interviews I had conducted that were based around questions I had developed from my observations and initial pilot interviews that followed a more structured format. Although the images showed specific physical objects such as rice growing in a field, cows grazing, friends and family, water, houses, the road, the pagoda, the school, money and so on, the participants were able to articulate a much deeper sense of meaning behind the photographs that went far beyond the initial literal interpretation of the images. I had been worried that it may have been difficult for the participants to

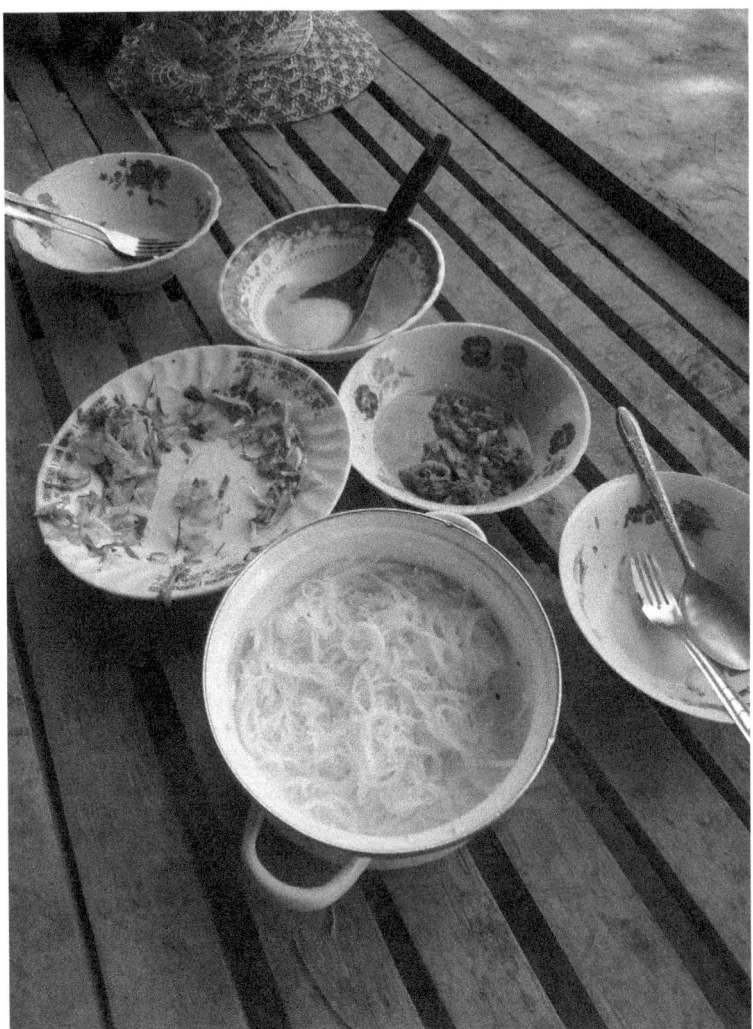

Figure 9.2 Cambodian noodles

take photographs that represented more conceptual aspects of wellbeing such as participation, health and relationships, but on that score I was proved very wrong. For example, the woman shopkeeper took a photograph of a tin of money (Figure 9.3). For her, money represented an important part of her life as it meant she could support her family, but it then led on to a discussion about the changes in the village that were

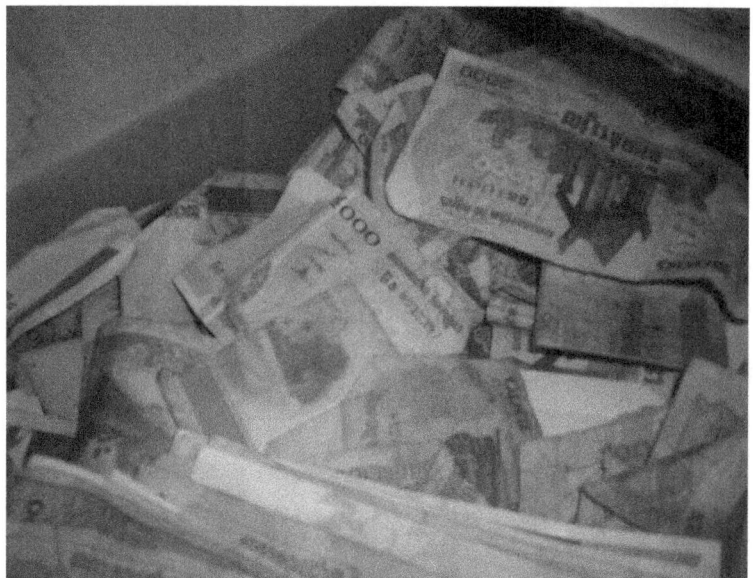

Figure 9.3 Tin of money

taking place and how so many people were leaving, which meant she was worried about her business. From there, she then spoke about the importance of health to her wellbeing which was suffering because she was so concerned about the situation in the village that it had led to her developing stomach problems. The discussion then went full circle back to money as she was worried that she would not have enough to pay for treatment.

The most common subject of the photographs was land and rice growing (see Figures 9.4 and 9.5). For the villagers, land is one, if not the most important aspect of their lives and is linked in numerous ways to other aspects of their wellbeing. Land provides security; it is the source of food for the family, but also means that if necessary they can borrow money against their land to buy seeds or other essential items such as paying for medical care. Without land there is no livelihood, and the clearance of landmines has meant that the participants now feel safe ploughing their fields and tending their crops, whereas in the past they were afraid, but had no choice but to walk and work on suspected hazardous land. Mr J had taken images of his children working on the land and making charcoal. For him, this represented the intertwined importance to his wellbeing of his family and the land as their source of livelihood. He

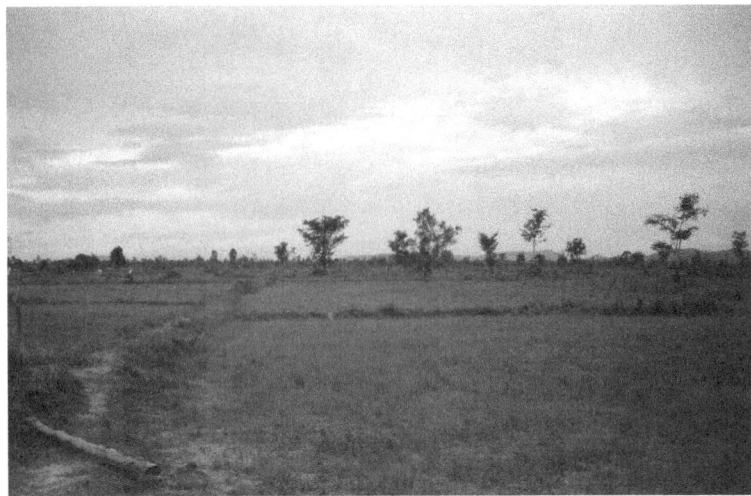

Figure 9.4 Rice fields

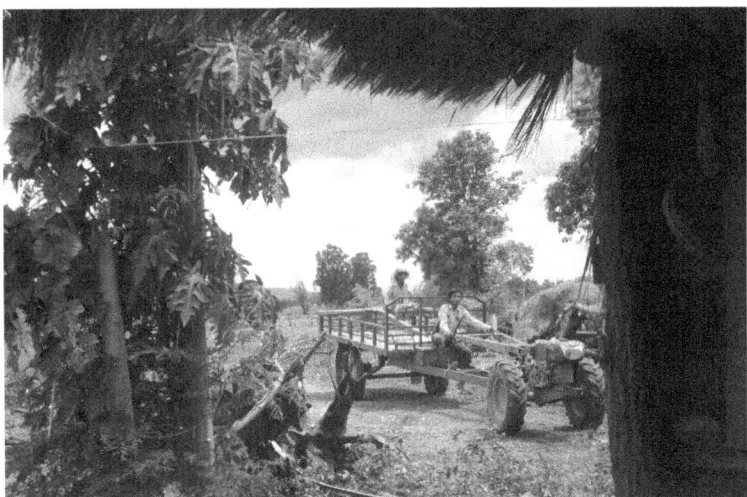

Figure 9.5 Going to the fields

spoke about the limitations that were placed on his life by the presence of landmines. In his words, 'Landmines make us poor.' They stop people accessing land, which means that people find it difficult to survive as they cannot grow enough rice to support their families. Especially in the early days, before much de-mining had taken place, the mines had also reduced the social connections he could make as people were afraid to walk along the path and very few people could live in such harsh conditions. He also talked about how he felt coming back to live in a place where he had been severely injured by an anti-tank mine explosion, and how that affected his mental and physical health. But, the overriding sense that he conveyed was that his life was improving. Despite the difficulties he continued to face, the physical changes in the village such as having a road that did not get muddy in the rainy season and having land that was free of mines meant that he was gently optimistic for the future wellbeing of himself and his family. Gradually, step by step, he was ensuring that he could plan for the future and would make sure that the lives of his children would be better than his own.

Another interesting aspect of wellbeing that was revealed through discussion of the photographs was the level of fear and constant stress that the participants felt as a result of living in a mine-contaminated landscape. Going back to the early days of settlement in the village, a number of the participants talked about the calculated risks they took every day to work on their land or to forage for firewood or vegetables in the surrounding forest. This situation severely restricted their lives and was detrimental to their wellbeing as it meant that they did not have the freedom to go where they wanted. Mrs P talked about the photograph she had taken of her husband standing in the rice field and explained that before clearance she could only go five metres from her house because she was afraid of the forest and the mines. The fear encroached on every aspect of her life and was the embodiment of the way that the presence of mines negatively affected her wellbeing. She told me that in the past, whether she was asleep or awake, she was always thinking about where she could go because if she went one way there were mines, and if she went another way, there were mines there too. Now, however, she said that her life is much better than before as she is no longer afraid and can go wherever she wants to without fear. Time and time again I heard the villagers say, 'Yes I was afraid of the mines, but I had no choice. I had to walk on the land. I had to take the risk.' These examples demonstrate some of the very real psychological and emotional impacts of living with landmines. What I found fascinating was that a photograph could prompt such insights into the lives of the participants. By taking a photograph of, for example, a field of rice, the participants were able to provide access to a myriad of memories about how their lives were in the past which then, for the most part, prompted a discussion of the improvements to their wellbeing that

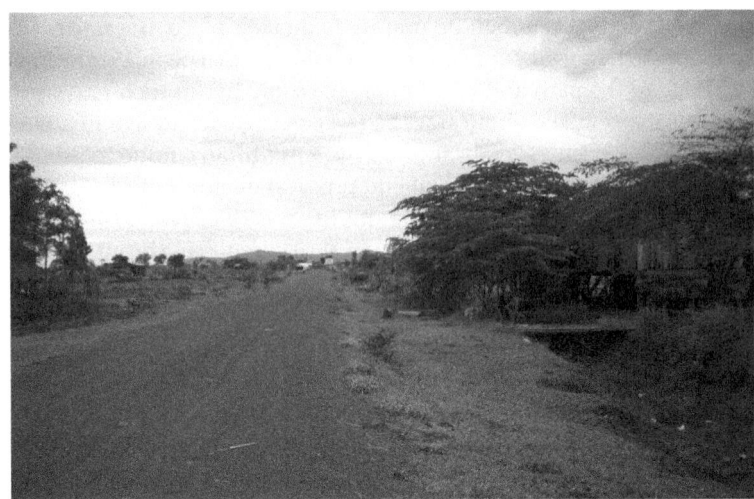

Figure 9.6 The road through the village

had taken place once the mines had been cleared, demonstrating a clear and intertwined relationship between people and the environment and highlighting the importance of place for wellbeing.

Several participants took pictures of the road in the village (see Figure 9.6). The man in the shop explained that when he first moved to the village ten years ago, it was densely forested and full of landmines. Following clearance (of both trees and mines), CMAC had built a road. This was important for him because it meant that he could now travel freely without fear of mines, that business people from the nearby town could come and buy his crops and that he could more easily access health services if the need arose. Mrs FL talked about the road in terms of increasing social connections and making it easier for people to visit one another. She told me that she was much happier now that a lot of people had come to live in the village. She also explained about the importance of the road for her children, as it meant that they could easily go to school and get an education. Education was deemed important to their lives and wellbeing, as in the words of Mrs FV, 'If we have education we can do everything; if we have no education we cannot do anything.'

Water was also a prominent facet of people's lives and wellbeing. Several participants took photographs of ponds and ditches. In the past, although there was a lot of rain, there was nowhere to store it. With the

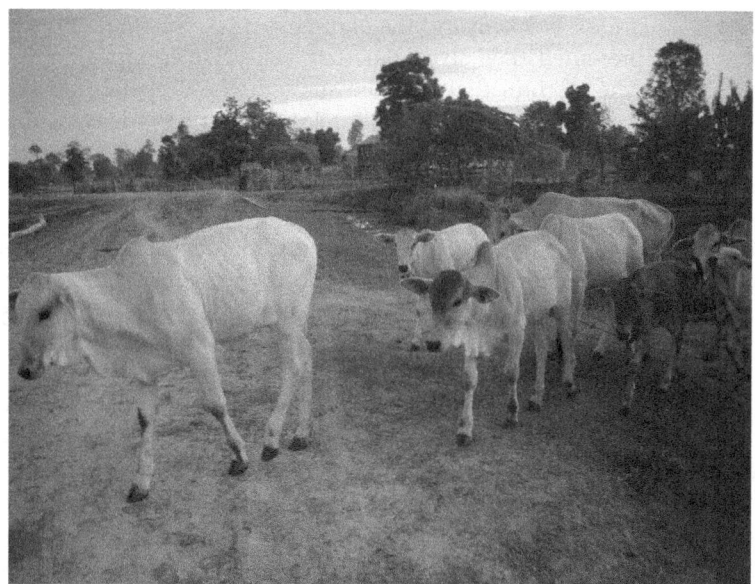

Figure 9.7 Cattle

integrated approach to mine clearance and development that CMAC has adopted, several communal ponds have been dug in the village, which means that villagers can safely and easily access water. Mr N talked about the long distance he had to travel in the past to fetch water and how because of the scarcity he could only use two cups of water to wash himself. Mrs FV explained about the ditch that CMAC had deepened for her which had significantly improved her life as it meant that she had enough water not only for herself and her family, but also her cows. Cattle (see Figure 9.7) were seen as an important aspect of people's lives as they represented security for the future, a form of insurance policy. By breeding livestock, several of the participants were able to profit from selling the calves, and in addition, if a family member became ill, they were able to sell the cows to pay for treatment. Additionally, as Mrs FL explained, cows were a means of production and helped her to plough her rice fields and could also be a source of food if the need arose.

Practical lessons learned

Photographic images can therefore be seen as an interesting way of accessing people's knowledge and understandings about their past and present situations. Not only did the participants take photographs that they felt represented their lives, but they were able to articulate stories around the pictures that revealed some of the deeper issues that affect their wellbeing. The most abiding lesson that I learned was that images and photographs provide participants with the opportunity to show wellbeing through their eyes. It was an enjoyable experience for all concerned and resulted in some wonderful pictures and some fascinating discussions that were focused and in depth. In fact, this part of my research prompted me to consider my own wellbeing in a mine-affected landscape and how I would picture it. That, however, is a story for another time.

Throughout my research, ethics played an important role. As a reflexive person I constantly assess the way I act, speak and behave, and I carried this through into the way I conducted my research. The core principle underpinning my ethical approach was 'Do no harm' (Anderson 1999), and as such I was sensitive to the impact that my presence and my research was having on the villagers. The participatory photography added another ethical element as the villagers invariably took pictures of other people as well as places and objects that were important to them. I therefore made sure to ask all the people captured in the images if I could use the photographs of them in my thesis and any subsequent publications. I also ensured, as part of the informed consent process, that the villagers involved in the participatory photography were made aware and agreed that I could use their pictures to illustrate my research. In this way we had joint ownership of the images, although where people were easily recognisable, I chose not to include them in this chapter in order to maintain anonymity.

Participatory photography, although not without its challenges, represents an interesting and rewarding way of capturing wellbeing from a visual perspective. A simple image can generate a wealth of meaning when used as the basis for discussions about wellbeing. As a reflexive tool, photo-taking and photographs have the ability to provide people with a different space and perspective from which to think about their lives and tell their stories. Firstly, by giving people cameras, it allows them time to think about what is important to them rather than being faced with an immediate interview question, and enables them to frame the images in a way that is meaningful to them, which can then be discussed during interview. The images provoke memories of their past experiences as much as their present realities, and produce much more focused, detailed discussions that presented a three-dimensional way of assessing wellbeing that recognises the intertwining of person with environment, as well as past, present and future with material, subjective and relational aspects of wellbeing.

Conclusion

For the participants, wellbeing and having what they need for life to be good revolves around land. From land they have sustenance and security, which relates to family and close relationships. Growing crops is dependent on water, and having the ability to store water was another key facet of wellbeing. The relatively new village ponds that a number of participants took photographs of meant that they no longer had to travel for long distances to carry water, but instead could use that time to work in the fields or to do other jobs that would enable them to earn more income. Relating to this are the many images of the road that the participants took that showed not only a means of getting from A to B more quickly, but represented freedom of movement and freedom of choice. Children can now safely go to school, which gives them more opportunities for the future. Both villagers and people from surrounding villages can now safely travel to the pagoda for ceremonies, fostering greater social connections and participation while allowing people to worship and practise their religion in order to increase their spiritual wellbeing.

Despite the variations in age and gender of the participants, the photographs the villagers took revealed marked similarities in what was viewed as important for life to be good. This was useful in building up a composite picture of what wellbeing meant for people living in this community. Additionally, through the discussions about the photographs I was able to track the changes in wellbeing from living an almost claustrophobic, isolated life during the time of heavy landmine contamination, to a much freer and less fearful existence post-mine clearance. The images also captured the small everyday occurrences that make a difference to people's lives: being able to collect water from a clean, nearby pond, allowing their children to walk to school on the safe road, while the subsequent interviews provided people with the space to explain why these small changes made so much improvement to their lives and wellbeing.

Ultimately, the participatory photography proved to be a positive experience for everyone involved. As a process it also provided villagers with an opportunity to reflect on their situations and how these had changed with the clearance of the majority of the landmines from their everyday landscape. Ultimately, all the participants concluded that although life had been very difficult in the past, they had seen a significant improvement in their lives and wellbeing and were cautiously optimistic for the future.

References

Anderson, M. B. (1999) *Do No Harm: How Aid Can Support Peace – Or War.* Boulder, CO: Lynne Rienner Publishers.

Banks, M. (2007) *Using Visual Data in Qualitative Research.* London: Sage Publications.

Camfield, L., Crivello, G. and Woodhead, M. (2009) Wellbeing Research in Developing Countries: Reviewing the Role of Qualitative Methods. *Social Indicators Research* 90(1): 5–31.

Collier, J. and Collier, M. (1986) *Visual Anthropology: Photography as a Research Method.* Albuquerque: University of Mexico Press.

Davies, G. M. (2015) *Living with Landmines: Mine Action, Development and Wellbeing in Post-Conflict Society – A Case Study in Cambodia.* PhD thesis, University of Bath.

Denzin, N. K. and Lincoln, Y. S. (2005) Introduction. pp. 1–42 in N. K. Denzin and Y. S. Lincoln (eds.) *The Sage Handbook of Qualitative Research.* 3rd ed. London: Sage Publications.

Gough, I. and McGregor, J. A. (eds.) (2007) *Wellbeing in Developing Countries: From Theory to Research.* Cambridge: Cambridge University Press.

Harper, D. (2002) Talking About Pictures: A Case for Photo Elicitation. *Visual Studies* 17(1): 13–26.

Harpviken, K. B. and Millard, A. S. (2000) *Reassessing the Impact of Humanitarian Mine Action: Illustrations from Mozambique.* PRIO Report 1/2000. Oslo: PRIO.

Lacey, N. (1998) *Image and Representation: Key Concepts in Media Studies.* Basingstoke: MacMillan Press Ltd.

McGregor, D. P., Morelli, T. P., Matuoka, J. K. and Minerbi, L. (2003) An Ecological Model of Wellbeing. pp. 108–128 in H. A. Becker and F. Vanclay (eds.) *The International Handbook of Social Impact Assessment: Conceptual and Methodological Advances.* Cheltenham: Edward Elgar.

Millennium Ecosystem Assessment (MEA) (2005) *Ecosystems and Human Well-Being: Synthesis.* Washington, DC: Island Press. Available at: http://www.millenniumassessment.org/documents/document.356.aspx.pdf.

Noland, C. M. (2006) Auto-Photography as Research Practice: Identity and Self-Esteem Research. *Journal of Research Practice* 2(1): Article M1.

Panelli, R. and Tipa, G. (2007) Placing Well-Being: A Maori Case Study of Cultural and Environmental Specificity. *EcoHealth* 4(4): 445–460.

Prosser, J. and Schwartz, D. (1998) Photographs within the Sociological Research Process. pp. 101–115 in J. Prosser (ed.) (2001) *Image-Based Research: A Sourcebook for Qualitative Researchers.* London: Falmer Press.

Roberts, R. and Littlejohn, G. (2005) *Maximizing the Impact: Tailoring Mine Action to Development Needs.* PRIO Report 5/2005. Oslo: PRIO.

Thomas, M. E. (2009) Auto-Photography. pp. 224–251 in R. Kitchen and N. Thrift (eds.) *International Encyclopedia of Human Geography.* London: Elsevier.

United Nations Development Programme (UNDP) (2013) *Human Development Index*. Available at: http://hdrstats.undp.org/en/countries/profiles/KHM.html [accessed 27 September 2013].

Wellbeing Pathways (2013) *An Integrated Approach to Assessing Wellbeing*. Briefing Paper 1. Revised ed. Available at: http://www.wellbeingpathways.org/images/stories/pdfs/briefing_papers/BP1rev-web.pdf.

White, S. C. (2009) *Analysing Wellbeing: A Framework for Development Practice*. WeD Working Paper 44. Available at: http://www.welldev.org.uk/wed-new/workingpapers/workingpapers/WeDWP_09_44.pdf.

White, S. C. and Jha, S. (2014) *Social Protection and Wellbeing: Food Security in Adivasi Communities, Chhattisgarh, India*. Wellbeing and Poverty Pathways; Briefing No. 3, Centre for Development Studies, University of Bath. Available at: http://www.wellbeingpathways.org/images/stories/pdfs/briefing_papers/India_BP_for_website_LARGER.pdf.

10
Authorised Voices in the Construction of Wellbeing Discourses: A Reflective Ethnographic Experience in Northern Mexico

Juan Loera-González

Introduction

There is now quite widespread recognition of the difference between global and local understandings of wellbeing. What is less commonly recognised is the diversity *within* local understandings of wellbeing. This chapter explores some dimensions of this, emphasising in particular the way that such understandings may be obscured by inter-ethnic and intra-ethnic power relations at the local level (Mathews and Izquierdo 2009).

Researching wellbeing amongst indigenous people and ethnic minorities in situations of oppression requires particular attention being placed on the implications of power relations for constructions of wellbeing. Such constructions are influenced by the historic, cultural and collective experiences of the social group in question. In trying to capture a collective sense of wellbeing for the group as a whole, there is a danger of building a unified and clean narrative which fails to consider that indigenous or ethnic groups are not homogeneous or isolated units defined only by cultural difference, nor should they be understood as such. Instead they should be located in a complex and intricate web of inter-ethnic power relations, mobilising discourses of ethnicity and enacting ontological differences that depart from a homogenising political project of modernity (Blaser 2012). While recognising such groups' disadvantaged positions in relation to national majorities however, it is also important to identify forms of exclusion within these marginalised groups. This draws attention to the politics involved in the representation of emic understandings of wellbeing as political discourses of identity and ethnicity (see Rodríguez, this volume).

Latin America is experiencing a shift in development thinking informed by indigenous notions of wellbeing. In line with a critique of neo-liberal policies and counter-hegemonic development approaches, the region is considered by some as 'the very center of world resistance against this pattern of power and of the production of alternatives to it' (Quijano 2008: 3). These alternatives go beyond the so-called turn to the Left, where many newly elected governments have adopted leftwing policies that urged for a re-orientation of the course followed over the past three to four decades. Whereas these government-led initiatives have focused on following progressive agendas by fostering rights-based approaches and economic redistribution, keeping extractive economic models intact, the discourses and strategies of some social movements suggest radical possibilities towards post-liberal and post-development political projects (Escobar 2010). One such radical possibility is the *Buen Vivir* political project, or the Good Life in English, that speaks of a need to revalue indigenous knowledge in terms of what a good life is and how to harness wellbeing in the light of new social, environment and political contexts. Overall, most studies have focused on the political mobilisation of discourses of wellbeing with respect to the *Buen Vivir* within the Andean region known as *Sumak Kawasay* (in the Kichwa language) or *Suma Qamaña* (in the Aymara language). However, little has been said about how related ideas are shaping indigenous discourses in other Latin American countries, or how to study such discourses.

This chapter reflects on methodological challenges involved in documenting local perceptions and notions of wellbeing, drawing on my experiences of, and reflections on, ethnographic fieldwork in Northern Mexico amongst the Rarámuri (Tarahumara) indigenous people (Loera-Gonzalez 2013). Specifically, it considers the risks of overlooking marginalised voices within the communities that we, as researchers, visit and study. These may tell a different story to the one expressed by the most visible, and often privileged, members of the locality. In doing so, I illustrate the importance of a reflexive ethnographic approach that looks at how we insert ourselves into the field in order to avoid representing a homogenous narrative based on what might be a false sense of shared community that hides a diversity of positions within a social group (Cooke and Kothari eds. 2001, White and Pettit 2004).

Discourse and voice

Before proceeding, it may be helpful to review the key terms that I will be drawing on. Firstly, I will refer to discourses as forms of representations, ideas and habits that produce culturally and historically located meanings of wellbeing that are politically enacted through the medium of individual accounts, or voices. I will use Nancy Fraser's (1992) work on how discourses and counter-discourses are formulated in the ways citizens deliberate their common affairs in an institutionalised public sphere. I will present specific accounts of my informants in order to incorporate their voices and exemplify how they inscribe themselves into different discourses of wellbeing portrayed by the Rarámuri people.

Acknowledging the importance of reflexivity when doing fieldwork, I conclude that there is not just one single discourse of how Rarámuri people conceptualise wellbeing, but a diversity of them. In this chapter I will explore only two such discourses, one that is rather common amongst their communities and a second that is articulated in a more hidden way. This first Rarámuri discourse of wellbeing is intrinsically normative and is often framed in terms of ethnic identity. It was identified in most of the empirical accounts and information gathered, but it was especially evident amongst Rarámuri individuals (men and women) who are currently, or were previously, in positions of authority in the socio-political structure. A second Rarámuri discourse of wellbeing was vocalised in young people's accounts and in the voices of individuals who were not always associated with or seen as role models by the rest of the people, and who were therefore not legitimised by the Rarámuri political context. Both discourses represent how wellbeing is understood and performed, sometimes in a competing fashion, as a discursive tool that expresses ethnicity and reinforces cultural adscription to the Rarámuri people in differentiating them from the wider society.

I will refer to these discourses using the terms 'authorised' or 'unauthorised', depending on whether they are referring to a hegemonic discourse, the one I found more frequently enacted by figures of political power within the community studied, or the counter-dominant discourse, the one enacted mostly by younger people. This is done in order to express how wellbeing plays out in contested and asymmetric scenarios, namely in relation to ethnic adscription. Whether certain voices are authorised depends on if they are considered legitimate according to the current norms held by the Rarámuri political system. The issue of legitimacy is inherently cultural and context-specific. It denotes the normative status expressed through signs, arguments and actions conferred by a group of people upon their governors' institutions. I will explore these discursive differences and the dilemmas I experienced in deciding how to document and make sense of them. By presenting Rarámuri wellbeing discourses, this chapter helps to exemplify one of the main points of this book: that constructions of wellbeing are intrinsically connected to the context in which they are articulated and the research methods used to capture them.

Ethnographic fieldwork

The main fieldwork was undertaken in two localities between January and December in 2010. Laguna de Aboreachi has a mainly *mestizo*[1] population (315) and Aboreachi has a Rarámuri population (120). Both are in the Guachochi municipality of the state of Chihuahua. These localities are closely linked in terms of commercial and administrative ties. The Rarámuri people living in Aboreachi regularly travel to the *mestizo* locality to supply their households with groceries and arrange administrative processes such as government hand-outs and social-protection transfers. As I was interested in comprehending local constructions of wellbeing within a particular contextual perspective, I undertook long periods of fieldwork in order to perform ethnographies, participant observation, surveys and in-depth semi-structured interviews. This set of techniques and instruments aimed to capture voices concerning ideas of wellbeing and how to live a good life amongst the Rarámuri people in Mexico. To complement the ethnographic research, I carried out interviews and surveys with 30 self-identified Rarámuri and 30 *mestizo* inhabitants of the selected localities. Secondary sources of information ranged from a variety of government documents, research projects, reports written by organisations, academic studies, dissertations, journal articles, books, etc. Additionally, archival research included two historic collections: the Archive from the Coordination Centre of Guachochi for Indigenous Action of the National Institution of Indigenous Affairs (INI) and the Smithsonian Institution Archive Section of the Tarahumara Region. These complemented the above research methods by adding a diachronic perspective.

In my approach to fieldwork, I was largely inspired by Stephen Gudeman and Albeto Rivera's (1990) *Conversations in Colombia*, a text which focuses on the domestic economy of daily life in order to understand social process and dynamics from a local perspective. I aimed to build up a conversational community with informants, not only to obtain information from them, but also as a way to verify and validate sources of information. This was done to try to prevent the usual asymmetries that occur in subject/object relationships during fieldwork research (Fals-Borda and Rahman 1991). Living with the people enabled me to get good quality information. I sought to engage with people wherever possible in their everyday activities and with ideas produced within that context, rather than limiting myself to questionnaires and surveys. Later, I used a data-analysis approach influenced by constructivist grounded theory to build up concepts and arguments based on the elements and emic categories that the people in the Sierra Tarahumara themselves considered to be important. I then related the developing categories to key concepts identified in the literature. The combination of empirical and grounded facts with bibliographical accounts provides robustness to the claims presented. Throughout the process, reflexivity was key and I tried to pay attention to my own positionality. This was done by reflecting constantly on my role as an ethnographer in the field, the assumptions and expectations local people had regarding my presence and being attentive to how people performed their ethnicity. Often, I reflected on this while writing my ethnographic diary at nights.

The process of gathering information was a good opportunity for me to learn about the culture and context in which I was inserted; this implied adapting to it. For instance, I learned that asking questions one after another, directly and persistently, is not considered polite amongst the Rarámuri people. It was therefore essential to bring together what people told me in interviews, what I gathered from informal conversations and everyday activities about how ideas of wellbeing are constructed. Specifically, I wanted to discover what matters to Rarámuri people, how they make sense of their living conditions and the factors that contribute to their wellbeing. In doing so, I began to use my own concepts and terms in interviews and conversations, such as poverty and wellbeing, and soon – as described later – people began elaborating and sharing their own ideas of what it is to live a good life in their own terms. As an ethnographer I aimed to generate understandings of culture through representation of what is called an *emic* perspective, the emphasis in this representation being on allowing crucial categories and meanings to emerge from the ethnographic encounter.

At the same time, I tried to engage myself with collective practices. Rarámuri, men and women alike, frequently attend gatherings around the highly demanded drink made of fermented maize called *teswuino*. These *teswuino* gatherings are deeply embedded in the group's culture and constitute an important part of social co-operation networks consisting of family members, neighbours and close friends (Kennedy 1963, 1978, Saucedo 2003, Urteaga 1998). *Teswuino* is also intrinsically related to festivities and ceremonial practices used to perpetuate the farming cycle and forms part of the traditional welfare system. Therefore, *teswuino* gatherings were essential spaces to learn about many aspects of life, including livelihood strategies, visits to the community by medical staff, or the occasional stopover of political candidates during election time. Hence, participating in as many of these gatherings as possible became vital to the progress of my fieldwork. During these gatherings, I spent time mingling in group conversations, hearing and participating in individual dialogues, learning new facts, corroborating information, identifying conflicting versions of stories and having the chance to meet potential informants.[2]

However, what became clear as my fieldwork progressed was that I was not in contact with all members of the community. This became progressively evident for instance while participating in the *teswuino* gatherings. I was consistently introduced and encouraged to talk to people that had experience in the Rarámuri political system. They were sometimes considered to be cultural warrants of the group and therefore expressed rather eloquently the distinctions between the Rarámuri and the non-Rarámuri. In other words, I was presented with a homogenised ethnic representation that tended to emphasise certain legitimate elements over others, while at the same time masking less visible variations and contradictions. The way I entered the community influenced who I interacted with and this therefore shaped the type of wellbeing accounts I had more contact with at the beginning of fieldwork.

Approach to the site

Being no stranger to the region of North Mexico, I approached the Rarámuri communities in the usual way most anthropologists and researchers – including myself – had approached the local population previously; through the traditional Rarámuri leader of the community, the *Seriame*. In other words, I entered the community through the traditional channels of authority, and it was through those channels that I obtained permission to perform interviews and undertake fieldwork.

In line with usual practice, my first contact occurred in the form of an informal visit to the *Seriame's* house. After talking to the *Seriame* about myself, the weather and other apparently irrelevant topics of the day, my intentions and presence in the community were explained along with the larger research aims. After that, the *Seriame* gave initial clearance for me to enter into the community, and his willingness and interest to participate in the proposed research became evident. The subsequent step was for the *Seriame* to introduce me collectively to the rest of the people in one of the regular public gatherings taking place in the church courtyard every other Sunday. This was a helpful opportunity that allowed me to talk publically about my research interests and objectives, and people were able to ask questions about my work. It also let people know about my presence in the community. As a result, most of the residents had been aware of my intentions as a researcher since the beginning of fieldwork and the first image they had of me was by the side of the *Seriame*, the authority in the region.

What I did not fully understand at that moment was how the associations that people had of me with the traditional channels of authority would play out further on during fieldwork or the implications for the information I could gather. Being introduced by the authority figure and standing at his side was in itself an act of legitimisation on my part and a positioning that publically associated me with the *Seriame* and the political power he represents. On the one side, this positioning gave me the opportunity to meet further people and set the conditions for creating trust and confidence amongst men and women whose perceptions I was trying to document. On the other hand however, as later became evident, this association granted me greater access to those informants in positions of power within the Rarámuri society, leaving behind marginalised individuals and those who did not see eye to eye with the Rarámuri political leadership.

However, intensive and enduring fieldwork enabled me to explore the 'hidden transcripts' (Scott 1990) through the establishment of friendship ties with the people of Aboreachi and therefore be receptive to their thoughts and opinions. The following sections of this chapter set out some of what I learned when I moved away from this association with the dominant groups and began to listen to more hidden voices.[3]

Authorised voices

My first informants in the early stages of fieldwork were mostly elder men and women who enjoyed a high social status at the community level, some having been figures of authority within the Rarámuri political structure in previous years. They in turn introduced me to people who thought in a similar way to themselves. They presented to me a common perception of wellbeing as being associated with maintaining an ethnic identity in the form of cultural institutions, practices and structures of authority in contrast to the prevailing non-indigenous influence in their territories.

The accounts of wellbeing presented by these elder individuals of high socio-political status were framed in terms of a normative discourse based on the idea of *Gara wachi inaropo nai gawich* in the Rarámuri language, or 'living on the right path' in English. The questions I asked that made these voices visible concerned mainly ideas of what is a plentiful life, how it could be harnessed and what constituted a good life within the Rarámuri context. I understood that the idea of living on the correct path relates to the ideal of how to be a Rarámuri, the normative guidelines for everyday behaviour which stress differences between the Rarámuri and the *mestizos*. For the elder individuals, the search for living well implies maintaining living conditions that allow them to live *well*; this does not necessarily imply improving conditions through material accumulation and commodities in order to live *better*, as the non-indigenous lifestyle generally assumes. This discourse is based on a desire and ideal of homogeneity in living conditions and a collective ability to control their own cultural practices and spaces (Chambers 1983, Li 1996).

In a sense, this discourse mirrors the way wellbeing is positioned in the Latin American *Buen Vivir* discourse as expressed by a number of Latin American authors, such as Acosta and Martínez (2009), Dávalos (2008) and Huanacuni Mamani (2010). Firstly, it aims to preserve cultural and political distinctiveness from the non-indigenous wider world through the recognition of collective rights in addition to individual rights. Secondly, it emphasises contentment with securing a livelihood that provides certain essentials as the basis for a meaningful life rather than continuously improving one's life condition. Ultimately, it questions the way wellbeing as the aim of mainstream development processes is understood.

There are two main dimensions in the discourse found amongst the Rarámuri; first, the significance of farming; and second, the importance of having a strong sense of community rooted in solidarity and co-operative practices. I mention the significance of farming because it refers not only to access to the land as a physical asset; it concerns having access to good quality land and seeds, and involves religious rituals, traditional knowledge and community exchange practices inherent in the act of farming. The second dimension, having a strong sense of community, has to do with community cohesion and effective social ties between families and friends which support the structures of social and political authority amongst the Rarámuri.

These two dimensions also suggest that, for an important segment of the Rarámuri, living well is accomplished by pursuing the right strategies with which to maintain their livelihood, such as subsistence agriculture; communal rather than individual ownership of the means of production; social systems that are heavily reliant on kin relations; and culturally embedded forms of sharing and reciprocal exchange – such as *teswuino* gatherings – which entail collective returns rather than focusing on individual accumulation (Kennedy 1963, 1978, Saucedo 2003, Urteaga 1998). In this way, the articulation of the discourse on living well supports social and cultural mechanisms that maintain ethnic differentiation (Gluckman 1958, Grinker 1994).

The following examples show how these two dimensions were expressed:

> If a Rarámuri household works its plot of land well, that is, according to group traditions and as the ancestors used to do, then you will be fine and won't be deprived.
>
> (Interview, Aboreachi, México, July 2010)

> As long as we have land to work on and to leave as inheritance to my offspring there is no problem about poverty, with maize it's enough, is the base to have *pinole*, *teswuino* and tortillas; food can be complemented by other vegetables gathered seasonally, like *quelites*, mushrooms and such.... And if you have friends and family to help you that's also helpful. That's why we must make *teswuino* to offer it to *Tatadiosi* [God] and to your friends for helping you when you need it.... If you have money and a lot of possessions people will have envy and that's not good, they will tell that you don't need help, you have too many things.
>
> (Interview, Aboreachi, México, June 2010)

This clearly normative discourse expressed by elderly authority figures appeals to the importance of maintaining traditional practices, of securing economic sufficiency rather than accumulation, which is perceived to threaten the continuity of community relations amongst people and deities. In this sense, material accumulation is not only seen as unnecessary but also discursively considered undesirable, an argument that clearly goes against assumptions of mainstream development thinking. This discourse draws some parallels to what Scott-Villiers (2011) finds in her ethnographic analysis of a policy meeting between development agencies and pastoralist communities in the Horn of Africa. She describes how the village elders' view of what constitutes poverty contests the understandings of non-governmental organisations (NGOs) and state agents. The elders' view referred to enhancing the local capacity of sustaining their community's social-protection mechanisms, production system and the quality of their knowledge, while for development actors it was to secure economic production and distribution of aid through channels and networks controlled and defined by them. Scott-Villiers understands the elders' view as a counter-discourse compared to the universalising discourse performed by the development industry on the terrain of moral responsibility. In the same way, the wellbeing discourse expressed through authorised Rarámuri channels positions itself in a contrasting position to the non-indigenous wider society.

This Rarámuri discourse also emphasised social homogeneity. When asked about the poorest or most marginalised households in the locality, these interviewees tended to state that everyone enjoys roughly the same quality of life, mentioning for instance that all households maintain their families by working hard on their farms, and that risks and harsh conditions affecting the locality are shared amongst all. Even where differences in family size or the size of the farm are evident from household to household, the majority of the Rarámuri population living in Aboreachi choose not to recognise or express this openly. Where particular hardship is admitted, it is seen as something temporary, not evidence of a more sustained social difference:

> Here [in Aboreachi], we all live the same, we suffer from the same things (...) is not like in Chihuahua [city] or in other places. If somebody needs something, we must help him as it could be ourselves that might be in that situation tomorrow.
> (Interview, Aboreachi, Mexico, February 2010)

This tendency to express collective uniformity reflects a social ideal that is part of Rarámuri ethnic identity: the oneness of the community is linked to their social and economic homogeneity. Their unity was expressed by invoking their common exposure to environmental conditions, kinship links and their practice of sharing key livelihood resources between themselves. An example of such a narrative is the following:

> All of us are related somehow; we share farming tools or even animals for our plots.... If it doesn't rain we all suffer equally; if it rains and the crops grow well we are all happy.
> (Interview, Aboreachi, Mexico, February 2010)

This emphasis on shared experience is also intended to maintain communal cohesion and avoid confrontation, coercion or envy. This is an issue of significant importance to the traditional authorities to preserve their status amongst the community. As with other rural populations, the Rarámuri recognise that envy and conflicts which originate from bragging about being relatively better off, or showing off material assets, produce a negative effect that endangers the sense of cohesion and homogeneity within the locality.

> God wants us to live happily without conflict; if we keep fighting and shouting at *teswuino* gatherings – as some young teenagers do – we only create problems.
>
> (Interview, Aboreachi, Mexico, June 2010)

This picture of social homogeneity is not shared by everyone, however. Other, more hidden voices emphasise unequal living conditions and disparities in a way that suggests the representation of community cohesion is a myth. As Li (1996) argues, such idealised representations of community stressing harmony, equality and tradition have material outcomes. They enable a range of strategies to obtain or retain access to key resources and are 'capable of producing strategic gains, as they counter prevailing development orthodoxies, open up opportunities, and provide a legitimating vocabulary for alternative approaches' (Li 1996: 502).

When I encountered the first discourse of wellbeing during fieldwork it was appealing to document it as the only collectively shared construction of wellbeing amongst the Rarámuri, one which appeared to unify them and present their ethnic identity as a ready political tool. It had clear resonance with the collective construction of wellbeing and the resilience of ethnic identity framed by the long political struggles of indigenous people and ethnic minorities in Latin America. However, when living amongst the Rarámuri it became clear to me that this was not the only reality, and that as an anthropologist I had a responsibility to bring out contestations in that construction of wellbeing and the hidden voices that this politically authorised discourse obscured. I thus had to reflect on the implications of the approach I had followed thus far, and question whether there were other voices that would provide greater nuance to the understandings of wellbeing. I am referring to these other voices as unauthorised as they occupy a subordinate position within the Rarámuri context, in the same way Nancy

Fraser (1992: 123) uses the term as a 'counter-discourse that formulates oppositional interpretations'.

Unauthorised voices

During fieldwork there were distinctive voices that were more hidden and less openly expressed by community members; these represented the aspiration and desire to live a life similar to that displayed by the wider society and the *mestizo*. The voices of these often-marginalised individuals stressed the importance of securing a family income throughout the year instead of relying on subsistence agriculture. Justified by precarious and often vulnerable livelihoods, these voices were more publically open to including material assets and accumulation in the calculation of wellbeing. And, crucially, they prioritised improving one's quality of life in its individual dimension over preserving and maintaining shared cultural institutions, practices and traditions. This alternative discourse represented marginal voices in contrast to the first discourse, which enjoyed a more dominant position within Rarámuri society, especially amongst elders and privileged individuals.

Amongst these hidden voices were recently formed households of newly married people, some single-headed households, teenagers and young men, who – at least in part – were engaging in seasonal migration to the cities, a practice expected for males of that age. I was not encouraged by the elderly traditional leaders to talk to these people about how a Rarámuri should live or what their aspirations were as they were seen as 'not being Rarámuri enough'. They were not considered to be role models in the eyes of most Rarámuri people and they were marginalised and stigmatised by traditional Rarámuri authorities when it came to enunciating wellbeing scripts. In a sense, they constituted illegitimate voices of the Rarámuri ethnicity and collectiveness. I was only able to access these accounts at a later stage when I started to reflect on my approach to the field. I started to look at issues of legitimacy and to question who possesses the authorised voice of the collective. Consequently, I began to visit each household within the community and have one-to-one conversations with members who had not been considered key informants until that moment. This created, over time, a space of trust that allowed them to speak more freely in a private context.

Many of the teenagers and young people who migrated seasonally to work in agricultural fields or to neighbouring cities were vulnerable to accusations of creating envy due to their new experiences and new material possessions. Some of these individuals were accused of fighting in collective gatherings, disrupting the social norms of the community. It is important to note that being marginalised and not seen as a legitimate conveyor of the idea of what is to be a Rarámuri and how his or her life should be does not necessarily imply that these individuals were socially marginalised from the community as a whole. They might be actively participating in other solidarity networks or collective festivities.[4]

It is important to capture the full spectrum of wellbeing understandings and how they form different discourses, in this case, that depart from the authorised voice of Rarámuri ethnicity. Hearing other voices adds nuance and texture to the existing differences and avoids homogenising social groups. In addition, these voices express more openly the need to claim equal opportunities within labour and commercial markets available in larger non-indigenous towns or cities, and in a way, to claim for redistribution over recognition (Fraser 1997). While the authorised discourse conjures the sufficiency of subsistence agriculture, this one emphasises its insufficiency and limitations. Finding an alternative source of income then becomes a priority. This next account provides an example.

> Here in Aboreachi, one has so few desires and cravings; for instance one can be happy with just enjoying a coke bought at the store – or if someone gives it to you as a gift, even better!.... But sometimes I get bored here, there's nothing here so I need to work in the city, to earn money for the family, this year we did not harvest half of what we need.... I would be happy if I can only pay all my debts and have money so I can buy things, that's why *Oportunidades* [the social-protection programme] is important, perhaps with time I can move to the city and make my life there.
>
> (Interview, Aboreachi, México, October 2010)

This testimony of a young man shows how, for some individuals, their aspirations distance them from the legitimate Rarámuri voices shown earlier. Suddenly, options appear which offer the possibility of a life outside of the one dictated by the Rarámuri guidelines of their elders. Migration becomes an option. This leads young people from their late teens to migrate in search of temporary employment and experiences in urban settings within the wider society.

In place of an emphasis on tradition and common life, young people emphasise the hope of a better future for themselves and their families.

The experience of working, at least temporarily in the city, brings aspirations of new possibilities beyond the context of the scarcity of the Tarahumara region, and beyond the shared normative values that discourage material accumulation and promote communitarianism, which are the building blocks of the legitimate discourse seen earlier. Migration thus seems to provide a new path to wellbeing which many young people identify with as a means to improve standards of living, with potential benefits at both the individual and the collective level. For further discussion of wellbeing in the context of mobility as part of the search for getting ahead, please see Huovinen and Blackmore (Chapter 7, this volume).

The testimony above and other similar accounts documented in fieldwork uncover the tensions between living in the urban or rural setting and the different livelihoods this implies: the rural livelihood practised by the dominant sector of the Rarámuri does not fit easily with the comparatively individual, profit-oriented, commoditised way of living within large cities. Ironically, those voices that remain hidden, and – in a way – illegitimate, within the Rarámuri community are linked to what is considered mainstream in the wider society. The relative position of discourses, whether authorised or unauthorised, depends on the context of specific struggles and their competing norms and representations of community across a range of levels and settings.

Making sense of the clash between authorised and unauthorised voices

I frame the discordance of voices as an acknowledgement of the complexity of human society. The discursive clash reflects a struggle for political representation and cultural identity of the Rarámuri that express how life should be, what aspirations and expectations are involved and how wellbeing is signified. The authorised voices are articulated into a discourse that portrays identity and claims recognition and distinctiveness in a way that is necessarily homogenised and ideal. Ultimately, it draws parallels to the *Buen Vivir* discourse portrayed by other indigenous people in Latin America in that it departs from mainstream global society in the construction of wellbeing and development. In contrast, the unauthorised voices represent a discourse that stresses the need to secure a livelihood focusing on all socio-economic and cultural opportunities available, aligned or not to aspirations from Rarámuri political leadership. It therefore links to the struggle for redistribution and inclusion in wider development policies. This constitutes, in the terms of Nancy Fraser (1992), the struggle between hegemonic and subaltern understandings in order to formulate oppositional interpretations of identities, interests and needs. These discourses also show differentiated ways of conceiving and achieving livelihoods, aspirations and ways of relating with land and society, and ultimately wellbeing. Both discourses seek to endure and make do with what one faces in life, an aspect encountered by Jackson (2011) amongst the Kuranko people in Sierra Leone.

The discourse expressed by traditional leaders of the Rarámuri – the idea of *Gara wachi inaropo nai gawich* – maintains that there is a correct path to live. However, the second discourse expressed by other Rarámuri claims that another path exists. This discourse exists at the margins, and is justified by an appeal to precarious and vulnerable livelihoods that demand alternative ways of living, aspirations and constructions of what it is to live well. It is not that unauthorised voices articulate a competing vision of community to the idealised harmony and equality of living conditions presented in the legitimate discourse, but they appeal more to the economic vulnerability implied within it. Fraser (1992) sees that counter-discourses can partially offset, although not wholly eradicate, the participatory privileges enjoyed by members of dominant social groups in stratified societies. Consequently, unauthorised voices often say nothing to disagree with the traditional leaders when they share a public scenario. It is only when approached by someone non-Rarámuri in a private context that they express their opinion more freely. This is what James Scott (1990) called the 'hidden transcript' of discourses.[5]

This shows that wellbeing discourses – and the way we approach them – are always located in a particular historical and political context. Which discourse is legitimate and which one not of course depends on the scope of analysis. If we focus within the context of the Rarámuri community, certain ideas of what is valued and how one should live in relation to land, farming and community co-operation are clearly dominant over others. If we focus beyond the local context, on the wider sphere of political relations at the state level, the Rarámuri discourse based on the idea of 'living your life on the correct path' would be in a subaltern position. In other words, both discourses are located within an uneven terrain where wider power relations shape livelihoods and ways of living. The uneven terrain where discourses are located enables and opens up the Rarámuri–non-Rarámuri political arena to articulate day-to-day struggles over key resources that constitute the 'practical political economy' through which different parties defend their interests and advance their claims (Chambers 1983, Li 1996).

This reflects the larger picture, that indigenous lifestyles are constantly open to new influences at the individual and collective level: the education system, mass media, new technologies and infrastructure in their localities, and greater commoditisation of everyday life. In this sense, it could be argued that the unauthorised discourse introduces new subordinations of modernity into the local context.[6] It opens up the broader political context of how indigenous people engage with the mainstream of Mexican society. If we consider the full complexity of the social and political realms surrounding Rarámuri–non-Rarámuri relationships, I see both discourses not necessarily in opposition to one another, but rather their relationship can be more accurately described as strategically complementary. In some moments, depending on specific political and social arenas, Rarámuri people articulate and reconfigure one discourse over the other without ruling it out completely.

In this sense, I argue that wellbeing amongst the Rarámuri can be understood as the balance of two forces: the discourse of communal rights of recognition and the discourse of the rights of distribution (Fraser 1997). On the one hand, living well is harnessed by the collective right to maintain a livelihood based on subsistence agriculture, their distinctive set of cultural and religious beliefs, communal rather than individual ownership of the means of production, social systems based heavily on kin relations and the practice of culturally embedded forms of sharing and reciprocal exchange which entail collective returns rather than focusing on individual accumulation. In short, the right to live differently from what the mainstream Western idea of development stands for through control over those everyday mechanisms that help reinforce Rarámuri identity and self-definition. This, of course, refers to the importance of having an indigenous rights framework where Rarámuri people and others not only participate actively in the development of approaches that affect them, but also recognise a differentiated citizenship that grants them distinctiveness from the rest of society.[7]

Conversely, living well for the Rarámuri does not limit itself to the right to maintain autochthonous practices of self-consumption and collective networks; it also implies the right to build reciprocal relations with the state and wider society which entails having income-generating activities and access to basic services and benefits from social-protection programs. In this sense, the unauthorised voices are articulating the right to distribute opportunities to engage with broader economic, social and political institutions to make their way in life. Crucially, this participation in the wider non-indigenous world must occur in equal circumstances, without being characterised by current conditions of exclusion and discrimination that build up persistent asymmetries between groups.

It is within the fluctuation between these two forces that wellbeing understandings are articulated, sometimes switching between these two sides, alternatively emphasising one or the other. I believe the balance between subsistence agriculture and having the possibility of engaging with the state and local markets through, for instance, temporal migration to agricultural fields away from their communities is important. In a way, having a mixed economy of subsistence and market participation and sharing socio-political spaces with the broader society ensures they are able to adapt in the face of vulnerabilities and manage their dual claims to rights of recognition and redistribution. It seems that the overall Rarámuri idea of wellbeing consists precisely of maintaining this balance. It is therefore in the spaces between these forces that wellbeing ideas construct their meaning.

Learning

The learning that I extract from my research experience amongst the Rarámuri people relates directly to the discussion of wellbeing addressed in this book. I acknowledged that human interactions are always dynamic, constantly constructing themselves, suffused with power relations and uneven positions that constantly define aspirations and understandings, including those of ideas of wellbeing. In recognition of this, it is vital to consider our positionality as researchers by being sensitive to our incursion into a pre-existing social and cultural setting, and possibly being associated with local figures of power – traditional authorities, NGOs, official institutions, or otherwise that might influence how we are perceived in the field.

Finally, this experience appeals to the usefulness of ethnographic methods in qualitative research in exploring the politics of representations of wellbeing. Ethnographic methods provide depth to the exploration of a wide range of social realms including relational dimensions. By acknowledging the variability and contentious views of wellbeing that emerge from diverse cultural and socio-economic contexts, we can prevent dominant social orders from legitimising well-established power symmetries by re-inscribing homogenised ideas of wellness. Heterogeneity of human experiences and collective political aspirations are at the heart of constructions of wellbeing and the research methods we use can help us document and capture them. At the same time, the in-depth description of everyday life and practice that constitutes the ethnographic approach enabled me to understand the complex and subtle dynamics of how ethnicity is represented and their effect on the constructions of wellbeing discourses amongst the Rarámuri people. Following Ahmed's (2010: 13) comment mentioned in Introduction to this book, that happiness shows us different values and orientations, we can argue that within the Rarámuri context, ethnicity is crucially valued and oriented in diverse and dynamic ways. These dynamic ways emerged from the ethnographic encounter as crucial understandings and meanings that became central to identifying the balance of having the right to live differently and the right to distribute opportunities and to participate actively within the nation state and wider society. In effect, these learnings relate to the argument presented in the book that how we capture and understand constructions of wellbeing is intrinsically connected to the broader cultural and social context and the methods used to document them. Within this, the research is a key element.

Notes

1. Non-indigenous people living in the same geographical area.
2. It is important to mention that although the fermented *teswuino* plays a major role in these gatherings, alcohol intake is not that high and is certainly not the main objective of the gatherings. In a way, the opposite holds true, as it is not socially acceptable to get drunk and generate problems for others. Therefore, participation in these gatherings did not usually pose an obstacle in terms of recording data or the reliability of the data itself.
3. I recognise that nonetheless my age and gender meant that there remained some discourses that were more available to me, and others that were less so. For instance, I am conscious that it was much easier for me to approach and build trust with males than females, and that my gender played an important part in the dynamics of participation in the *teswuino* gatherings and therefore in terms of the information I collected, since these gatherings usually occur in physically divided groups of women and men.
4. See Virtanen (2012) on how young indigenous Amazonian people create their social worlds differently from other members of the localities and the need to incorporate their silent voices into the existing anthropological literature.
5. Scott (1990) distinguishes between the 'public transcript' which is the discourse shaped by the dominant group performed openly to any observer, and the critical discourse of the subordinated group that appears in the 'hidden transcript' as space outside the reach of the dominant group.
6. While discussing encounters between modernity – the mainstream Western worldview – and the indigenous people in the Americas, Blaser (2009: 883) mentions, 'modernity implies first and foremost, a language of exclusion and,

only then a promise of inclusion – of course, always demanding that non-moderns reform themselves to be modern. In other words, the alternatives offered to the non-modern [is] in many cases, "convert and we will not only give you the carrot [of modernity] but also will stop using the stick", or "if you don't pursue the carrot we will entice you to it with the stick."' It could be argued that the two discourses explored here represent the language of exclusion/inclusion in the larger battle between forms of worldviews.

7. Iris Marion Young (1990) has labelled differentiated citizenship in which citizens' rights are conceived around their social and cultural differentiation rather than conceiving all citizens as the same.

References

Acosta, A. and Martínez, E. (2009) *El Buen Vivir: Una vía para el desarrollo*. Quito: Abya-Yala.
Ahmed, S. (2010) *The Promise of Happiness*. Durham and London: Duke University Press.
Blaser, M. (2009) Political Ontology. *Cultural Studies* 23(5): 873–896.
Blaser, M. (2012) Ontology and Indigeneity: On the Political Ontology of Heterogeneous Assemblages. *Cultural Geographies* 21: 49–58.
Chambers, R. (1983) *Rural Development: Putting the Last First*. Harlow, UK: Longman.
Cooke, B. and Kothari, U. (eds.) (2001) *Participation: The New Tyranny?* London: Zed Books.
Dávalos, P (2008) El 'Sumak Kawsay' ('Buen vivir') y las censuras del desarrollo. *Boletín ICII-Rimay* 10(110): 17–24.
Escobar, A. (2010) Latin America at the Crossroads: Alternative Modernizations, Post-Liberalism, or Post-Development? *Cultural Studies* 24(1): 1–65.
Fals-Borda, O. and Rahman M. A. (1991) *Action and Knowledge: Breaking the Monopoly with Participation Action-Research*. New York: Intermediate Technology Publications and Apex Press.
Fraser, N. (1992) Rethinking the Public Sphere: A Contribution to the Critique of Actually Existing Democracy. pp. 109–142 in C. Calhoun. Habermas and the Public Sphere. Cambridge, MIT Press.
Fraser, N. (1997) *Justice Interruptus: Critical Reflections on the Postsocialist Condition*. London: Routledge.
Gluckman, M. (1958) *Analysis of a Social Situation in Modern Zululand*. Paper No 28. Manchester University Press for Rhodes Livingstone Institute.
Grinker, R. (1994) *Houses in the Rainforest; Ethnicity and Inequality among Farmers and Forages in Central Africa*. Berkeley: University of California Press.
Gudeman S. and Rivera A. (1990) *Conversations in Colombia: The Domestic Economy in Life and Text*. Cambridge: Cambridge University Press.
Huanacuni Mamani, F. (2010) *Buen Vivir/Vivir Bien. Filosófica, políticas, estrategias y experiencias regionales andinas*. La Paz: Coordinadora Andina de Organizaciones Indígenas (CAOI).
Jackson, M. (2011) *Life within Limits, Wellbeing in a World of Want*. Durham and London: Duke University Press.
Kennedy, J. (1963) Tesguino Complex: The Role of Beer in the Tarahumara Culture. *American Anthropologist* 65: 620–640.

Kennedy, J. (1978) *Tarahumara of the Sierra Madre: Beer, Ecology and Social Organisation*. Arlington Heights, III: AMH Publishing Corporation.

Li, T. M. (1996) Images of Community: Discourse and Strategy in Property Relations. *Development and Change* 27(3): 501–528.

Loera-Gonzalez, J. (2013) *Conflicting Paths to Wellbeing: Raramuri and Mestizo Inter-Ethnic Relations in Northern Mexico*. PhD thesis, Institute of Development Studies, University of Sussex.

Mathews, G. and Izquierdo C. (2009) *Pursuits of Happiness: Well-Being in Anthropological Perspective*. USA: Berghahn.

Quijano, A. (2008) *Des/colonialidad del poder: el horizonte alternativo*. Unpublished manuscript, Lima.

Saucedo, E. (2003) Reciprocidad y Vida Social en la Tarahumara: El Complejo del Tesguino y los Grupos del Sur de la Sierra. pp. 217–267 in S. Millán y J. Valle (eds.) *Etnología de las regiones Indígenas de México en el Nuevo Milenio: La comunidad sin Límites*, Vol. III, México: INAH.

Scott, J. C. (1990) *Domination and the Arts of Resistance: Hidden Transcripts*. New Haven, CT: Yale University Press.

Scott-Villiers, P. (2011) We Are Not Poor! Dominant and Subaltern Discourses of Pastoralist Development in the Horn of Africa. *Journal of International Development* 23: 771–781.

Urteaga, A. (1998) We Semati Ricuri: Trabajo y Tesgüino en la Sierra Tarahumara. In Sariego, J. L. (ed.) *Trabajo, Territorio y Sociedad en Chihuahua durante el siglo XX*. México: Universidad Autónoma de Ciudad Juárez.

Virtanen, P. K. (2012) *Indigenous Youth in Brazilian Amazonia: Changing Lived Worlds*. New York: Palgrave Macmillan.

White, S. C. and Pettit, J. (2004) *Participatory Approaches and the Measurement of Human Well-Being*. WeD Working Paper 08. ESRC Research Group on Wellbeing in Development Countries.

Young, I. M. (1990). *Justice and the Politics of Difference*. Princeton: Princeton University Press.

11
Historical Reconstruction and Cultural Identity Building as a Local Pathway to 'Living Well' amongst the Pemon of Venezuela

Iokiñe Rodríguez

> The problem with development is not that we don't know enough. It is that we don't do enough.
>
> Sarah White,
> Wellbeing and Subjectivity Conference,
> Oxford, January 2014

Introduction

Indigenous people in Latin America have their own way of talking about wellbeing. The Quechua from Ecuador call it *Sumak Kawsay*, the Aymará, *Suma Gamaña*, the Guaraní from Paraguay, *Teko porâ o teko kavi*, and the Mapuche from Argentina call it *Kyme Mogen*.[1] Inspired by indigenous notions of Living Well, many Latin American countries including Ecuador, Bolivia and Venezuela, which are undergoing processes of re-conceptualisation of development, have incorporated the notion of Good Living into national development plans, goals, discourses and legal frameworks such as national constitutions. Although this is a major breakthrough in terms of recognising cultural difference in the frameworks of nation states, there is still a considerable gap between the discourse and practice of pluri/interculturality. Narratives of national identity and modernity are deeply rooted in Latin American society even within emerging pluri-cultural nation-state models such as those present in Venezuela, Bolivia, Mexico, Paraguay, Guatemala and Ecuador (Méndez 2008).

Indigenous peoples themselves, despite their varied conceptualisations of Living Well, have been subject for a long time to intense processes of cultural change and shifting local identities, which puts them under very inequitable conditions to engage in intercultural dialogues with other actors about their, or the wider society's, goals of wellbeing or development in more general terms. There has been a paucity of discussion about creating the conditions for intercultural dialogues to take place effectively. A necessary starting point is for indigenous peoples to have the opportunity to critically analyse their own situations and to define their own wellbeing agendas in a way that can help them to face and confront the multi-dimensional pressures being exerted upon their cultures and ways of life.

This paper tells two stories in one:

a) the story of Kumarakapay, a small Pemon/Taurepan indigenous community from Canaima National Park and World Heritage Site in south-eastern Venezuela, and its experience of confronting the strong power asymmetries that prevent intercultural dialogues about wellbeing between indigenous peoples and other actors, and
b) to a lesser extent, my experience of facilitating part of this process and observing its development over time.

In 1999, after feeling increasingly disoriented and concerned about their sense of loss of cultural identity, Kumarakapay took the lead in initiating a variety of processes of community-wide critical reflection on their history and processes of cultural change as part of the definition of the community's *Life Plan (Plan de Vida)*. The final aim of this process was to help the people from Kumarakapay clarify their views of a desired future and thus strengthen their capacity to engage in dialogue and negotiations with other actors about the present and future management of their territories. This triggered a variety of processes of cultural reassertion, including the publication of a community-authored book about the oral history of the Pemon from Kumarakapay. It also had a knock-on effect on how the Pemon now wish to define conservation and development agendas more broadly with external actors on their lands.

The most distinctive aspect of the way in which the Pemon reflected about their wellbeing is the attention paid to reconnecting with identity and with the past, an aspect of wellbeing that is not sufficiently accounted for, neither in Western ways of conceptualising wellbeing, nor in more alternative 'ethnic' ways, such as *Buen Vivir*. In the former, culture is practically absent and in the second it is simply taken for granted.

The Pemon story serves as an example of how culture and its complexities could be more thoroughly integrated into the way wellbeing is being broadly conceptualised, but also, and perhaps most importantly, of how indigenous people themselves can take the lead in talking about wellbeing in their own terms. As will be shown, such a people-centred approach for conceptualising and thinking about wellbeing can have great impact, not only in promoting community reflexivity about their current situation, but also in terms of doing something about it.

Setting the scene: Canaima National Park, a land of conflicts, exclusion and cultural violence

Canaima National Park (CNP) is located in south-eastern Venezuela, near the border with Brazil and Guyana (see Figure 11.1). It protects the north-western portion of the Guyana Shield, an ancient geological formation shared with Brazil, the Guyanas and Colombia. CNP was created in 1962 with an initial area of 10,000 km. It was extended to 30,000 km in 1975 to protect its watershed function: the Guri Dam, which generates 70 per cent of Venezuela's electricity, and is located 300 km downstream of the north-western border of the CNP. The best-known landscape components of the CNP are the 'tepuyes', ancient mountains

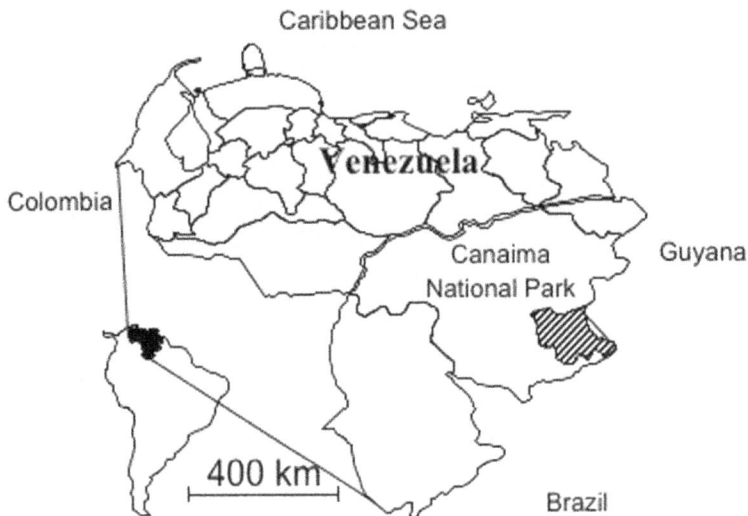

Figure 11.1 Location of Canaima National Park (highlighted in the black and white shaded area)

in the form of a plateau, receiving their name from the indigenous word *tüpü*. CNP's vegetation is markedly divided between a forest-savannah mosaic in the eastern sector known as the *Gran Savana* and an evergreen forest in the western zone. In recognition of its extraordinary landscapes and geological and biological values, CNP was registered on the list of the United Nations Educational, Scientific and Cultural Organisation (UNESCO) Natural World Heritage Sites in 1994.

A wide variety of conflicting demands enter into tension in CNP, largely because the protected area was established on a territory occupied ancestrally by the Pemon people, who are the main occupants of this vast area. With an estimated population of 20,000 people, most of the CNP Pemon live in settlements of 100 to 1,000 inhabitants, although some still maintain the traditional system of scattered nuclear-family settlements. Their lifestyle is based largely on traditional activities: agriculture, fishing, hunting and gathering, although there is increasing work in tourism and associated activities (e.g. handicrafts), as well as in public administration posts (teachers, nurses, community police, municipal staff, etc.).

Despite the strong cultural bonds that the Pemon have with their land, their relationship with the CNP has not been a happy one. The very name of the park symbolises a long history of antagonism between the Pemon people and the environmental managers of this area. To the detriment of the park management, *Canaima* in Pemon means 'spirit of evil' and 'refers to [a person who perpetrates] sorcery, using secret methods that we call witchcraft' (Butt-Colson 2009). The name of the park was inspired by the novel *Canaima* by Venezuelan author Rómulo Gallegos. The novel, written in 1935, is set in ancestral Pemon lands (north of CNP), and represents a strong complaint against abusive leadership and the domination and control of man over nature characteristic of that time. A much more appropriate name would have been Makunaimö National Park, or *Makunaimö Kowamüpö Dapon*, which means 'the Land of Makunaimö' (the supreme cultural hero of the Pemon).

The lack of sensitivity in naming the park is one of the many ways in which the Pemon have been made to feel like strangers in their own land. Although the park has helped protect this part of the ancestral Pemon territory, the Pemon have largely experienced the park as a threat to their existence. This is due to a style of environmental management and development planning in the southern part of the country which has systematically excluded the Pemon's cultural values, knowledge and notions of authority and territorial property.

The result has been local territorial management with a high level of conflict. On the one hand, there are long-standing conflicts over land use, fundamentally due to the use of fire in *conucos* (slash and burn) agriculture and in savannah burning, both indigenous practices considered by environmental managers as a threat to the conservation functions in the watersheds of the CNP. Despite a variety of strategies developed by the government to change or eliminate the use of fire in agriculture and the savannahs (repression in the 1970s, environmental education, introduction of new farming techniques and a fire-control program), many Pemon, especially the elders and those living in more isolated communities, have continued using fire extensively. By contrast, younger Pemon generations have become gradually critical of the use of fire and, as a result, inter-generational tensions are increasingly common on this topic.

Tourism activities have also generated major confrontations between the Pemon and the government, fundamentally because of pressures by non-indigenous tourism companies to establish themselves in the protected area. Using political demonstrations and taking the law into their own hands, the Pemon have so far managed to retain their right to provide tourism services in the CNP, especially in the *Gran Sabana*. However, conflicts over tourism management have continued due to unresolved struggles over different notions of authority and land ownership with the National Institute of National Parks (INPARQUES). Furthermore, there are conflicts over projects of national strategic interest implemented within the park's boundaries, such as the building of a high-voltage power line to export electricity to Brazil (1997–2000) and the installation of a satellite sub-base (2007). Although the Pemon insisted on a commitment from the part of the government to recognise their territorial property rights as a condition for agreeing to the completion of both projects (stated in the 1999 National Constitution), to date no territorial rights have been granted to them. Therefore, the Pemon remain actively in conflict with the government over this issue.

These various conflicts have been developing within a context of rapid cultural change resulting from educational and national integration policies implemented systematically since 1940. As a result, and despite their varied resistance strategies and struggles for self-determination and cultural recognition, the Pemon have increasingly experienced a feeling of disorientation about who they want to be in the future and how they wish to live as a people. In particular there is great concern over the loss of self-esteem of younger generations, as well as over the loss of Pemon knowledge and tradition. Furthermore, these processes of cultural change have led to increasing tensions between young Pemon and elders over current ways of life. This combination of factors has systematically placed the Pemon at a great disadvantage, leaving them vulnerable when they engage in dialogue with other stakeholders about development and territorial management of their land. The greatest threat is the imposition of other people's wellbeing agendas over theirs.

Grounding a Pemon pathway for 'Living Well'

I started working in CNP in 1995, coordinating a conflict-resolution project for a national non-governmental organisation (NGO). My frustration at seeing only minor progress in fostering dialogue between the Pemon and the park managers forced me to take a step back in 1997 and try to understand the conflicts better before attempting to engage with them. Later, in 1999, I went back to CNP in order to carry out my PhD fieldwork.

My plan was to carry out ethnographic research, simply observing how conflicts evolved and were negotiated on the ground. I had no intention of using participatory research in order to avoid getting into messy ground or reviving my frustration from previous years about trying to foster dialogue in the park. However, reality pushed me in another direction.

When I approached the village chief of Kumarakapay, Juvencio Gomez, in order to seek permission to base myself in his village to study and analyse conflicts in the CNP, his response was:

> You can stay as long as you help me and my village reflect about who we are and who we want to be in the future. We – the Pemon – don't know where we are going because of all the projects that are being imposed on our territory; we are totally disoriented. We need to be clear about who we are and who we want to be as a people.

This response startled me. Of course, for him, conflicts are part of his daily life, and because of that he was very much aware of those dimensions of conflicts that are invisible to the stranger's eyes, those dimensions that end up making dialogue impossible as a starting point. He knew that any attempt at fostering dialogue with other actors had to start with the Pemon confronting their own internal tensions over cultural identity. This was something I had completely overlooked, both in my years trying to help 'solve' conflicts in the park and in the design of my fieldwork research protocol.

Another thing he said was, 'Studying conflicts is fine for you, but we don't have time, we need to act now, in two or three years' time, it might be too late for us.' The image I had of myself, working from the comfortable position of a detached academic, was shattered in a matter of minutes. What surprised me the most was his capacity to see that despite the fact that the previous work I had carried out in the park had contributed little to solving conflicts, there was still a role for me to play in fostering dialogue, only it had to be from a different standpoint. I accepted the challenge of working together to design and develop this process of self-reflection alongside my wider research objectives.

As an indigenous leader, Juvencio Gomez had participated in a number of international indigenous rights forums, and heard that indigenous peoples in Colombia were conceptualising development (or wellbeing) in their own terms through the construction of *Life Plans* (*Planes de Vida*). Claudino Pérez, Indigenous Representative from Corpoamazonas, Colombia, defines a *Life Plan* in the following way:

> The 'plan de vida' is a plan made by indigenous organizations and communities in an effort to survive and to maintain traditions, customs, and the hope of having a society with its own identity based on the traditional knowledge of its people. It is a means of guaranteeing better conditions and a better quality of life for indigenous communities. However, it is also a document to be used in negotiations with both the regional and national government. It includes the issues of health, education, territory, the environment, natural resources, the economy and production, government, justice, youth, and women's and gender issues, among others.
>
> (Perez 2009)

Thus, the Colombian experience became an inspiration and a path to follow in the search for a self-defined society and future. It was Juvencio Gomez's view that the starting point for conceptualising this local pathway to wellbeing was to confront themselves with their identity, reconnecting with their past and analysing their current situation. Promoting and constructing this process of personal and collective confrontation with cultural identity became our joint endeavour.

The result was a year-long participatory process of self-reflection which we conducted in conjunction with a group of approximately 30 people (about half elders and half youth). We focused on discussing and researching the following topics:

- Who are we? The origin of the Pemon according to mythological beliefs.
- Where do we come from? Historical and ancestral settlement areas.
- Community history: important historical figures, events, foundation processes of the village.
- How has our community and territory changed over time? Discussion of social and environmental change.
- Things that we need to solve to improve our living conditions and environment.
- Views of development.
- Good and bad things of the past and of the present.
- Vision of a desired future.

As part of this process, we also carried out participatory research on the Pemon's vision and uses of fire in order to help clarify internal tensions about this local activity and encourage dialogue about fire with external stakeholders under conditions of greater equity (Rodríguez 2007).

Community meetings and workshops were used to adapt the process of reflexivity and enquiry to the deliberative, oral-based decision-making structure of Pemon society (Thomas 1982). Different participatory tools were used in these meetings and workshops, including oral testimonies, timelines, territory and community mapping, matrices, brain-storming, group and plenary discussions (Davis 1992). When necessary, assemblies were held to validate information and have the community's consent to continue carrying out the process of self-enquiry.

Of all the points and issues discussed, the one in which the most concrete conceptualisation of wellbeing was achieved was when discussing an ideal vision of the future. Yet, reflexivity about the origin, past, identity, changes and current situation of the Pemon was crucial for grounding this final discussion.

The discussion about the future addressed three main questions:

a) How should the Pemon from Kumarakapay be in the future?
b) What has to change to achieve this?
c) What can we count on in order to achieve this change?

These three questions were then used as a base to collectively construct a vision of the ideal type of society that the Pemon from Kumarakapay wanted to have; in essence, a local construction of wellbeing. A summary of this discussion can be found in Boxes 11.1 and 11.2.

> **Box 11.1 The ideal vision of the future for the Pemon from Kumarakapay**
>
> **How should the Pemon from Kumarakapay be in the future?**
> We should:
> - Be the owners of our knowledge, history, territory and destiny.
> - Write about our history and cosmogony and make it known to others. Others should not have to come to write about the life of our People.
> - Be a society educated in the pedagogic principles of our education and own ancestral knowledge, but also according to the principles of the wider Venezuelan society.
> - Practise and apply the knowledge acquired to help others.
> - Be formed and trained in diverse disciplines and specialties.
> - Practise good manners, be respectful and obedient to our parents: we should practise the Pemon culture, loving each other and not making fun of others, specially our elders.
> - Live and recreate our community in our land, without having to emigrate to the cities.
> - Have a spirit of collaboration and put into practise the knowledge we have acquired in the construction of our society, seeking always to be better.
> - Speak well our own indigenous language, as well as Spanish.
> - Improve and consolidate our tourism lodges and restaurants in order to improve the quality of our service.
> - Dedicate ourselves to agriculture and cattle grazing.
> - Have our own university and hospital administered by the Pemon.
> - Be prepared to confront the pressures of the wider society which harm our society.
> - Be aware that we belong to the Pemon society with our own millenary culture which exists from the times of our ancestors.
> - Defend our rights, above all our land.
> - Value and cherish our culture, especially our dances and songs.
> - Be always Pemon, even though there might be differences among us.
> - Develop and look for productive alternatives to ensure our food security: agriculture, cattle grazing and fishing.

- Practise traditional medicine without undervaluing occidental medicine.

What has to change to achieve this?
We have to:

- Overcome the differences that create rivalries, through dialogue and being aware of the principles and values that have allowed us to coexist in harmony until the present.
- Eliminate bad manners, such as theft, laziness, gossip, envy, selfishness and disobedience.
- Avoid using enchantments (*taren*) to harm other people.
- Avoid the irrational exploitation of natural resources.
- Be protagonists of our own process. Don't wait for others to come and solve our problems. The participation of everyone is important, especially the youngsters.
- Value and respect our elders as our source of knowledge and not make fun of them.
- Demand our parents to be an example to the children, and be responsible in their homes.
- Make use of time to discuss important problems, to look for alternatives and find solutions to our problems.
- Avoid the vice of alcohol consumption because it destroys our future.
- Practise good manners and traditions.
- Create spaces for conversation between elders and youngsters, for the elders to teach and train the young ones about traditional farming, hunting, fishing and other types of knowledge necessary for life.
- Ensure the participation of all in the solution to our problems, especially our women.
- Develop our own education systems, based on our ancestral pedagogic principles, for an integral education of the Pemon.

What can we count on in order to achieve this change?

- With institutions whose objectives are to form, train and orient the inhabitants of our community to improve their quality of life (e.g. educational, health and the church).

Box 11.1 (Continued)

- With the presence, support and disposition of our elders, knowledgeable of the principles of life and history of the Pemon. With their wisdom and knowledge we can recover stories, legends, histories, songs, values and ancestral knowledge of other aspects of our lives.
- With natural resources to generate and diversify our production alternatives.
- With people who have specialised knowledge (mechanics, carpenters, builders) who can be facilitators in the integral formation of the Pemon.
- With parents who have knowledge of astronomy, botany and other subjects, who are willing to teach their children and descendants.

Source: Roraimökok Damük (2010).

Box 11.2 The type of society that the Pemon of Kumarakapay want to have

- A Pemon society with awareness of who we are, and with a sense of identity and of belonging.
- Knowledgeable about our history, culture, tradition and language.
- Owners of our land – territory, knowledge, culture and destiny.
- A society educated with ancestral and modern knowledge.
- A society that values its wise people (parents and grandparents).
- A respectful, hard-working, obedient, kind, courteous, cheerful, generous, harmonious, understanding society where there is love.
- A productive, autonomous society.
- A society that defends its rights and is ready to confront pressures from Venezuelan society.

Source: Roraimökok Damük (2010).

The variety of reflexive processes carried out had different types of impacts. First of all, the reconstruction of Pemon historical roots (both in terms of mythological and factual history) made both elders and youth revalue the importance of their cultural heritage. Important aspects of their past that were starting to be erased from the community's oral memory were discussed and made visible through this process. As a result, the elders issued a request to the younger generations to put this history into writing in order to make it known to the younger Pemon and wider Venezuelan society. This request effectively materialised in 2010 (see below). Secondly, reflections on their situation and socio-environmental changes led the Pemon from Kumarakapay to consider their livelihood potential and options for the future. A critical issue they face is food security. The shift in the settlement pattern experienced since 1950, from semi-nomadic to a permanent village, is depleting their farming land. Taking this situation into consideration, in 2000, the Pemon of Kumarakapay decided to focus on becoming a tourist community and since then have been training more actively in this activity. They are also trying to find agro-ecological alternatives for slash and burn agriculture.

The reflections derived from the participatory research project on the use of fire in Kumarakapay fostered discussions amongst the Pemon about traditional use of fire, prompting a revaluation of the ancestral lore underpinning this practice (Rodríguez *et al.* 2013). These reflections led Pemon youth to reconsider their criticisms of the use of fire, seeing instead the urgent need to learn from their grandparents about the use of fire in order to guarantee that they can continue to manage the landscape dynamically in the future.

Under their own initiative, the inhabitants of Kumarakapay also started undertaking a series of activities to revalue their identity, such as reconstructing the Pemon calendar, carrying out educational workshops, cultural activities, fairs of the Pemon culinary culture and native sports competitions.

With further external assistance between 2000 and 2004, they implemented a project for self-demarcation of the Pemon territory in the eastern part of the CNP (Sletto 2009). This has now been issued as part of a formal claim for territorial property rights. In 2010, following the request of the elders made back in 1999, they published a book entitled *The History of the Pemon of Kumarakapay*, which is used in schools and other communities of the *Gran Sabana* as a guide for developing *Life Plans* (Roraimökok Damük 2010). This book expresses the need to reconstruct the past and revalue the Pemon identity to be able to visualise a desired future. It includes much of the information compiled during community reflection on the past, present and future of Kumarakapay. By putting their history in writing, the Pemon of Kumarakapay have not only become more visible, showing the wider society that they exist as a people, with their own knowledge, language, culture and traditions, but at the same it has generated local commitment to collectively start building their desired future. As a result of this publication, the community began a new series of cultural reassertion activities such as workshops and seminars on community philosophy with the guidance of elders (grandmothers and grandfathers), in order to orient their development, education and organisational-building.

The knock-on effect: The Pemon *Life Plan* and intercultural dialogues

This process of internal strengthening amongst the Pemon of Kumarakapay about their cultural identity has played an important part in levelling power relations in the CNP's conflicts. With visions more clearly articulated regarding their current situation and visions for the future, the people from Kumarakapay have enhanced their capacity for public deliberation with environmental managers regarding pressing issues of CNP management, such as the use of fire. They have reinforced their organisational capacity to build the future they want. They have also taken strategic advantage of a number of recent governmental social policies for the area (e.g. funding for local development by setting up community councils) to empower productive activities such as tourism.

However, in addition to the value of this experience for the people of Kumarakapay, the process of cultural reaffirmation was also key in reasserting Pemon cultural identity at a wider level, and in particular with regard to the need to advance the construction of a Pemon *Life Plan*. Over the last two decades, territorial property rights and the *Life Plan* have become two interdependent pillars upholding the struggle for cultural reaffirmation, environmental integrity and defence of the Pemon territory (García 2009). While territorial property rights are conceived of as the primary material basis for cultural survival, the *Life Plan* is viewed as its ideological, spiritual and philosophical foundation. The *Life Plan* has also gradually come to be acknowledged as a platform for intercultural dialogue with external actors about the current and future wellbeing of the Pemon, as well as for articulating different institutional agendas.

Juvencio Gomez played a key part in pushing forwards the *Life Plan* agenda into the public policy arena. In 2001, for instance, a collaboration involving the Ministry of Education and Sports, the Indigenous Federation of the State of Bolivar (FIEB), Econatura and the Nature Conservancy carried out a project to evaluate Pemon public policies in the socio-economic and environmental arenas. This generated a series of intra-community dialogues about the Pemon people's socio-cultural vision in order to inform a definition of public policies 'by and for the Pemon'. This provided an opportunity for reflection amongst the Pemon about the need to play a more active role in their relations with the government, and to orient both public policy formulation and the construction of a Pemon *Life Plan*.

> We the Pemon have been passive... we have accepted projects and programs without analysing their pros and cons. It is time for us to react and begin rebuilding our lives as the Pemon People, based on our past and present, so the future will be clearer.... In response to the need of the Pemon People to set our own policies in order to cope with the pressure constantly applied, to this day, by governmental and non-governmental institutions, we have decided to take part in Evaluating Public Policies involving the Pemon People.... Recognising the effort made to gather information and data supporting the Pemon Life Plan, we expect progress to be made in developing more correct, fair, realistic, participatory policy, by exercising our own rights.
>
> (Gómez 2004)

Since then, the *Life Plan* agenda has been incorporated into the political discourse of most Pemon leaders and forms an important part of the wellbeing agendas of some Pemon villages (Pizarro 2006). The Pemon *Life Plan* is viewed as a critical self-analysis of their current situation, their changes but also their cultural values, in order to help them reflect about who they are, and who they want to be in the future, as a people. As a Pemon leader from the village of Kavanayen stated, 'Perhaps the *Life Plan* can become our space to think and reflect about ourselves. Just as Western people have universities, we also need a space to think and mature our ideas as a society.' By developing a clear vision of their identity, needs and desires, a *Life Plan* seeks to allow them to negotiate more strategically with state and other external institutions: 'our own Life Plan will not only strengthen us as a people, but also facilitate the necessary interactions with the institutions with which the Pemon interact, helping such institutions structure their initiatives and activities with the communities' (World Bank 2006).

This has led to a series of projects to advance the development of an overarching *Life Plan* for the Pemon in CNP. This began during the preparatory phase of the global environmental facility (GEF) of the World Bank 'Canaima Project' in 2004–2006. In response to the need for a collaborative strategy to manage CNP, a six-million-dollar project was formulated in 2006 for GEF-World Bank funding. At that time, one of the Pemon's conditions for taking part in the participatory management of CNP was that the project would be implemented in coordination with communities' *Life Plans*. A series of workshops defined a preliminary version of the Pemon *Life Plan*, emphasising the following components: indigenous territory and habitat; education and culture; organisation-building; health and culture; social infrastructure; and production and economic alternatives (Pizarro 2006). However, although the World Bank approved this project, it was never implemented because of changes in the Venezuelan government's political priorities and the decision to cut off ties of cooperation with the World Bank.

In collaboration with external actors, the development of community *Life Plans* continued in 2008 through a new multi-disciplinary, inter-institutional project entitled 'Risk Factors in Reducing Habitats in the Canaima National Park: Vulnerability and Tools for Sustainable Development' (Bilbao and Vessuri 2006). Here, the *Life Plan* was used as a platform for dialogue between the academic sector and the Pemon about the current and future situation of the CNP. The work has concentrated on two communities: Kumarakapay, resuming the process begun in 1999, and in Kavanayen, where, in addition to conducting a participatory evaluation of socio-environmental changes and visions of the future, an intercultural research team was formed to probe the following themes:

a) Historical reconstruction.
b) Reconstruction of cultural traditions and practices where the use of fire plays an important role.
c) Use of land and food security.
d) Social and political organisation.

In 2010, another multi-disciplinary research project adopted the *Life Plan* process as a platform for knowledge articulation and intercultural dialogues with the Pemon: the 'Impact of Climate Change and Human Occupation in Savannah-Forest Mosaics in the Orinoco Water Basin: An Interdisciplinary Project'. Here, the community of Kavanayen was assisted by external facilitation to carry out an in-depth reconstruction of its history as part of the development of its *Life Plan*. As in the case of Kumarakapay, the final aim is to produce a community-authored book of the history of the Pemon/Arekuna of Kavanayen. This process of self-enquiry into the community's past in turn helps to shed light on important questions about the historical and archaeological patterns of human occupation in the CNP and their links with climate and landscape change.

However, although the concept of the *Life Plan* as an alternative to conventional development approaches is increasingly anchored in the Pemon discourse as an ideal to pursue, progress in developing concrete *Life Plans* is fundamentally circumscribed to two of the 30 communities comprising the CNP. A challenge therefore is to spread this process to other communities.

Furthermore, in the last decade, environmental policy has continued to favour a highly centralised management style, ignoring the area's cultural diversity. What may be more alarming for the purposes of achieving intercultural environmental management is that, over the last ten years, park management has been severely constrained by dwindling funding, insufficient personnel and lack of inter-institutional coordination and will from the national government to support the national system of protected areas (Bevilacqua *et al.* 2009, Novo and Díaz 2007). Environmental policies have been upstaged by social policies geared towards hard-core development, which jeopardises the Pemon *Life Plan* by emphasising rather than reducing the historical relationship of dependence on the government.

So how much time and space do the Pemon actually have to clarify their inward visions of wellbeing and how much of this process must be constructed alongside agendas already decided by the government regarding their territories? This is not clear. In any event, progress can hardly be made without the Pemon remaining on the scene as political actors continually pressing for the recognition of their cultural differences in their dealings with the government and other actors. Since collaboration between the Pemon and environmental managers is still weak, external collaboration from academia and civil society has a major future role to play in legitimising and helping to facilitate intercultural dialogue in the park.

Conflict and contestation over local constructions of wellbeing

The story of Kumarakapay reasserting a local pathway to wellbeing in the CNP would be incomplete without a mention of the internal tensions and frictions in the making of this process. I do not wish to give the false impression that local constructions of wellbeing in contexts of strong cultural change and shifting local identities, such as the one discussed here, can be easily articulated without local dissent and contestation. On the contrary, this experience, alongside its positive outcomes, revealed important challenges in constructing local conceptions of wellbeing due to the local frictions and resistances that it triggered.

Despite paying great attention to avoiding a gender or age bias in the community self-reflection process, as well as respecting community decision-making procedures and structures, it was impossible for the process to be free of conflicts. Resistance arose on two fronts. Firstly, from different community fractions and leaders, who self-defined themselves as more 'modern' or less 'indigenous'. To them, the process of self-reflection, rather than strengthening their sense of identity, was a threat to it, and thus they opted not to participate. Secondly, resistance arose from certain elders who saw the process of self-reflection as something foreign, which, contrary to its aims, would weaken the Pemon in their dealings with outsiders. This group, led by one particular elder, claimed that the information gathered through the self-reflection process was of more use to me than to them, and feared that I would betray the community, publishing the results for my own interest. On several occasions, this group tried to sabotage the process by raising doubts and fears amongst the elders who formed part of the research group. Additionally, given that the process took place over a period of ten years, local leadership changed, and thus so did the support for the process. Progress was made mostly during the periods in which Juvencio Gomez was community chief (1999 and 2009–2010).

Dealing with the fears, doubts and rejection that the self-reflection process raised amongst certain groups and fractions of the community was an intrinsic part of the construction of local conceptions of wellbeing. On some occasions, special assemblies were organised in order to dissipate doubts and ensure local consent to continue the process. On other occasions, differences and fears were dealt with through internal and private conversations amongst the team members and their families. The group of elders who were suspicious of the process were also systematically invited to the research meetings and informed about the progress being made, despite their resistance to participate.

All these strategies for dealing with local conflict were devised and put into practice by the team members, with guidance from Juvencio Gomez and the elders. Although internal differences amongst different community fractions were always present, the self-reflection process made its progress thanks to the persistence at dealing with and clarifying the suspicion and fears that emerged as the processes unfolded. In the end, it was the successful completion of the project and the publication of the community-authored book that truly dissipated suspicions about the intention behind the self-reflection process. So much so that the elder who had attempted on several occasions to sabotage the community self-reflection process was the main speaker in the launching of the book.

Final reflections and lessons

The story of Kumarakapay can teach us important lessons relevant to the discussion of wellbeing addressed in this book. First of all, the articulation of local constructions of wellbeing can play an important part in helping indigenous people deal with conflicts with external actors on their territories. The pressures exerted by an ever-increasing number of development and conservation projects being carried out on their lands can have a profound effect, fracturing indigenous people's identities. This in turn puts them in a very disadvantaged position in policy-making, planning and implementation. As shown in the Kumarakapay story, local discussions about wellbeing can provide a platform for indigenous peoples to reconnect with their identity and thus be in a stronger position to analyse and assess their current situations, articulate their desires and visions for the future and define the rules and conditions of interactions with outsiders. In other words, local constructions of wellbeing can help level the playing field in conflicts.

Linked to this, the second important lesson is that culture is a central part of local conceptualisations of wellbeing. Hence, if conflict and the loss of a sense of identity that comes with it are endangering indigenous people's cultural and physical survival, then cultural identity building and revival must be an intrinsic part of the way that wellbeing is conceptualised and constructed at the local level. Special attention must be paid to creating opportunities for indigenous people to feel sufficiently secure so that they can be profoundly honest with themselves and with others about their fears, hopes, pains and responsibilities. Without feeling secure, honest discussions about identity are very unlikely to emerge.

A third lesson relates to the importance of the past in constructions of wellbeing. As the Kumarakapay story showed, although local constructions of wellbeing are very much an exercise of visualisation of a desired future, in order to be able to look towards the future, it is essential to look to the past. Reflexivity about the origin, past, identity, changes and current situation of the Pemon were crucial for grounding the discussion of a desired future.

Fourth, respect for local autonomy is essential in the construction of local conceptions of wellbeing. The impact of the processes carried out in Kumarakapay in terms of reviving cultural identity and positioning the *Life Plan* agenda, both amongst the Pemon and as a platform for dialogue with outsiders, is without doubt related to the fact that the process emerged and evolved as a local initiative. Local control of the process not only ensured the design of a process that was relevant and meaningful to the Pemon, but also that the local conflicts that arose in the making of the process were dealt with successfully by the Pemon themselves, following their own customary procedures and strategies.

Fifth, and linked to the above, relates to our role and place as 'academics' in this process. As shown in my account of the reflexive process carried out in Kumarakapay, although local control and autonomy are central to the construction of local conceptualisations of wellbeing, there is a huge scope for collaboration with social scientists in developing this process, particularly in providing methodological assistance. However, a people-centred approach to conceptualising wellbeing such as the one discussed here requires an important degree of role reversal in the social research process. Rather than acting as detached researchers, where local people are seen as objects of study, we need to be willing to move towards a more engaged role, one in which we can play an active part in helping others to do their own research.

This takes me to my sixth and final lesson. Academia can play an important part in helping to build intercultural relations as part of a local agenda of wellbeing and of a wider contribution to the transformation of conflicts. But this requires taking interculturality seriously. As Katherine Walsh (2005) says, building intercultural relationships 'is not solely a matter of acknowledging, discovering or tolerating the other or cultural difference. It is neither about making identities static. It is about actively promoting processes of exchange that allow building spaces of encounter amongst different beings, knowledge, logics and practices.' This requires an openness of mind on the part of academics to critically consider the what, why and what for of knowledge production in order to ensure its local relevance. This involves being willing to help revitalise indigenous knowledge, reconstruct collective memory and to promote confrontation, exchange and negotiation of Western knowledge with that of indigenous peoples as part of the overarching process of knowledge production.

Note

1. The literal translation of 'Living Well' in Quechua and Aymara languages is 'To Live in Plenitude'. The Guari version, *Teko porâ*, literarily means, 'a good way of being' or 'a good way of life', but as stated by the Aymara writer Fernando Huanacuni, from Bolivia, none of the literary translations of the term does justice to the depth of its meaning from an indigenous perspective. Living Well is a holistic concept rooted on principles and values such as harmony, equilibrium and complementarity, which from an indigenous perspective must guide the relationship of human beings with each other and with nature (or Mother Earth) and the cosmos.

References

Bevilacqua, M., Medina D. A. and Cardenas L. (2009) Manejo de Recursos Naturales en el Parque Nacional Canaima: desafíos institucionales para la conservación. pp. 207–221 in J. C. Senaris, D. Lew and C. Lasso (eds.) *Biodiversidad del Parque Nacional Canaima: Bases Tecnicas para la Conservacion de la Guayana Venezolana*. Caracas: La Salle Natural Science Foundation and The Nature Conservancy.

Bilbao, B. and Vessuri H. (2006) *Factores de Riesgo en la Reducción de Hábitats en el Parque Nacional Canaima y Herramientas para el Desarrollo Sostenible*. Caracas: FONACIT, USB-IVIC-UNEG-Parupa Research Station Group.

Butt-Colson, A. (2009) *Land. Its Occupation, Management, Use and Conceptualization. The Case of the Akawaio and Arekuna of the Upper Mazaruni District, Guyana*. Somerset, UK: Last Refuge Publishing.

Davis, D. (1992). Herramientas para la comunidad. Conceptos, métodos y herramientas para el diagnóstico, seguimiento y la evaluación participativos en el Desarrollo Forestal Comunitario, Manual de Campo No 2. Rome: FAO.

García J. (2009) Materiales para una Historia Pemon. *Antropologica* 52(111–112): 225–240.

Gómez, J. (2004) *Aproximación Pemon para la Formulación de Políticas Públicas. Relatorías de las Asambleas Generales y Comunitarias*. Caracas: Ministry of Education and Sports, Federation of Indigenous of the State of Bolívar (FIEB), Econatura and The Nature Conservancy.

Méndez, A. I. (2008) Los Derechos Indígenas en las Constituciones Latinoamericanas. *Cuestiones Políticas* 24(41): 101–125.

Novo I. and Díaz, D. (2007) *Final Report on the Evaluation of the Canaima National Park, Venezuela, as a Natural Heritage of Humankind Site. Project on Improving Our Heritage*. Caracas: Vitalis.

Perez, C. (2009). El Plan de Vida- What Is a Life Plan? *Acción Colombia*, Colombia Support Network, Spring, 2009. pp. 3–4. Available at: http://colombiasupport. net//wp-content/uploads/2012/02/CSN_Spring_09_Newsletter1.pdf (accessed 15/7/2015)

Pizarro, I. (2006) El Plan de Vida del Pueblo Pemon. In J. Medina and A. Vladimir (eds.) *Conservación de la Biodiversidad en los Territorios Indígenas Pemon de Venezuela: una Construcción de Futuro*. Caracas: The Nature Conservancy.

Rodríguez, I. (2007) Pemon Perspectives of Fire Management in Canaima National Park, Venezuela. *Human Ecology* 35(3): 331–343.

Rodríguez, I., Bjørn, S., Bilbao, B., Sanchez-Rose, I. and Leal, A. (2013) Speaking about Fire: Reflexive Governance in Landscapes of Social Change and Shifting Local Identities. *Environmental Policy Making*. DOI: 10.1080/1523908X.2013.766579.

Roraimökok Damük (2010) *La Historia de los Pemon de Kumarakapay*. p. 124 in I. Rodríguez, J. Gómez and Y. Fernández (eds). Caracas: Ediciones IVIC. Instituto Venezolano de Investigaciones Científicas, Caracas.

Sletto, B. (2009) Autogestión en Representaciones Espaciales Indígenas y el Rol de la Capacitación y Concientización: el Caso del Proyecto Etnocartográfico Inna Kowantok Sector 5 Pemon (Kavanayén- Mapauri), the Grand Savannah. *Antropologica* 113: 43–75.

Thomas, D. (1982) *Order without Government. The Society of the Pemon Indians of Venezuela*. Chicago: University of Illinois Press.

Walsh, K. (2005) Interculturalidad, Conocimientos y De-colonalidad. *Interculturalidad, Conocimientos y Revist: Signo y Pensamiento*, XXIV(46): 39–50.

World Bank (2006) Annex 20. Project brief on a proposed grant from the Global Environment Facility Trust fund in the amount of USD 6 million to the government of Venezuela for a Venezuela-expanding partnerships for the National Parks System Project. World Bank, May 2006.

Index

Note: Locators followed by n refers to notes.

acceptance, 22–3, 112, 115
accounts of wellbeing, 2–3, 20
activity (physical), *see* exercise
adaptation, 18–19, 52
Adivasi, 150
affect, 17, 18, 31, 35
   'affective turn' in social science, 118
   see also emotion; distress; love
age, 115
   and ageing, 10
   and appropriate behaviour, 100
   and life-course, 30
   structuring views of wellbeing, 51, 248, 251–3, 264
   see also children
agency, 9, 121, 128, 130, 132, 136, 144, 184–5, 262
   and close relationships, 147, 153
   indicators of wellbeing domain, 128, 159–60
   see also autonomy
Ahmed, S., 18, 22, 24, 27, 30, 120, 147, 257
alcohol, 98, 102, 103, 106, 109–11, 113–15, 177, 202, 205, 209
'anchoring routines,' 180
'art of listening', 67, 81–3, 89
aspiration, 5, 14, 17, 39, 51, 56, 84, 251–4, 256
assets, 9
Atkinson, S., 2, 29, 31, 32
'authentic happiness' (Seligman), elements of, 10
authority
   authoritative accounts of wellbeing, 2
   science as, 4
   see also discourses; power
autonomy, 20, 21–2, 24, 40n, 145
   local, 278

Bangladesh, 146, 152
   conceptions of wellbeing in, 30
basic needs, 9
   threshold, 127
Battambang (Cambodia), 220–1
behaviour change, 10
   see also 'health behaviour'
'beyond GDP', 8, 13
Bhutan, 11
Brazil, 262, 264
bricolage approach, 219, 223–4
buen vivir (living well), 15, 37, 118, 241, 247, 260, 261
   discourse, 253
   political project, 241
   see also indigenous

Cambodia, 3, 36, 219–38
Cambodian Mine Action Centre (CMAC), 221–2
   infrastructure and community development projects, 222
Cameron, D., 66, 67, 77
Canaima, 263
Canaima National Park (CNP), 262–5, 271, 272, 274–6
   conflicts in, 263, 265
Canaima Project, 274
capability approach, 8–9, 29, 121
Cape Town, 33
care, *see* 'taking care'
case studies, 96, 113
Chhattisgarh (India), 144, 165, 168
Chiawa (Zambia), 124–5
children
   care for, 134, 135, 136–7, 151, 156
   care given by, 181, 187, 189, 191
   'circulation' of children (Zambia), 137
   'circulation' of children (Peru), 182–7

children – *continued*
  child poverty, taxonomy of (Ethiopia), 57–62
  see also age
choice, 5, 13, 22, 23, 34
  of indicators of wellbeing, 10
churches (African independent)
  in Huila (Angola), 204–6
  as resource for healing, 210–12
close relationships, 35
  constructing items for assessment of, 151–4
  ideologies of, 157
  and wellbeing, 114, 145–8
  see also family; 'happy family'; marriage
clothing and self-esteem, 58
CMAC, *see* Cambodian Mine Action Centre (CMAC)
CNP, *see* Canaima National Park (CNP)
coding traps, 75, 83, 91
cognitive debriefing, 47, 52–7, 62
collective
  identities, 29, 272
  rights, 15, 264, 270, 271, 272, 273
  wellbeing, 32, 38, 248, 249, 250
  see also discourses; indigenous
community, 6, 14, 30, 39n, 246–54, 261, 263, 267, 271–7
  -based research, 61
  of believers, 211
  conflicting views of wellbeing within, 242–3, 253–4, 276–7
  conversational, 243
  identities, 30
  need to share resources with, 135
  relations in urban Peru, 180
  rural, 182
  self-reflection process, 265–72
  as territory, 110
competence, 21, 121, 132, 145
comprehensive wellbeing, 8–10, 16, 33
concepts of wellbeing, 16–22
  see also culture; discourses
conflict, 245, 250, 262, 263, 264, 265, 26, 272, 276, 277, 278
conservation, *see* environment

context
  importance of grounding in, 3, 4, 18, 19, 167, 254
  policy, 20
Craib, I., 23–5, 118
crime, 69, 96, 99, 100, 103, 110, 113, 115
cross-cultural analysis of wellbeing, 18, 22
  see also culture
culture, 277
  constructing views of wellbeing, 272–3, 277–8
  culture-based syndrome, 138
  cultures of wellbeing, 2, 22–3, 25, 29
  cultural change, 261, 264–5
  cultural difference, 18, 80, 240, 260
  cultural identity, 260–79
  cultural reaffirmation, 272
  inter-cultural dialogue, 261, 278–9
  religion and, 209
  curandeiros (traditional healers), 208, 210–11

Deci, E. L., 21, 121, 145, 185
deslocados (internally displaced people), 203, 211
development, 125, 140, 200–2, 263, 272, 275, 277
  development alternative, 14–15, 37, 241, 260–1
  and religion, 212
  wellbeing and, 5, 8, 11, 48, 265, 266
Diener, E., 16–18, 29, 120, 127, 146
discourse analysis, 67, 89
discourses
  authorised/unauthorised, 242–3, 253–4
  buen vivir, 253
  dimensions in, 247
  discursive dominance, 5
  'hidden transcript' of, 254
  indigenous, 242, 247, 249
  normative, 247, 248–51
  unauthorized, 251–2
  and voice, 242–3

distress, 103, 112, 198
　concepts of, 198
　perceptions of, 203
　spiritual dimensions of, 199
drug abuse, 106

Easterlin, R. A., 13, 126, 127
'Easterlin paradox', 13–14, 17
Economic and Social Research Council (ESRC), 223
economics
　economics and subjective wellbeing/happiness, 34, 126–7, 256
　behavioural, 49
　as expressive idiom, 137–9
　of happiness, 13, 118
　and inner wellbeing, 126–33
　affecting other dimensions of wellbeing, 160
　and subjectivities, 133–141
　see also food; land; livelihoods; love; moral economy
economic sufficiency, 125–6
economy, definition of, 119
　see also economics
EFA, *see* exploratory factor analysis (EFA)
Ehrenreich, B., 18, 23, 31
emic perspectives, 244
emotion, 35–6, 56
　see also affect; distress; love; *pena*
empowerment, 5, 121, 144, 146, 147, 162
entrepreneurs in South Africa, 52–7
environment, 2, 11, 14, 36, 224, 234, 237, 263–4, 271, 272–3, 274–5
　policy, 275
　see also sustainability
epistemology, 3, 20, 26–8
ERW, *see* explosive remnants of war (ERW)
ESRC, *see* Economic and Social Research Council (ESRC)
ethical issues, 67, 81, 201, 236
Ethiopia, 3, 32, 48, 53, 58

ethnography, 202, 240–1
　ethnographic fieldwork, 243–5
　introduction to the site, 245–6, 265–6
　revealing politics, 256–7
eudaemonic wellbeing, 18, 20, 22
evaluation (of policy), 7, 12, 19
exercise (physical), 98, 100, 108, 109, 115
　see also sport
experience sampling, 17
expert knowledge, 2, 76, 95, 115
　expertise in research teams, 33
exploratory factor analysis (EFA), 152
explosive remnants of war (ERW), 221

FA, *see* factor analysis (FA)
factor analysis (FA), 127–8
faith, *see* religion
faith-healers, 208
　see also healing
faith-healing, 205, 207, 210
　see also healing
family, 56, 60
　ideologies of, 148, 156–7
　in India, 147
　nuclear-family settlements, 263
　social importance of, 147
　support from, 101, 104, 105, 107, 146, 176, 180
　see also children; close relationships; 'happy family'; marriage; siblings
female headed households, *see* single women
Five Ways to Wellbeing (Thompson), 10
food, 101, 102, 108–9, 111, 114, 125, 135, 140, 231
forced choices, 79–81
'Fourth world', *see* indigenous
free text fields, 68–76, 79–81, 82–90
freedom, *see* autonomy
functionings, 9
fundamental attribution error, 138

Gallup World Poll, 16, 17, 39, 40
GDP, *see* gross domestic product

gender, 22, 34, 35, 115, 124, 132, 134–5, 193
  in Adivasi society, 150
  and life cycle, 182
  norms, 100, 144, 148, 156
  responsibilities, 176, 186, 190
  structuring experience of wellbeing, 193
  violence, 166
  see also masculinity; women
Global Agewatch Index, 10
Global North and Global South, 5
Global Person Generated Index (GPGI), 53
GNH, *see* Gross National Happiness (GNH)
gospel of prosperity, 206
GPGI, *see* Global Person Generated Index (GPGI)
Graham, C., 14, 17, 29, 51, 52, 118, 120, 127, 147
gross domestic product (GDP), 7, 8, 9, 14, 15, 39
Gross National Happiness (GNH), 11

happiness, 5–6, 118
  critiques of use in policy, 22–5
  emotion-based assessments of, 17
  'faces' of, 15–16
  and inner wellbeing, 129–31
  and personal wellbeing, 10
  political manipulation of, 27
  variability in views of, 24
  see also wellbeing
'happy family', 6, 35, 147, 152, 153, 154, 156–7, 159, 162, 164, 165
'happy peasant', 18, 152
'happy planet index' (HPI), 9
HDI, *see* Human Development Index (HDI)
healing
  perceptions of, 203
  practices, 199
  spiritual dimensions to, 201–2, 206–7, 210–12
  strategies and resources for, 202
health, 3, 4, 6, 10, 104–5
  'behaviours', 95–6, 102, 113, 114–16
  domain of, 132

mental, *see* mental health
public, *see* public health
reporting on, 113–14
hedonic wellbeing, 8
hidden transcripts, 246
  of discourses, 254
hierarchy of needs, 126
history
  community, 261, 278
  of international development, 5
Horn of Africa, 248
household, 48–51, 58, 62, 83, 107, 123–5, 132, 133, 135, 146, 147, 150, 153–5, 157, 158, 160, 162–4, 183, 186, 187, 189–91, 193, 221, 226, 248, 249, 251
  taxonomy of, 57–62
Human Development Index (HDI), 9
human needs, 9, 13, 127
human rights, *see* rights
humanitarian aid, 198, 200–2

illness, 189
  cause of, 207
  conceptualisations of, 206–10
  spiritual dimensions of, 199
  and stigma, 105
  see also health
income, 6, 9, 14, 17, 39, 114
  and SWB, 126–7, 133
India, 3, 9, 22, 35, 36, 121, 138, 144–68
indicators of wellbeing, origins of subjective indicators, 13
indices of wellbeing, 9–10
indigenous
  identities, 276
  relations with dominant society, 255
  views of wellbeing, 14–15, 37–8, 247, 260
  see also collective; discourse
individual, critique of individualized approaches to wellbeing, 10–11, 21, 29–30
inequality, 13, 18, 23, 39, 51, 63, 90, 118, 261

Index

inner wellbeing (IWB), 121–2, 149
  domains, regressions of, 132
  economics and, 126–33
  economic status indicators and, 131
  happiness and, 129–30
  inter-cultural research, 2
  intercultural dialogue, 260, 261, 272–5
  inter-disciplinary nomad, 223–4
  inter-disciplinary research, *see* mixed methods
  international migration, 175
  interviews, 96, 149–50, 155, 161, 162–3, 177–9, 225–6
  sequencing within, 105
  see also photo-elicitation interviews
  intimacy, 161, 167
IWB, *see* inner wellbeing (IWB)

justice, *see* social justice

knowledge, 235–7
  balancing 'expert' with local people's, 115
  forms and sources of, 113
  wellbeing, 202–3
Kumarakapay (Venezuela), 261, 265, 267, 271–2, 274–7

land, 36, 124, 125, 222, 224–5, 231, 233, 237, 247, 248, 264, 268, 271, 272
landmines, 220–3
Langa (Cape Town, South Africa), 98
Language, 50, 54, 57, 80, 96, 268
Law, J., 67, 78, 79, 82, 88, 89
Layard, R., 10, 11, 29, 78
Legatum Institute, 10
life cycle, 182, 193
  see also age
life satisfaction, 6, 9, 13–20, 48
  cultural interpretations of l.s.questions, 56, 99, 103, 105–6
Life Plan (Plan de Vida), 261
Likert scale, 27
Lima (Peru), 176–81, 183–5, 187–92
literacy, 150
livelihoods, 34, 123–5, 149, 175, 251, 253, 254

living well, Latin America, 260–2
  conflicts, exclusion and cultural violence, 262–5
  local constructions of wellbeing, 276–7
  Pemon pathway for, 265–72
  reflections and lessons, 277–9
  see also buen vivir
love, 30, 105, 134–5, 146, 151, 156, 157, 180, 182, 184

market, 37
  as model of society, 20, 23
marriage, 12, 19, 137, 138, 144–8, 150, 151, 155, 156, 158, 162–4, 186, 205, 209
  and PWB, 146
  social importance of, 147
  and wellbeing, 134, 135, 145–6, 148
  see also close relationships; family; 'happy family'
masculinity, 34, 54, 134–5, 182, 189–90
  machismo, 190, 193
  see also gender
MEA, *see* Millennium Ecosystem Assessment (MEA)
measurement of wellbeing, 48, 62–3
Measuring National Well-Being (MNW) programme, 66
  art of listening, 81–3
  composition of programme, 68–9
  'findings from the debate,' 73–7
  free text *versus* forced choices, 79–81
  matter of understanding of, 83–8
  matters of debate, 68–73
  methodological alternatives, 81–3
  methodological issues, 77–9
  shifts in questionnaires, 68–73
Measuring What Matters, 66
men, *see* gender; masculinity
mental health
  concepts of, 198
  evidence-based approach to, 201
mestizos, 247
  inhabitants, 243
Mexico, 3, 37, 240–58
migration, 175–6, 251, 252–3
  see also mobility

286 Index

Millennium Ecosystem Assessment (MEA), 224
mine contamination, 219, 222, 223
mixed method research, 2, 25, 32–35, 47, 61, 113–15, 144, 145
MNW programme, *see* Measuring National Well-Being (MNW) programme
mobility in Peru, 35, 175–6
 relational dynamics of, 176
 mobility stories 176–9
modernity, 5, 23, 24, 118, 200, 214, 240, 255, 257–8n, 260, 270, 276
moral economy, 5, 135–6
MPI, *see* Multi-dimensional Poverty Index (MPI)
Multi-dimensional Poverty Index (MPI), 9

National Well-Being Debate report, 68
NCDs, *see* noncommunicable diseases (NCDs)
neo-liberal, 200, 241
New Economics Foundation (NEF), 9, 10
NGO, *see* non-governmental organisation (NGO)
noncommunicable diseases (NCDs), 95, 102, 115
 prevention policy, 114
non-governmental organisation (NGO), 31, 97, 149, 249, 265
normative discourse, 247, 248
North-South politics, 5
Nussbaum, M., 22, 52

objective wellbeing, 28, 149
 see also subjective and objective
Office for National Statistics (ONS), 9, 33, 66–9, 73, 75–8, 80, 88, 89
 personal finance, 75
 questionnaires, 69–72
 reports on MNW programme, 73
ontology, 3
ONS, *see* Office for National Statistics (ONS)
Organisation for Economic Co-operation and Development (OECD), 4, 9, 12, 28

PADHI, *see* Psycho-social Assessment of Development and Humanitarian Intervention (PADHI)
participatory research, 37–8, 78, 278
 see community, self-reflection process
participatory photography, 36, 220, 225–7, 229–37
 practical lessons, 235–7
Pemon people (Venezuela), 261–77
 personal finance, 75, 77
pena (sorrow, extreme sadness), 180, 181, 186, 190, 193
perceptions, 20
personal wellbeing, 10–11, 23
Personal Wellbeing Index (PWI), 16, 17
Peru, 35, 36, 51, 175–93
 photo-elicitation interviews, 225–7
 timing and location of, 229
place, 2, 14, 29, 31, 35, 37, 120, 148, 153, 157, 159, 161, 167, 176, 178, 180, 236, 248, 263
 displaced, 198–9, 215
pluri-cultural nation-state models, 260
policy, 5–15, 24, 95
 policy implications, 34–6
 using relational wellbeing in policy, 31–2
 see also evaluation; politics
politics
 of research methods, 33, 67–8, 75–6, 77, 78–9, 82
 of wellbeing, 3, 19, 37, 67, 253, 256–7
 use of Life Plan to assert collective rights, 272–5
positive attitude, 99, 114
positivist approaches, 18, 26
poverty, 9, 32, 48, 51, 61, 73, 146, 150, 175, 177, 180, 182, 193, 202, 204, 206, 214, 220, 223, 244, 248
 child, 57–62
power, 26, 37, 167, 213–14
 and close relationships, 157
 and discourses of wellbeing, 5, 213, 215, 246–56
 in professional relationships, 201

spiritual, 110, 114
wellbeing as a field of, 38–9
see also politics
practical political economy, 254–5
process
  research as social process, 27–8, 265–72, 278
  wellbeing as process, 26–7, 30–31
Prospective Urban and Rural Epidemiological (PURE) study, 96, 115
Prosperity Index, 10
psychological wellbeing (PWB), 20–2
  critiques of, 21
  domains of, 20
  scholars of, 30
Psycho-social Assessment of Development and Humanitarian Intervention (PADHI), 121
psychosocial wellbeing, 198–200
  conceptualisations of wellbeing and illness, 206–10
  description of, 198–9
  development, humanitarian aid and religion, 200–2
  dominant conceptualisation of, 199
  evidence-based approach to, 201
  independent churches, 204–6, 210–12
  instrumental view of religion, 212–14
  interventions, 36
  marriage and, 146
public health, 3, 34, 95–116
public policy, wellbeing in, 6–15
PURE study, *see* Prospective Urban and Rural Epidemiological (PURE) study
PWB, *see* psychological wellbeing (PWB)
PWI, *see* Personal Wellbeing Index (PWI)

QoL, *see* quality of life (QoL)
qualitative research, 20, 26, 28, 48, 50, 62, 95
  analysis, 74, 75
  combining with quantitative data, 61, 62, 100, 113–14, 155–6, 159–64, 167
  discrepancies with quantitative data, 53, 99–100, 101–2
  see also discourse analysis; ethnography; interviews; participatory research; subjective and objective
quality of life (QoL), 8, 12, 31
quantitative research, 18, 26, 28–9
  analysis, 129
  economic dimensions in, 127
  see also subjective and objective

Rarámuri people, 242–56
reciprocities, 135–6, 190
reflexivity, 26, 38, 242, 244, 262, 267, 278
  community self-reflection, 265–77
  importance of, 242
  see also research relationships; researcher identity, researcher role
reification, 3
relatedness, 21, 121, 145
relational anchoring, 35, 179–82
  importance of, 180
relational wellbeing, 29–32
  concern for social welfare, 75, 76
relationships
  anchoring points, 187–92
  children's, in contexts of mobility, 182–7
  conflicting demands of, 176, 187, 189, 192
  importance of, 10, 11, 17, 21, 146, 179
  and mobility stories, 177–9
  quality of, 151
  and relational anchoring, 179–82
  as source of strength, 106
  see also children; family; marriage; close relationships; relatedness; taking care
religion, 34, 36
  and culture, 209
  and development, 200–1, 212, 214
  as power for change, 110

religion – *continued*
 and psycho-social work, 201–2, 213
 religious beliefs, 114, 201–3, 205, 208, 225, 255
 and spirituality, 198–206
 and wellbeing, 211–12
research methods, 2, 3, 14, 26
 bricolage and inter-disciplinary nomad, 223–4
 research relationships, 158, 162–4, 167, 245
 researcher identity, 158, 163, 257n
 researcher role, 265–6, 278–9
 see also case studies; ethical issues; ethnography; mixed methods; participatory research; qualitative research; quantitative research; subjective and objective
rights
 collective, 37, 38, 247, 255
 human, 13
 to political inclusion, 14, 15
Rivers, W. H. R.
 fieldwork in Solomon Islands, 1, 26–7
Ryan, R., 21, 121, 145, 177, 178, 185
Ryff, C. D., 20, 21, 40n.13, 145

safety, 99–100
Sahlins, M., 23, 28, 30, 40n.17
santa, 210–12
Sarkozy Commission, 66
 see also Stiglitz Report
satisfaction with life
 Satisfaction with Life Scale (SWLS), 16
 see life satisfaction
science of wellbeing or happiness, 4, 28–9
SDT, *see* self-determination theory (SDT)
secularism, 200
security, 30, 39n
self as perfectible project, 23
self-determination theory (SDT), 21, 145
 argument for cross-cultural applicability, 22

self-reflection process, 276–7
self-reported data
 defined, 48
 influences on, 49–52
Sen, A., 8–9, 18, 22, 29, 90n.3, 91n.8, 121, 157, 18
 see also capability approach
sharing, 35, 157, 222, 244, 249, 255, 256
 culturally-embedded forms of, 255
sibling relationships, 111, 134, 191–2
silence, *see* voice
single women (women heading households), in Zambia, 123, 132, 133, 135, 137–8
smoking, 109, 114
social capital, 121
 instrumental concepts of, 176
social desirability bias, 27
social justice, 14
 approach to wellbeing, 121
Social Progress Index/Imperative, 10
social resources, instrumental concepts of, 176
sociology, 95–116
somatization, 139
South Africa, entrepreneurs in, 52–7
Soweto, 54
spirit exorcism, 209
'spirit of evil,' 263
spiritual healing, 208–9
spirituality, religion and, 198–206
sport, 108–9
 see also exercise (physical)
'stages of progress' method, 58
state, 15, 24
STEPS study, 54
Stiglitz Report, 8
subjective and objective, 6–8, 14, 17–18, 20, 27–9, 30, 32–3, 47, 48–49, 149
subjective wellbeing (SWB), 16–20, 220
 critiques of, 18–20, 62–3
 cross-cultural analysis of, 18
 description of, 16
 and economic status, 126–7
 and inner wellbeing, 129–31
 manipulation of, 19

quantitative measures of, 16–20
robustness of data on, 19
scholars of, 30
self-assessment, 18
and subjectivity, 119–20
use in policy, 32
utility and, 12–14
see also, happiness; life satisfaction
subjectivities, 7, 23–5, 26, 27–8, 35, 119–21
  foregrounding economic aspects of, 137–9
  re-thinking, 133–4
survey methods, 53–7, 58–62
  design of, 69–73, 79
Sumak Kawasay (living in plenitude), 241, 279n
Suma Qamaña (living in plenitude), 241, 279n
sustainability, 11, 14, 15, 30, 36
sustainable development, 11
sustainable wellbeing toolbox, 31
SWB, *see* subjective wellbeing (SWB)
SWLS, *see* Satisfaction with Life Scale (SWLS)

'taking care,' gendered identities in, 134–5
  amongst siblings for parents, 187
  sibling responsibilities, 191
taxonomy
  categories, 58
  of child poverty, 57–62
  of household, 57–62
  and selection of indicators, 59–60
time, 30, 31, 37, 51, 62, 164, 193, 227
tourism, 264
transport, 103, 114

unauthorised voices, 251–3
  authorised *vs.*, 253–6
unemployment, 103, 106, 107, 110, 113, 115
United Nations Development Programme (UNDP), 9
United Nations (UN) Happiness Resolution, 11
United Nations (UN) Human Development Index, 220

United States of America (USA), 13, 15, 19, 23
universalist approaches to wellbeing, 21, 29, 39, 167
  see also context
utility, 12–14

values, 11, 14, 18, 21, 29, 38, 48, 50, 58, 79, 87, 95, 115, 138, 147, 160, 180, 181, 223, 224, 253, 263, 270, 273, 279
violence, 153–6, 162, 166, 177, 183, 193
  cultural, 262–5
visual explorations of wellbeing, 219–20
  methodology, 225
  participatory photography and photo-elicitation interviews, 225–7
  practical lessons, 235–7
voice, 240–57
  authorised, 253–6
  choosing not to speak, 148, 153, 157, 159, 161, 167
  unauthorised, 251–6

Warwick–Edinburgh Mental Wellbeing Scale (WEMWBS), 21
WeD, *see* Wellbeing in Developing Countries (WeD)
wellbeing
  accounts of, 2–3, 20
  close relationships and, 114, 144–71
  comprehensive, 8–10
  conceptualisations of, 16–25, 206–10
  conflict and contestation, 31, 276–7
  constructions of, 3, 25–9, 203, 219–20, 260, 278
  and development, 48
  economics and subjectivities, 118–43, 219–20
  field of, 4–6
  framing, 30
  and happiness, 5–6
  and harmony, 160
  indigenous discourses of, 242, 246–50, 261

wellbeing – *continued*
  inter-relations between components of, 30, 160
  knowledge, 202–3
  measurement of, 49–52
  multiple accounts of, 2–3
  personal, 10–11
  in public policy, 6–15
  relational, 29–32
  and relationships in mobility, 175–97
  and self-management, 30–1
  visual explorations of, *see* visual explorations of wellbeing
  see also specific types
wellbeing ecology, 224
Wellbeing in Developing Countries (WeD), 49, 121
  approach, 224
  concept of wellbeing, 224
  Research Group, 178, 223–4

wellbeing pathways
  definition, 223–4
  research, 149
women, 35
  women's wellbeing in India, 145–9
  case studies, 154–63
  and close relationships, 145–8, 151–4
  see also gender; single women
World Bank, 54, 274
World Health Organization (WHO), 20, 98, 133
World Values Survey, 9
work, 59, 60, 81, 153, 155, 156, 157, 180, 182, 183, 184, 185, 187, 188, 189, 191
  housework, 158, 160, 161, 166–7
  and migration, 253

Young Lives, 58, 63

Zambia, 118–41

Printed and bound by CPI Group (UK) Ltd, Croydon, CR0 4YY